Frontiers in Colorectal Surgery

Edited by
Robin KS Phillips & Sue Clark

tfm Publishing Limited
Castle Hill Barns
Harley
Shrewsbury
SY5 6LX
UK

Tel: +44 (0)1952 510061
Fax: +44 (0)1952 510192
E-mail: nikki@tfmpublishing.com
Web site: www.tfmpublishing.com

Design:	Nikki Bramhill, tfm publishing Ltd.
Typesetting:	Nikki Bramhill, tfm publishing Ltd.
	Ben Doyle, Derek Doyle & Associates, Stockport, Cheshire, UK

First Edition   © June 2005

ISBN 1 903378 33 8

The entire contents of *Frontiers in Colorectal Surgery* is copyright tfm Publishing Ltd. Apart from any fair dealing for the purposes of research or private study, or criticism or review, as permitted under the Copyright, Designs and Patents Act 1988, this publication may not be reproduced, stored in a retrieval system or transmitted in any form or by any means, electronic, digital, mechanical, photocopying, recording or otherwise, without the prior written permission of the publisher.

Neither the authors, the editors nor the publisher can accept responsibility for any injury or damage to persons or property occasioned through the implementation of any ideas or use of any product described herein. Neither can they accept any responsibility for errors, omissions or misrepresentations, howsoever caused.

Whilst every care is taken by the authors, the editors and the publisher to ensure that all information and data in this book are as accurate as possible at the time of going to press, it is recommended that readers seek independent verification of advice on drug or other product usage, surgical techniques and clinical processes prior to their use.

The authors, editors and publisher gratefully acknowledge the permission granted to reproduce the copyright material where applicable in this book. Every effort has been made to trace copyright holders and to obtain their permission for the use of copyright material. The publisher apologizes for any errors or omissions and would be grateful if notified of any corrections that should be incorporated in future reprints or editions of this book.

Printed by Gutenberg Press Ltd., Gudja Road, Tarxien, PLA 19, Malta.

Tel: +356 21897037; Fax: +356 21800069.

Contents

PART I: FRONTIERS IN NEOPLASIA

		Page
Chapter 1	Screening for colorectal cancer and high risk adenomas *David AL Macafee, Charles A Maxwell-Armstrong*	1
Chapter 2	Follow-up strategies for colorectal cancer (CRC) *Sanjay Purkayastha, Paris P Tekkis*	11
Chapter 3	Primary prevention of colorectal cancer (diet and chemoprevention) *Patrick M Lynch, Marina Wallace*	21
Chapter 4	Polyp management *Brian Saunders*	29
Chapter 5	Endoscopy training: state of the art *Siwan Thomas-Gibson, Margaret Vance*	45
Chapter 6	The evaluation of rectal cancer *Kirsten M Boyle, Dermot Burke*	55
Chapter 7	Invasive palliative therapies for colorectal cancer *Rakesh Bhardwaj, Michael C Parker*	69
Chapter 8	Colorectal liver metastases *Robert Hutchins, Jina Krissat, Satya Bhattacharya*	81
Chapter 9	Evaluation and management of local recurrence *Sue Clark, Sina Dorudi*	89
Chapter 10	The TME debate in light of the Dutch radiotherapy trial *Gisella Salerno, Brendan Moran*	101
Chapter 11	Chemotherapy trials in colorectal cancer *Gary Middleton*	113

PART II: FRONTIERS IN IBD

Chapter 12	Adjuvant treatment after Crohn's resection *Emma R Greig*	121
Chapter 13	New pharmacology *Anton Emmanuel*	131

Chapter 14	Management of the devastated perineum *Paul Hollington, Rajiv Grover, John MA Northover*	139
Chapter 15	Ulcerative colitis surveillance *Matt Rutter*	149
Chapter 16	Laparoscopy at the frontier of colorectal surgery *Timothy A Rockall*	161

PART III: FRONTIERS AROUND THE ANUS

Chapter 17	Frontiers in fistula *Gordon N Buchanan, C Richard G Cohen*	167
Chapter 18	Haemorrhoid surgery *Per-Olof Nyström, Roger Gerjy*	187
Chapter 19	The treatment of anal fissures *Philip J Conaghan, Ridzuan Farouk*	201
Chapter 20	Incontinence *Carolynne J Vaizey*	213

PART IV: FRONTIERS IN MANAGEMENT

Chapter 21	Multimodal strategies for peri-operative optimisation *Sarah C Mills, Alastair C Windsor*	221
Chapter 22	Anti-adhesion strategies *Michael C Parker*	231
Chapter 23	Should we sub-specialise further? *Omer Aziz, Paris P Tekkis*	243

PART V: GENDER ISSUES

Chapter 24	Fertility after pouch surgery *Kasper Ørding Olsen*	253
Chapter 25	Erectile dysfunction *Ian Lindsey*	261

Contributors

Omer Aziz BSc MRCS Research Fellow, Surgical Oncology, Imperial College, St. Mary's Hospital, London, UK

Rakesh Bhardwaj FRCS FRCS (Ed) Specialist Registrar, Darent Valley Hospital, Dartford, Kent, UK

Satya Bhattacharya MS MPhil FRCS Consultant Hepatopancreatobiliary Surgeon, Barts and the London NHS Trust, London, UK

Kirsten M Boyle MB ChB MRCS Clinical Research Fellow, Colorectal Surgery, The General Infirmary at Leeds, Leeds, UK

Gordon N Buchanan MSc MD FRCS (Gen) Specialist Registrar in Colorectal Surgery, St. Thomas' Hospital, London, UK

Dermot Burke PhD FRCS Senior Lecturer in Surgery and Consultant Surgeon, The General Infirmary at Leeds, Leeds, UK

Sue Clark MD FRCS (Gen Surg) Consultant Colorectal Surgeon, Barts and the London NHS Trust, London, UK

C Richard G Cohen MD FRCS (Gen) Consultant Colorectal Surgeon, St. Mark's Hospital, Harrow, Middlesex, UK

Philip J Conaghan MA MRCS Specialist Registrar, General Surgery, Royal Berkshire Hospital, Reading, UK

Sina Dorudi PhD FRCS Professor of Surgical Oncology, Barts and the London, Queen Mary's School of Medicine and Dentistry and Honorary Consultant Colorectal Surgeon, Barts and the London NHS Trust, London, UK

Anton Emmanuel MD FRCP Senior Lecturer Gastrointestinal Physiology and Honorary Consultant Gastroenterologist, St. Mark's Hospital, Harrow, Middlesex, UK

Ridzuan Farouk MCh FRCS (Glas) FRCS (Ed) FRCS Consultant in Colorectal Surgery, Royal Berkshire Hospital, Reading, UK

Roger Gerjy MD Registrar in Colorectal Surgery, University Hospital, Linköping, Sweden

Emma R Greig PhD MRCP Consultant Gastroenterologist, Taunton and Somerset NHS Trust, UK

Rajiv Grover BSc MD FRCS (Plast) Consultant Plastic Surgeon, St. Mark's Hospital, Harrow, Middlesex, UK

Paul Hollington MB BS PhD FRACS Consultant Surgeon, Colorectal Surgery, Flinders Medical Centre, Bedford Park SA, Australia

Robert Hutchins MS FRCS Consultant Hepatopancreatobiliary Surgeon, Barts and the London NHS Trust and Honorary Senior Lecturer, Institute of Cancer, London, UK

Jina Krissat MD Liver Surgeon, Centre Hepatobiliaire, Hopital Paul-Brousse, Paris, France

Ian Lindsey FRACS Consultant Colorectal Surgeon, John Radcliffe Hospital, Oxford, UK

Patrick M Lynch JD MD Associate Professor, University of Texas, MD Anderson Cancer Center, Houston, Texas, USA

David AL Macafee BMBS (Hons) MRCS Specialist Registrar in General Surgery, Queen's Medical Centre, Nottingham, UK

Charles A Maxwell-Armstrong DM FRCS (Gen Surg) Consultant Colorectal Surgeon, Queen's Medical Centre, Nottingham, UK

Gary Middleton MD MRCP Consultant Medical Oncologist, Royal Surrey County Hospital, Guildford, Surrey, UK

Sarah C Mills MRCS Colorectal Fellow, St. Mark's Hospital, Harrow, Middlesex, UK

Brendan Moran MCh FRCSI Consultant Colorectal Surgeon, North Hampshire Hospital, Basingstoke, UK

John MA Northover MS FRCS Consultant Surgeon, St. Mark's Hospital, Harrow, Middlesex, UK and Professor of Intestinal and Colorectal Disorders, Imperial College, London, UK

Per-Olof Nyström MD PhD Consultant Colorectal Surgeon, University Hospital, Linköping, Sweden

Kasper Ørding Olsen MD PhD Research Fellow, Colorectal Surgery, University Hospital of Aarhus, Aarhus C, Denmark

Michael C Parker BSc MS FRCS FRCS (Ed) Consultant Surgeon, Darent Valley Hospital, Dartford, Kent, UK

Robin KS Phillips MS FRCS Honorary Professor of Colorectal Surgery, St. Mark's Hospital, Harrow, Middlesex, UK

Sanjay Purkayastha BSc MB BS MRCS Research Fellow, Surgical Oncology, Imperial College, St. Mary's Hospital, London, UK

Timothy A Rockall MD FRCS Consultant Surgeon, Minimal Access Therapy Training Unit, Royal Surrey County Hospital, Guildford, Surrey, UK

Matt Rutter MD FRCP Consultant Gastroenterologist, University Hospital of North Tees, Stockton-on-Tees, Cleveland, UK

Gisella Salerno BSc MRCS Surgical Research Fellow, North Hampshire Hospital, Basingstoke, UK

Brian Saunders MD FRCP Senior Lecturer in Endoscopy & Consultant Gastroenterologist, Wolfson Unit for Endoscopy, St. Mark's Hospital, Harrow, Middlesex, UK

Paris P Tekkis MD FRCS Senior Lecturer, Surgical Oncology, Imperial College, St. Mary's Hospital, London, UK

Siwan Thomas-Gibson BSc MRCP Research Fellow, Gastroenterology, St. Mark's Hospital, Harrow, Middlesex, UK

Carolynne J Vaizey MD FRCS (Gen) FCS (SA) Consultant Colorectal Surgeon & Clinical Senior Lecturer, St. Mark's Hospital, Harrow, Middlesex, UK

Margaret Vance RGNDip MSc Nurse Consultant, Gastroenterology, St. Mark's Hospital, Harrow, Middlesex, UK

Marina Wallace FRCS Consultant Colorectal Surgeon, Watford General Hospital, Watford, UK

Alastair C Windsor MD FRCS FRCS (Ed) Consultant Colorectal Surgeon, St. Mark's Hospital, Harrow, Middlesex, UK

Foreword

While coloproctology has emerged and matured as a specialty, rapid progress continues, with subspecialist areas developing. This book is not designed to be an exhaustive textbook of coloproctology, but rather to cover a broad spectrum of topics where there has been recent advance, and exciting developments are likely.

The authors are active researchers and clinicians, who have been asked to summarise up-to-date concepts, and have also been invited to look to the future. This provides a fresh and highly relevant account of aspects of modern coloproctology, ideal for the practising consultant wishing to update and also the candidate approaching the end of higher specialist training. It also provides a stimulating and thought-provoking glimpse of what coloproctology might look like in years to come.

Professor Robin KS Phillips MS FRCS
Honorary Professor of Colorectal Surgery
St. Mark's Hospital

Miss Sue Clark MD FRCS (Gen Surg)
Consultant Colorectal Surgeon
Barts and the London NHS Trust

The Editors

Robin Phillips MS FRCS has been a Consultant Colorectal Surgeon at St. Mark's Hospital since 1987, where he is now Clinical Director. Building on the clinical advantage of the range of cases seen at St. Mark's, he has researched and written widely on all aspects of colorectal surgery. He is Honorary Professor of Colorectal Surgery, Imperial College, London and President of the British Colostomy Association.

Sue Clark MD FRCS (Gen Surg) qualified at Cambridge and St. Thomas's Hospital Medical School. She was a Higher Surgical Trainee in South West Thames, a Research Fellow with the Imperial Cancer Research Fund at St. Mark's Hospital, and a Resident Surgical Officer at St. Mark's. She is now a Consultant Colorectal Surgeon at Barts and the London NHS Trust. Her research interest is in familial adenomatous polyposis and other inherited colorectal cancer and polyposis syndromes.

PART I: FRONTIERS IN NEOPLASIA

Chapter 1

Screening for colorectal cancer and high risk adenomas

David AL Macafee BMBS (Hons) MRCS, Specialist Registrar in General Surgery
Charles A Maxwell-Armstrong DM FRCS (Gen Surg), Consultant Colorectal Surgeon
Queen's Medical Centre, Nottingham, UK

What is the issue?

Colorectal cancer (CRC) is the third most common cancer in the European Union, with over 217,000 cases annually and a lifetime risk of 3-5% [1]. There are 34,000 new cases per year in the UK and it remains the second commonest cause of cancer death [2]. Male CRC incidence rates have increased by 20% since 1970 (from 47 to 56 per 100,000 in the late 1990s) but female rates have remained stable [3]. Median 5-year survival remains static at 40-50% despite CRC mortality rates having fallen by 27% in men and 43% in women since 1972 [2, 4].

Genetic and environmental risk factors are currently being addressed through high risk family identification, anti-smoking and anti-obesity campaigns, and the "five a day" healthy eating programme [5]. These public health measures are important but are unlikely to have any impact on CRC incidence for decades.

Screening

Screening involves the investigation of asymptomatic individuals with the aim of identifying disease at an earlier, treatable and potentially curable stage. The process can be opportunistic (either instigated by the patient or their doctor) or centrally organised as a national screening programme.

For screening to be worthwhile the disease must be common, have a well recognised pre-malignant lesion and treatment of that pre-malignant lesion must reduce the risk of cancer. Of the various polyps in the large intestine, the adenoma has the most consistent link with later CRC development (adenoma-carcinoma sequence) [6]. Adenomas are common and few ever progress to cancer, so criteria for adenomas at highest risk have been developed and include: a diameter greater than 1cm; three or more adenomas; tubulovillous or villous histology, severe dysplasia or malignancy; and more than 20 hyperplastic polyps above the distal rectum [7].

The UK Breast and Cervical Screening programmes have been in place for some time, and as CRC is common and has an identifiable pre-cursor, it too is a suitable disease for screening. However, whilst there is only one currently accepted screening tool (mammogram or PAP smear) for the other diseases, CRC has a range of acceptable screening tools, each with potential pros and cons. Deciding which to use (on a national scale) must take into consideration: cost, patient acceptability, compliance and manpower implications. In the longer term, the programme must be sustainable and remain cost-effective.

Table 1. Current (2004) American Cancer Society recommendations for colorectal cancer screening for all men and women 50 years and over [9].

Faecal occult blood test	Annual
or	
Flexible sigmoidoscopy	Every 5 years
or	
Faecal occult blood test and Flexible sigmoidoscopy	Annual FOBT and flexible sigmoidoscopy every 5 years
or	
Double contrast barium enema	Every 5 years
or	
Colonoscopy	Every 10 years

Where are we now?

Screening for CRC has been shown to improve CRC mortality rates (presumably through the detection of earlier stage disease) but also has the potential to reduce CRC incidence, through the detection and excision of high risk adenomas. Although the evidence for a mortality reduction is robust, a reduction in incidence has not been consistently found in randomised trials.

Screening has been recommended in the US for some time using one of a variety of screening tools and uptake in adults ranges from 34% to 53% [8,9] (Table 1). A recent US review has suggested that CRC mortality could be reduced by 50%, whilst the UK government's current aim is a more conservative 15% [10,11]. Mass population screening of the average risk individual is a topical issue, with a national pilot (in Central England and Scotland, using biennial FOBT [faecal occult blood tests]) now complete, and a rolled out NHS Bowel Cancer Screening programme set to begin in April 2006 [12]. Unfortunately, it remains unclear which screening tool ought to be employed. The only test to have been rigorously assessed in a randomised trial setting is guaiac-based FOBT, although preliminary results from the "once only" flexible sigmoidoscopy trial have shown it to be an effective and acceptable screening tool [7]. These two tools appear the most likely contenders for a national UK screening programme.

The range of screening modalities is discussed below and compared in Table 2 [7,13–15]. In forming a decision on screening, it is worth considering that the best screening tool for an individual is not necessarily the optimal tool for screening a nation. This section focuses its discussion on a national screening perspective.

Guaiac-based faecal occult blood tests

The five most widely quoted trials of population screening for CRC using FOBT are listed in Table 3. A meta-analysis of the four randomised trials found a reduction in CRC mortality of 16% for those allocated to screening, rising to 23% in those who were actually screened [16-21]. To achieve this reduction, approximately 1254 individuals need to be offered screening (or 746 to accept screening) to prevent one CRC death with one major complication from colonoscopy (requiring surgery) occurring for every ten colorectal cancer deaths prevented [22].

Although the major trials stopped screening some years ago, most are continuing to follow their trial participants. Cumulative CRC incidence rates remain similar in both the screened and control groups after 8-13 years of follow-up in all the randomised trials [13]. There is therefore no clear evidence yet of a reduction in CRC incidence by FOBT screening.

In the UK national pilot study of FOBT screening using Haemoccult II, a higher FOBT positivity rate was observed in Scotland, in men and in individuals from more deprived areas. The positive predictive

Table 2. Comparing possible screening modalities.

Factors	Screening modalities			
	Faecal occult blood test	Flexible sigmoidoscopy	Colonoscopy	CT colonography
Setting	Home	Outpatient endoscopy	Outpatient endoscopy	Outpatient radiology
Method of detection of pathology	Microscopic blood from gastrointestinal tract	Visual identification of area reached (descending colon)	Visual identification of area reached (caecum)	Computed tomographic identification
Further test required	Colonoscopy	Colonoscopy	Barium enema	Colonoscopy
Referral rate (reason)	2% (positive test)	5% (positive test)	5–15% (incomplete colonoscopy)	Up to 20% (positive test)
Bowel preparation	No	Self-administered enema	Full bowel preparation	Full bowel preparation or faecal tagging
Oral preparation	Diet restriction	-	Clear fluids day before	Clear fluids day before
Sedation	No	No	Yes	No
Staff	Tester	Endoscopist (physician or nurse) Nurse	Endoscopist (physician or nurse) Nurse Pathologist	Radiologist Radiographer
Duration of procedure	3 separate stools (consecutive days)	5-10 minutes*	15-20 minutes*	10-15 minutes**
Compliance	51% (Towler 2000)	40% (UK Sigmoidoscopy 2002)	+	+
Day off work	No	No	Yes	No
Complications	None	Perforation (1 in 40,332) Bleeding (6 in 40,332) Mortality (6 in 40,332 at 30 days)	Bleeding (0.07%)^ Perforation (0.13%)^ Mortality (0.07%)^	Radiation exposure Drug reaction
Intestine visualised	No	Rectum, sigmoid, descending colon	Whole large intestine	Whole large intestine
Therapeutic ability	No	No	Yes	No

* Endoscopic procedures - time taken is generally experience and patient-dependent, taking longer in trainees
** CT colonography - mean examination time 9 minutes, time spent in CT suite 23 mins, reporting time 14 mins (Taylor 2003)
\+ No randomised screening trial has been performed to date
^ Recent UK figures for colonoscopy for symptomatic patients (not screened) (Bowles 2004)

value for neoplasia increased with advancing age and was higher in males. Stage distribution showed a shift towards earlier stages, with 72% of cancers being either Dukes' A or B disease [23].

The most persistent criticism of guaiac-based FOBT has been its low sensitivity for cancer and polyps (46-64% for cancer with biennial testing) and research has focused on improving this. The Minnesota trial used rehydrated FOBT samples and found that sensitivity rose to 92%, although this was at the expense of specificity (90%). When unhydrated, sensitivity fell to 80% but specificity rose to 98% [19]. The rehydration method (now not

Table 3. Five major trials of screening for colorectal cancer using faecal occult blood tests.

Characteristics	Lead author and date of population screening trial using FOBT				
	Mandel (1993)*	Hardcastle (1996)*	Kronborg (1996)*	Kewenter (1994)*	Winawer (1993)*
Location	Minnesota, US	Nottingham, UK	Funen, Denmark	Gothenberg, Sweden	New York, US
Study age group	50-80	45-74	45-75	60-64	>40
Trial basis	Intervention	Population	Population	-	Intervention
Unhydrated FOBT test	17.5%	Yes	Yes	Few	Most
Biennial screen	Yes (and annual)	Yes	Yes	16–20 months later	No
Percentage completing first screening round	90%	60%	67%	63%	80%
Test sensitivity for cancer	81%	64%	46%	81%	-
Proportion of cancers Dukes' Stage A	29%	21%	23%	26%	35%

* Randomised trials

recommended) led to a very high referral rate to colonoscopy (38% of the study population in 15 years) and it was suggested that the 33% CRC mortality reduction seen in this particular study (rehydrated annual FOBT) was attributable to the chance selection for colonoscopy [24]. Reducing the false positive rate was achieved in the Danish trial by diet restriction, with participants advised against consumption of red meats, fresh fruits, iron preparations, vitamin C, aspirin or other non-steriodals during the preceding three days [18].

Population compliance is also important for the success and cost-effectiveness of any screening programme. Although FOBT is technically harmless, complications do occur following referral to colonoscopy (in FOBT positive subjects). Handling faeces, person and physician preferences and repeated screening rounds are suggested reasons for a reduced compliance, although the national pilot found compliance was close to 60% with few adverse events [23].

The economic impact of FOBT screening in trial and population settings has also been examined [25-27]. Recently recalculated costs of the Nottingham FOBT trial found screening to cost £5290 per cancer detected and £1584 per life year gained (Table 4) [28]. In 1998, Garvican and colleagues examined the planning, projected costs and manpower requirements for a possible national screening programme [27]. Considering 50 to 69-year-olds, which at that time constituted 20% of the UK population, would result in 60,000 investigations annually. The cost estimate was over £40 million per year to detect 35% (5400) of the cases of CRC in the eligible population. The additional cost of a quality management system was approximately 3.8 million a year and so the cost-utility ratio rose to approximately £6500 per Quality Adjusted Life Year (QALY), whilst the recent national pilot found a cost per QALY of £2600 [23, 29]. Overall, CRC screening (with biennial FOBT) appears as cost-effective as the current breast and cervical screening programmes and lies well within the arbitrary thresholds of cost-effectiveness (circa £20,000-£30,000 per QALY).

Immunological tests

Immunological tests are diet-independent and highly selective for occult colorectal bleeding. The most

Table 4. Comparing the effectiveness and cost-effectiveness of screening modalities.

Factors	Screening modalities			
	Faecal occult blood test	Flexible sigmoidoscopy	Colonoscopy	CT colonography
Sensitivity for CRC	33%	95%	95%	100%
Specificity for CRC	97% Biennial unhydrated	100%	100%	99%
Sensitivity for polyps >1cm	10%	95%	95%	94%
Specificity for polyps >1cm	0.97	100%	100%	96%
References	Alexander (2004)	Hixson 1991, Wagner 1996	Hixson 1991, Wagner 1996	Fenlon 1999, Miao 2000, Pickhardt 2003
Cost				
Cost (cost year) of each test	£3.29	£56	£187	Estimate**
Mathematical modelling (Frazier)	$38	$279	$1012	-
Cost per person screened	£7.00	£82.20	-	-
Cost per cancer detected	£5,290	*	+	+
Incremental cost per life year gained				
Randomised trial (Whynes 2004)	£1584 (CI 717-8612)	*	+	+
Mathematical modelling (Frazier)	-	$1,200	$22,400	Not assessed
Mortality reduction	55%	16%	31%	Not assessed
Regimen used	Annual, unhydrated	One time at 55 yrs	One time at 60 yrs	Not assessed
References	Whynes 2004 Frazier 2000	Whynes 2003 Frazier 2000	Whynes 2004 Frazier 2000	-

CRC=colorectal cancer
Exchange rate £1 = $1.55 = €1.75 (2000 prices, discounted costs at 6% and benefits at 2%) (Model prices at 1998 prices, $ US dollars, discounted at 3%)
* Economic evaluation from randomised trial awaited
+ No randomised economic evaluation undertaken

commonly used tests are HemeSelect and FlexSure OBT, the former being based on reverse passive haemagglutination, the latter based on the specific binding of human haemoglobin to human haemoglobin antibody [30]. The additional benefit of these immunochemical tests has been to improve the sensitivity for cancer whilst retaining the benefits of a stool-based method. When HemeSelect (immunological) was compared with Haemoccult II (guaiac) in a non-randomised study, their sensitivities for detecting cancer were 69% and 37% respectively but their specificities were 94% versus 97% [31]. In the national pilot, the majority of positive FOBT tests came from repeat testing rather than the first screening round, which prompted the authors to conclude that immunological tests could be considered as a future alternative [23]. However, immunological tests have not been used in a randomised trial setting and the improved sensitivity is often at the expense of a higher false positive rate.

Whilst the guaiac-based tests provide a qualitative result which is reader-dependent, the immunological tests use agglutination tests, immunochromatography or ELISA to process results. Although this makes them more costly, there is the possibility that the reading could be automated in the future, which would have considerable manpower implications, particularly in a national programme. In addition, the result may be quantifiable, allowing a cut-off value for faecal haemoglobin to be set [32]. This would make such a test more versatile, enabling countries to set a value to suit the level of risk of CRC and adenomas in their population or setting the level in conjunction with their local resource availability.

Gene array tests

New tests designed to detect DNA shed from colorectal neoplasms are available but the two largest US multicentre trials are yet to report [33, 34]. One assay, for example, looks for 21 different point mutations in the APC, K-ras and p53 genes and for microsatellite instability (e.g. BAT-26). K-ras and p53 gene mutations have been the most frequently detected alterations in the stool of confirmed CRC patients, although DNA amplification is also of interest [35]. In a very small group of patients with CRC (n=9), SFRP2 methylation (DNA methylation) was found to be a sensitive (90%) and specific (77%) DNA-based marker for CRC [36]. Kahi et al estimate sensitivity at 70% for CRC and 30-40% for adenomas >1cm with screening intervals of 3-5 years and a charge of approximately $500 (£275) [37]. Most of these tests remain in the early research phases and are currently very expensive, but they do represent an exciting area of research and in the future may prove to be a most effective screening tool.

Flexible sigmoidoscopy

Flexible sigmoidoscopy (FS) allows examination of the distal 30-60cm (rectum to splenic flexure), where approximately 70% of CRC and adenomas are found.

Compared to rigid sigmoidoscopy, FS is more expensive due to the need for an enema, endoscopy time and equipment, but it is better tolerated and achieves greater yields [38].

There are currently four randomised trials underway worldwide, with the UK trial finding FS screening to be safe while achieving a sufficient yield of polyps and cancers to make it a worthwhile tool [7]. Although considerably more expensive per test than FOBT, £56 versus £3 (Table 4), the cost may be offset by the need to do the investigation only once (at age 50). This is a reasonable assumption considering the predominately left-sided position of cancers and adenomas, the high sensitivity of FS for these lesions and the long sojourn time (approximately 10 years) of the adenoma-carcinoma sequence. An additional hope is for the trial to detect a reduction in CRC incidence, due to the detection and excision of adenomas, although CRC mortality data from the trial have yet to be published (expected in 2006) and any fall in incidence may take considerably longer to detect.

A preliminary economic analysis of the trial has been published (Table 4) but an assessment of the cost-effectiveness awaits mortality figures [39]. Frazier et al predicted that one-time screening sigmoidoscopy at age 55 would enable a 14% reduction in incidence and a 16% reduction in mortality at a cost per life year gained of $1200 (1998 prices) [40]. In this mathematical model, one-time FS screening had the most favourable cost-effectiveness ratio of all the regimens tested.

The impact on local hospital services is also being assessed in the trial. Although the number of nurse endoscopists currently practising in the UK is low, expansion of their numbers would almost certainly be required for a national FS screening programme. In 6% of cases, a detected lesion (high risk polyp or cancer) on FS would require referral to colonoscopy [7]. Compared with colonoscopy, the complication rates, screening times and time to train endoscopists are less, but the cost of instrument maintenance and disinfection are the same and only a proportion of the large bowel is visualised. The most consistent concern with FS screening is the reliance on distal (left-sided) "marker polyps" for the identification of proximal (right-sided) pathology. These marker polyps have been shown to be indicators of potential synchronous, proximal lesions, and their presence should prompt colonoscopic examination. The problem is that one in 15 people without a marker polyp (distal adenoma) will have a proximal adenoma with one in 42 having an advanced proximal adenoma [41]. As with FOBT screening, public confidence would be affected by "missed lesions" on screening and this problem will only be compounded if a right-sided shift in CRC distribution proves to be real [42]. In addition, the referral rate to colonoscopy in the UK trial would probably be double that of the FOBT trial, placing additional pressure on endoscopy departments and increasing both the costs and the number of complications.

Combined faecal occult blood testing and flexible sigmoidoscopy

Using both tests at different times of a screening programme is a potential option for screening, with one test compensating for the limitations of the other [43, 44]. Although the sensitivity of FOBT for proximal lesions is low, the addition of a rehydrated FOBT test to sigmoidoscopy saw a rise in the detection of advanced neoplasia from 70% to 76%, in one case study [45]. Annual unhydrated FOBT with 5-yearly sigmoidoscopy is currently one of the suggested US screening regimens, although it has not been assessed in a randomised trial setting as yet (Table 1).

Colonoscopy

Colonoscopy is the gold standard investigation for high risk groups such as hereditary non-polyposis coli (HNPCC) and familial adenomatous polyposis (FAP), but it has also been recommended as a screening tool every 10 years by the American College of Gastroenterology [46]. Although it is both a diagnostic and therapeutic tool (polypectomy) with the added advantage of detecting right-sided lesions, these benefits do not necessarily make it the most appropriate population screening tool. Population screening by colonoscopy in the UK would be very expensive both in terms of the cost of the test (£187) and treating the complications such a programme would undoubtedly yield [44]. Extrapolating current endoscopy complication rates to a national level, would potentially see over 500 severe haemorrhages, over 150 perforations, and 50 deaths each year. Complications on this scale would probably make national headlines and affect screening compliance.

The UK currently has neither the manpower nor the necessary facilities to undertake national colonoscopic screening as at least a doubling of UK endoscopy facilities and manpower would be required. In addition, the standard of colonoscopy in the UK remains variable and, although steps are being taken to address this, we are a long way from providing a uniformly high quality diagnostic colonoscopy service [15].

Computed tomographic (CT) colonography

CT colonography after a decade of development has now achieved levels of sensitivity (94%) and specificity (96%) for large polyps that enable it to be considered as a screening tool. Compared to colonoscopy, it is better tolerated with less cardiovascular effects and a better complication profile [47]. In addition, it is more sensitive for colonic neoplasia than barium enema and, if electronically subtractable faecal markers are used, it is possible to avoid bowel preparation. The high sensitivities for cancer, which can reach 100% in certain studies, tend to be in symptomatic patients, but one additional benefit here is the ability to stage detected colorectal cancers at the same sitting, and also identify other occult malignancies.

As with any techniques there are drawbacks. The radiation dose is similar to that of a barium enema, although this is operator- and machine-dependent. It lacks the therapeutic potential of colonoscopy and concerns remain about low sensitivities for polyps under 1cm [14, 37]. It has also been predicted that even with a threshold of a 1cm polyp, one out of every 13 patients would require referral for colonoscopy, which is a high referral rate [48]. The availability of CT scanners, the cost, the additional pressure on radiology staff and high inter-observer variation even between colonographic experts are currently unresolved issues [49, 50].

Most of the studies to date have been small and trials currently recruiting tend to be considering symptomatic patients in the first instance (see Useful resources). The general consensus seems to suggest that this technique has great potential but that it is not currently ready for widespread clinical application [49].

Double-contrast barium enema

Prior to colonoscopy or CT colonography, this was the investigation of choice for large bowel examination and current methods achieve sensitivities for cancers or polyps greater than 1cm of 90% and 80% respectively [51]. Population screening using barium enema has been assessed in model settings and found to be cost-effective at screening intervals of 3-5 years but it has not been investigated by a randomised trial [40]. It is more costly and inconvenient than FOBT, requires full bowel preparation, lacks the therapeutic potential of colonoscopy and has considerable inter-observer variation even amongst experts [52].

Where are we going?

To screen or not?

Following the recommendations of the national pilot, which concluded that population-based screening was feasible and cost-effective, the Government has provided funding for a national roll out of screening [23].

However, a fall in CRC mortality has been observed since 1972 and this is without mass population screening. This fall is probably due to improved public awareness coupled with improvements in diagnostic and therapeutic interventions, but a change in the natural history of the disease cannot be excluded. One additional concern secondary to finite resource availability is that management of symptomatic patients may well be adversely affected by mass screening. Delays in radiological and endoscopic investigations were noted in trial and pilot settings, although these areas of potential delay are under investigation. The UK endoscopy service was recently reviewed and Ward *et al* concluded in their consultation document that there was a need for rapid expansion to meet demands, particularly if the chosen population screening tool was endoscopic [53]. What should not be allowed to happen is that available resources are shifted from the care of the sick or high risk to the low risk [54].

Which tool to use?

Although protagonists of endoscopic screening will quote the higher sensitivity and specificity of the investigations, confirmation within a trial setting is important. The randomised studies of FOBT published to date have provided valuable information about compliance rates, implementation and local resource issues and have confirmed that no obvious psychological harm comes from CRC screening [55]. FOBT also fits the WHO criteria of a screening tool which state that "a screening test should be inexpensive, rapid, and simple, and is not intended to be diagnostic; those with positive tests require further evaluation" [56]. However, despite 11 years of follow-up, the Nottingham FOBT trial has yet to find any reduction in CRC incidence. Whichever tool is chosen, it is vital that over the longer term the cost-effectiveness of screening is maintained and that lead and length time bias are not confounding the original results. These two biases are a major concern for non-randomised studies.

Hopefully, in 10 years time, the national screening programme will be well established and we will have a clearer picture of population compliance and detection rates. The process of comparing existing (flexible sigmoidoscopy) and future technologies (faecal DNA analysis) against biennial FOBT (the baseline test) should form part of the long-term research programme into the most effective and acceptable national screening programme.

We can be confident that screening for CRC has three real strengths:

1. It will reduce the mortality of this eminently treatable cancer.
2. It is cost-effective compared to other screening programmes.
3. It provides the best chance of reducing CRC incidence in the near future (although for FOBT this effect may take decades to be detected).

The combined effect of screening, new advances in adjuvant chemotherapies, improved surgical techniques and increased resections of metastatic deposits will hopefully have a marked effect on the mortality of this disease in the decades to come.

Conflict of interests

Neither author has any conflict of interest in this book section. The brand names mentioned are done to aid recognition and not to promote one test over another.

Useful resources

1. American Cancer Society Guidelines for the Early Detection of Cancer 2004 [9].
2. Implementing Colorectal Cancer Screening Group 2 Report [57].
3. World Cancer Report [58].
4. Evaluation of the UK Colorectal Cancer Screening Pilot [23].
5. Cochrane colorectal cancer group: www.cochrane.org/cochrane/revabstr/COLOCAAbstractIndex.htm. CT colonography trial www.htacolonography.com.

References

1. International Agency for Research on Cancer. Cancer incidence, mortality and prevalence in the European Union, EUCAN 1998 estimates. Brussels: International agency for Research on Cancer 1998; Accessed 29/12/2003.
2. Cancer Research UK. British Cancer Death Rates. *BMJ* 2004; 328: 303.
3. Cancer Research UK. Bowel Cancer Factsheet. *Cancer Research UK* 2003.
4. Maxwell-Armstrong CA, Scholefield JH. Colorectal cancer. In: *Clinical Evidence.* BMJ Publishing group, 2003; 10: 509-17.
5. NHS Direct. Making changes. NHS direct 2003.
6. Leslie A, Carey FA, Pratt NR, Steele RJC. The colorectal adenoma-carcinoma sequence. *Br J Surg* 2002; 89: 845-60.
7. UK Flexible Sigmoidoscopy Screening Trial Investigators. Single flexible sigmoidoscopy screening to prevent colorectal cancer: baseline findings of a UK multicentre randomised trial. *Lancet* 2002; 359: 1291-300.
8. Subramanian S, Klosterman M, Amonkar MM, Hunt TL. Adherence with colorectal cancer screening guidelines: a review. *Preventive Medicine* 2004; 38: 536-50.
9. Smith RA, Cokkinides V, Eyre HJ. American cancer society guidelines for the early detection of cancer 2004. *A Cancer Journal for Clinicians* 2004; 54: 41-52.
10. Walsh JM, Terdiman JP. Colorectal cancer screening: scientific review. *JAMA* 2003; 289: 1288-96.
11. Milburn A. Winning the fight against cancer. In: Britain against cancer conference. Department of Health, London, 2002.
12. Department of Health. www.dh.gov.uk/PublicationsAndStatistics/PressReleases 27th October 2004. Accessed 18/01/2005.
13. Towler BP, Irwig L, Glasziou P. Screening for colorectal cancer using the faecal occult blood test, Haemoccult. *Cochrane Database of Systematic Reviews* 2000; 2.
14. Taylor SA, Halligan S, Saunders BP, Morley S, Riesewyk C, Atkin W, et al. Use of multidetector-row CT colonography for detection of colorectal neoplasia in patients referred via the Department of Health "2-week-wait" initiative. *Clin Radiol* 2003; 58: 855-61.
15. Bowles CJA, Leicester R, Romaya C, Swarbrick E, Williams CB, Epstein O. A prospective study of colonoscopy practice in the UK today: are we adequately prepared for national colorectal cancer screening tomorrow. *Gut* 2004; 53: 277-83.
16. Towler BP, Irwig L, Glasziou P, Kewenter J, Weller D, Silagy C. A systematic review of the effects of screening for colorectal cancer using the faecal occult blood test, Hemoccult. *BMJ* 1998; 317: 559-65.
17. Hardcastle JD, Chamberlain JO, Robinson MHE, Moss SM, Amar SS, Balfour TW, et al. Randomised controlled trial of faecal-occult-blood screening for colorectal cancer. *Lancet* 1996; 348: 1472-7.
18. Kronborg O, Fenger C, Olsen J, Jorgensen OD, Sondergaard O. Randomised study of screening for colorectal cancer with faecal occult blood test. *Lancet* 1996; 348: 1467-71.
19. Mandel JS, Bond JH, Church TR. Reducing mortality from colorectal cancer by screening for faecal occult blood. *N Engl J Med* 1993; 328: 1365-71.
20. Kewenter J, Brevinge H, Engaras B. Results of screening, rescreening and follow-up in a prospective randomized study for detection of colorectal cancer by faecal occult blood testing. Results for 68,308 subjects. *Scand J Gastroenterol* 1994; 29: 468-73.
21. Winawer SJ, Flehinger BJ, Schottenfield D, Miller DG. Screening for colorectal cancer with faecal occult blood testing and sigmoidoscopy. *J Natl Cancer Inst* 1993; 85: 1311-8.
22. Robinson MHE, Hardcastle JD. *Screening for colorectal cancer - who, when and how.* 1st ed. Blackwell Science, Oxford, 2000.
23. Alexander F, Weller D. Evaluation of the UK Colorectal cancer screening pilot. Edinburgh: Department of Community Health Sciences; 2003.
24. Lang CA, Ransohoff DF. Fecal occult blood screening for colorectal cancer. *JAMA* 1994; 271(13): 1011-3.
25. Whynes DK, Walker AR, Hardcastle JD. Cost-effective screening strategies for colorectal cancer. *J Public Health Med* 1992; 14(1): 43-9.

26. Whynes DK, Walker AR, Chamberlain JO, Hardcastle JD. Screening and the costs of treating colorectal cancer. *Br J Cancer* 1993; 68: 965-8.
27. Garvican L. Planning for a possible national colorectal cancer screening programme. *J Med Screening* 1998; 5(4): 187-94.
28. Whynes DK. Cost-effectiveness of screening for colorectal cancer: evidence from the Nottingham faecal occult blood trial. *J Med Screening* 2004; 11(1): 11-5.
29. Robert G, Brown J, Garvican L. Cost of quality management and information provision for screening: colorectal cancer screening. *J Med Screening* 2000; 7(1): 31-4.
30. Allison JE. Review article: faecal occult blood testing for colorectal cancer. *Alimentary Pharmacology and Therapeutics* 1998; 12(1): 1-10.
31. Allison J, Tekewa I, Ransom L, Adrain A. A comparison of faecal occult-blood tests for colorectal cancer screening. *N Engl J Med* 1996; 334: 155-9.
32. Young GP, Rozen P, Levin B. *How should we screen for early colorectal neoplasia.* Martin Dunitz, London, 2002.
33. Traverso G, Shuber AP, Levin B, Johnson C, Olsson L, Schoetz Jr DJ, et al. Detection of APC mutations in fecal DNA from patients with colorectal tumours. *N Engl J Med* 2002; 346: 311-9.
34. Ahlquist DA, Shuber AP. Stool screening for colorectal cancer: evolution from occult blood to molecular markers. *Clinica Chimica Acta* 2002; 315: 157-68.
35. Calistri D, Rengucci C, Bocchini R, Saragoni L, Zoli W, Amadori D. Fecal multiple molecular tests to detect colorectal cancer in stool. *Clin Gastroenterol Hepatol* 2003; 1(5): 377-83.
36. Muller HM, Oberwalder M, Fiegl H, Morandell M, Goebel G, Zitt M, et al. Methylation changes in faecal DNA: a marker for colorectal cancer screening? *Lancet* 2004; 363: 1283-85.
37. Kahi CJ, Rex DK. Current and future trends in colorectal cancer screening. *Cancer and Metastasis Reviews* 2004; 23: 137-44.
38. Robinson MHE. NNTs and NNHs - an individualised way to present benefit and risk. *Colorectal disease* 1999; 1: 45-6.
39. Whynes DK, Frew EJ, Edwards R, Atkin WS. Costs of flexible sigmoidoscopy screening for colorectal cancer in the United Kingdom. *International Journal of Technological Assessment in Health Care* 2003; 19(2): 384-95.
40. Frazier A, Colditz G, Fuchs C, Kuntz K. Cost effectiveness of screening for colorectal cancer in the general population. *JAMA* 2000; 284: 1954-61.
41. Lewis JD, Ng K, Hung KE, Bilker WB, Berlin JA, Brensinger C, et al. Detection of proximal adenomatous polyps with screening sigmoidoscopy. *Arch Int Med* 2003; 163: 413-20.
42. Rabaneck L, Davila JA, El-Serag HB. Is there a true "shift" to the right colon in the incidence of colorectal cancer? *Am J Gastroenterol* 2003; 98(6): 1400-9.
43. Atkin WS, Northover JMA. Population-based endoscopic screening for colorectal cancer. *Gut* 2003; 52: 321-2.
44. Macafee DAL, Scholefield JH. Population-based endoscopic screening for colorectal cancer. *Gut* 2003; 52: 323-6.
45. Lieberman DA, Weiss DG. One time screening for colorectal cancer with combined faecal occult blood testing and examination of the distal colon. *N Engl J Med* 2001; 345(8): 555-60.
46. Rex DK, Johnson DA, Lieberman DA, Burt RW, Sonnenberg A. Colorectal cancer prevention 2000: screening recommendations of the American College of Gastroenterology. *Am J Gastroenterol* 2000; 95: 868-77.
47. Taylor SA, Halligan S, O'Donnell C, Morley S, Mistry H, Saunders BP, et al. Cardiovascular effects at multi-detector row CT colonography compared with those at conventional endoscopy of the colon. *Radiology* 2003; 229: 782-90.
48. Rabaneck L. Is computed tomographic colonography effective for colorectal cancer screening. *Can Med Assoc J* 2004; 170(9): 1392.
49. Cotton PB, Durkalski VL, Pineau BC, Palesch YY, Mauldin PD, Hoffman B, et al. Computed tomographic colonography (virtual colonoscopy). A multicenter comparison with standard colonoscopy for detection of colorectal neoplasia. *JAMA* 2004; 291(14): 1713-9.
50. Johnson CD, Harmsen WS, Wilson LA, MacCarty RL, Welch TJ, Ilstrup DM, et al. Prospective blinded evaluation of computed tomographic colonography for screen detection of colorectal polyps. *Gastroenterology* 2003; 125(2): 311-9.
51. Ferrucci JT. Screening for colon cancer: programs of the American College of Radiology. *Am J Radiol* 1993; 160: 999-103.
52. Halligan S, Marshall M, Taylor S, Bartram CI, Bassett P, Cardwell C, et al. Observer variation in the detection of colorectal neoplasia on double-contrast barium enema: implications for colorectal cancer screening and training. *Clin Radiol* 2003; 58: 948-54.
53. Ward S, Cowan J. Analysis of the potential cost impact of the guidance on cancer services: "Improving outcomes in colorectal cancer" Expansion in Endoscopy capacity - Draft for 2nd consultation. School of Health and Related Research, University of Sheffield, Sheffield, Sept 2003.
54. Coebergh JWW. Colorectal cancer screening in Europe: first things first. *Eur J Cancer* 2004; 40: 638-42.
55. Parker MA, Robinson MHE, Scholefield JH, Hardcastle JD. Psychiatric morbidity and screening for colorectal cancer. *J Med Screening* 2002; 9: 7-10.
56. Wilson JMG, Jungner G. *Principles and practice of screening for disease.* World Health Organisation, Geneva, 1968.
57. Rozen P. Implementing colorectal cancer screening: group 2 report. *Endoscopy* 2004; 36: 354-8.
58. World Health Organisation. World Cancer Report. World Health Organisation, New York, 2003.

Chapter 2

Follow-up strategies for colorectal cancer (CRC)

Sanjay Purkayastha BSc MB BS MRCS, Research Fellow, Surgical Oncology
Paris P Tekkis MD FRCS, Senior Lecturer, Surgical Oncology
Imperial College, St. Mary's Hospital, London, UK

What are the issues?

CRC will affect approximately 5% of the western population [1]. Approximately two out of five patients with CRC will die from the disease [2]. However, over three quarters may present with potentially curable disease within 5 years of the original diagnosis [3]. Follow-up aims to identify cancer recurrence at an early, potentially curable stage. Eighty percent of recurrences are seen during the first 2 years after primary tumour resection, thus there has been discussion to suggest the intensity of the follow-up regimen should be highest in the first few years [4, 5, 6].

It seems logical that patients with higher staged disease are at greater risk from recurrence. But once these patients are treated with surgery with or without chemoradiotherapy, what is the most appropriate and effective surveillance necessary to increase survival as much as possible? Indeed, is surveillance necessary at all? If so, what modalities should be used? Who is best suited to carry out this surveillance and in what setting? How cost-effective are such strategies? What evidence is there to answer the above questions? These are the issues that will be discussed in this chapter.

Is surveillance necessary and what should be the aims? (Table 1)

As surgical clinicians, it seems intuitive that CRC patients should be followed-up after treatment: firstly, to monitor progress and post-surgical complications; and secondly, to monitor individuals to promptly assess the possibility of tumour recurrence - the latter may be for local or distant disease. There have been several randomised studies to look at CRC follow-up and none has shown evidence that there should be no post-treatment surveillance, although it must be noted that there are very few studies with "no follow-up" as the control arm. Most studies compare aggressive follow-up with less aggressive strategies. Increased surveillance has a positive trend towards survival advantage [7, 8, 9] and this may be due to earlier discovery of treatable recurrences amenable to curative re-resection. However, there is meta-analytical work that suggests that, although intense follow-up may pick up some asymptomatic recurrences, the numbers needed to treat are very high which leads to high labour intensity and poor cost-effectiveness [10]. From the same work, the author suggests that the focus of colorectal cancer follow-up should shift from the early detection of recurrence towards quality

> **Table 1. Aims of CRC follow-up.**
>
> - Management of postoperative complications
> - Early detection of recurrence
> - Early detection of new primary tumour
> - To aid decision-making for possible adjuvant therapies
> - Audit of outcomes
> - Assess quality of life
> - Patient reassurance

assessment and patient support. At present there is little valuable evidence on quality of life data with regards to long-term CRC follow-up, although there are trials in progress attempting to evaluate such factors.

Looking to the positive evidence for more intense follow-up, a Cochrane review of this subject [9] performed a meta-analysis of five randomised trials and concluded that there was indeed an overall survival benefit for intensifying the follow-up of patients after curative surgery for colorectal cancer. However, the trials used in the review had a wide variation in follow-up strategies and thus it was not possible to elucidate the most effective protocol or the cost-effectiveness of CRC follow-up.

Modalities that may be used in follow-up

Clinical review

Several randomised studies have shown possible benefits but because of relatively small sample sizes the results were not statistically significant. However, a meta-analysis by Rosen et al [7] pooled these results to show that more intensive follow-up leads to an increase in 5-year survival. A previous meta-analysis by Bruinvels et al [11] was unable to show a significant increase in 5-year survival rate for intensive follow-up of patients with colorectal cancer operated on for cure, but this study did not include the use of CEA for early detection of recurrence and also included two non-randomised trial data as part of the results.

Furthermore, Rosen et al [7] showed that patients who were in the intensive follow-up group were 2.5 times more likely to have a curative re-resection than those patients in the control groups (five studies: two randomised, three comparative cohort studies). Likewise, in the single-cohort studies, those patients with intensive follow-up were almost twice as likely to have a curative resection for recurrence than patients in the historic control group - thus strongly advocating the benefit of a more intense follow-up strategy, which also allows a higher chance of picking up recurrence in those patients at higher risk.

However, as already discussed above, other authors advocate less intense follow-up [10, 11], stating that the numbers needed to treat are far too high and that there is no adequate curative treatment for most recurrences anyway, especially if total mesorectal excision (TME) was performed correctly in the first instance [10].

The question as to who should be carrying out the follow-up process is a contentious one. Advocates of intense follow-up recommend surgical teams, which seems logical in the immediate and short-term postoperative period. But in the long term there are questions as to which healthcare professional should be the key contact. Should there be more primary care involvement, for example? Which clinicians would provide quicker diagnosis of recurrence but also have a more positive effect on the quality of life of the patients? Although these questions are contentious, currently each patient's situation should be considered individually as there is no real hard evidence to answer them one way or the other.

Blood tests: serum tumour markers (Table 2)

Serum carcinoembryonic antigen (CEA) has been used extensively both in the USA and Europe for follow-up for many years now, with the prospect that it is able to detect recurrence perhaps up to 6 months before symptoms develop. There is evidence that this relatively simple test leads to earlier diagnosis and more re-operative management [12]. But does this mean more cure of recurrence? This is unlikely and there is little evidence to suggest that salvage surgery changes survival rates on the whole. Moertel et al [13] showed that at any one time a vast

Table 2. Serum markers investigated for a role in CRC recurrence.

- Carcinoembryonic antigen (CEA)
- Carbohydrate antigen (Ca 19-9)
- Tissue polypeptide (TPA)
- Alpha-1-glycoprotein (AGP)
- Alpha-1-antitrypsin (AAT)
- Retinol-binding protein (RBP)
- Haptoglobin
- Caeruloplasmin
- Neopterin
- Protein-bound Hexose (PHex)

number of patients may be undergoing serial CEA measurements which undoubtedly has cost implications. The same study showed a false positive rate of 16% for CEA levels and recurrence. These findings led the investigators to conclude that patient survival from salvage surgery attributable to CEA monitoring is, at best, infrequent. Moertel et al [13] continued to question whether this small gain justified the substantial financial cost and physical and emotional stress that this intervention may cause for patients.

Against this view, a Dutch meta-analysis, published more recently, suggests that CEA should in fact be used as a primary means for the early diagnosis of recurrence. But this study also suggests that the number needed to treat (NNT) is high (360), which means that it still may not be cost-effective [10]. These contentious issues may be resolved should the results of the St. Mark's randomised trial on CEA levels during follow-up be published.

Other markers have been studied, for example, Ca 19-9 (carbohydrate antigen) and TPA (tissue polypeptide), and compared to CEA, but the latter seems to be the most sensitive. Furthermore, combinations of measured markers do not seem to change the overall sensitivity and specificity [14]. More recently studies have looked at newer possible markers, such as alpha-1-glycoprotein (AGP) and alpha-1-antitrypsin (AAT), both of which were not as sensitive as CEA for recurrence and both of which were also raised in patients with diverticulitis and therefore not useful for follow-up. It should be noted that as a routine, CEA is the only serum marker used extensively; this is because all the other markers above have been shown to be less specific and less sensitive for recurrence of CRC.

Colonoscopy

Colonoscopy has two important roles:

- Recognition of recurrence.
- Detection of metachronous tumours.

Endoscopic techniques are relatively insensitive for detecting recurrences, but this is because the majority of recurrences do not originate from within the bowel lumen. Thus its main use is that of diagnosing metachronous lesions and polyps. Guidelines set out by The American Society of Colon and Rectal Surgeons recommend surveillance colonoscopy 1 year postoperatively, then every 3 years if the colon is normal [15].

Scalmati et al [16] have demonstrated altered epithelial cell kinetics in colorectal mucosa after resection for cancer, thus suggesting a possible mechanism for predicting metachronous neoplasia. In this study, patients who went on to develop recurrence demonstrated a hyperproliferative colorectal mucosa, whereas in others the colorectal mucosa seemed quiescent. Patients with hyperproliferative mucosa developed metachronous adenomas, whereas those with the quiescent type did not. The study concluded that "until clinically feasible indicators of hyperproliferative colorectal mucosa are identified, periodic colon surveillance needs to continue for all cancer patients." The data from Khoury et al [17] reported the findings of annual surveillance colonoscopy in colorectal cancer patients, and concluded the following:

- The chance of a positive initial postoperative colonoscopy was 18.3%.

- After a normal colonoscopy, the chance of finding a neoplastic polyp on the next annual examination was 10.4%.
- After a positive colonoscopy, the chance of finding a neoplastic polyp on the next annual examination was 43%.
- The chance of a positive examination after finding multiple neoplastic polyps was 70.4%.

The investigators concluded that annual follow-up colonoscopy for 2 years after colorectal cancer surgery is beneficial for detecting recurrent and metachronous neoplasms and that the interval between subsequent examinations may be increased depending on the result of the most recent examination. It must, however, be remembered that these are the results of a retrospective review.

Atkin et al [18], discuss colonoscopic surveillance for patients with sporadic adenomas in the absence of a previous colorectal cancer. This paper formulated algorithms for low, intermediate and high risk patients with adenomas. Suggestions were made as to the optimum time for colonoscopic re-examination. Surveillance for metachronous tumours following CRC with its attendant resection might follow the high risk arm of this algorithm. Perhaps also CRC patients should be sub-grouped depending on their risks for a metachronous tumour.

Imaging

Ultrasonography has long been used to image the liver accurately with regard to metastases. Generally, it is sensitive and specific for even small lesions (e.g. 1cm in diameter), although it is highly operator-dependent. It was even recommended as part of the follow-up process from Keivit's meta-analysis [10] as the primary investigation (along with CEA levels) for useful surveillance.

Besides imaging the liver, ultrasound scanning (USS) has also been used to assess local recurrence of rectal cancer using endoluminal ultrasound (EUS) techniques [19]. This study showed a sensitivity of EUS and CT for recurrence of 100% and 86% respectively with a specificity of 89% and 93% respectively. Overall, the accuracy for both imaging techniques was found to be 93% and 83% respectively. However, because of the small study size, the findings were not statistically significant.

Computed tomography (CT) has long been considered to be effective in the diagnosis or CRC recurrence but with varying sensitivities. Along with Magnetic resonance imaging (MRI), it undoubtedly is the diagnostic tool of choice for delineating recurrence in the surrounding pelvic cavity. But its limitations must be noted:

- Lesion diameter.
- Low sensitivity for lymph node recurrence.
- Artifacts from surgical clips.
- Difficulty in differentiating between post-operative scarring and recurrence.

MRI has proved to be superior to CT for tissue characterisation, even in the presence of surgical artifact, enabling just as high, if not higher, sensitivities and specificities compared to CT. However, availability, cost and patient factors (e.g. metal prosthesis, claustrophobia) make this investigation less usable on occasion. MRI may also be used endoluminally and this may yet yield better results, possibly because of its deeper focal length.

One of the difficulties of both CT and MRI lies in differentiating between recurrence and scar tissue; this issue may be improved by the use of serial scanning rather than just one-off imaging. Other imaging modalities that allow differentiation of recurrence from postoperative surgical change include:

- Positron emission tomography (PET).
- Radio-immunoscintigraphy (RIS).

Where are we now?

This section supplies an overview of what is in place in different geographical regions, and what is advocated by various well known colorectal organisations.

United Kingdom: Association of Coloproctologists of Great Britain and Ireland (ACPGBI 2001) recommendations

- "The evidence to support or refute any survival value for regular follow-up is not available. In the absence of hard evidence it is reasonable to offer liver imaging to asymptomatic fit patients during the first 2 years after resection for the purpose of detecting operable liver metastases.
- There is no evidence that colonoscopic follow-up improves survival, but it has been shown to produce a high yield of treatable adenomatous polyps and cancer. If such a policy is pursued, it is recommended that a "clean" colon should be examined by colonoscopy at 3-5 year intervals. Patients should be counselled as to the risks from colonoscopy.
- In the absence of evidence from randomised trials, the most persuasive arguments for routine follow-up are patient support and audit. Evidence suggests that patients' preference is for follow-up but by whom and where may depend on local circumstances. Audit should be structured with particular reference to outcome measures, and should be regarded as a routine part of a consultant's work. It may be facilitated by use of a database, such as that promoted by the Association of Coloproctology [20]. If other 'local' databases are used it is recommended that field definitions should match those of the Association's data dictionary to ensure conformity of data collection."

The executive summary by Scholefield *et al* on the *Guidelines for follow-up after resection of colorectal Cancer* [21] stated that:

- "Although there is no evidence that intensive follow-up for the detection of recurrent disease improves survival, it is reasonable to offer liver imaging to asymptomatic patients under the age of 70 in order to detect operable liver metastases once during the first 2 years after resection. (Recommendation Grade: A).
- Although there is no evidence that colonoscopic follow-up improves survival, it does produce a yield of treatable tumours. It is recommended that a 'clean' colon is examined by colonoscopy 5 years after surgery and thereafter at 5-yearly intervals up to the age of 70 years. (Recommendation Grade: B).
- In the absence of randomised trials, the only realistic argument for routine follow-up is patient support and audit. Audit should be focused on outcome measures."

National Institute for Clinical Excellence (NICE 2004) [22]

From the recent randomised studies and meta-analyses discussed in this chapter, intense follow-up, especially for the first 2 years, increases diagnosis of recurrence and new tumours and may have positive effects on overall survival. All centres should recruit for the FACS trial (follow-up after colorectal surgery), the details of which are outlined below. NICE also commented on considering a primary care setting for follow-up but will await the outcomes of the FACS. With regards to cost, NICE concluded that costs per patient were calculated to be £4,758 for intensive follow-up and £2,279 for conventional follow-up, both for 5 years. This represented an incremental cost per life-year gained by intensive follow-up of £3,007. These results suggest that the cost-effectiveness of intensive follow-up after surgery for colorectal cancer compares favourably with that of other interventions which are currently widely used in the NHS.

The NICE guidelines also addressed psychological factors for patients, stating "follow-up may have positive or negative psychological outcomes. Positive outcomes include reassurance and support. Negative outcomes include false reassurance, increased anxiety, fear associated with early detection of an incurable recurrence, morbidity and mortality associated with operations done in response to abnormal test results, and distress caused by false-positive results. Recurrence of colorectal cancer is usually symptomatic. Around 75% of recurrences produce symptoms between follow-up appointments, even if these are scheduled at 3-monthly intervals. There is

Table 3. Proposed CRC follow-up for patients undergoing surgery with curative intent performed for Dukes' A-C cancers. Defining possible guidelines if investigations are normal at each stage post-resection.

	6 weeks	6 months	1 year	Yearly up to 5 years	Discharge after 5 years*
Reasons for follow-up	Post op problems	Early recurrence	Recurrence†	Recurrence†	
	Audit	Audit	Audit	Audit	
	Reassurance	Reassurance	Reassurance	Reassurance	
	Early adverse events	Late adverse events	Late adverse events	Late adverse events	
			Metachronous	Metachronous	
		Psychology	Psychology	Psychology	
Clinical tasks	Clinical history and examination	Clinical history and examination	Clinical history and examination	Clinical history and examination	
				Leaflet	
	Rectoscopy	Rectoscopy	Rectoscopy	Rectoscopy	
	CEA	CEA	CEA	CEA	
			Liver USS	Liver USS	
		Colonoscopy††	Colonoscopy††		5-yearly Colonoscopy†† to the age of 70

* Discharge after 5 years unless symptomatic
† If at any point ? recurrence - CT pelvis + follow on to MRI if suspicious
†† If at any point - adenomas - refer to surveillance guidelines after removal of colorectal adenomatous polyps [18]

evidence that reassurance at follow-up consultations can lead some patients to fail to report symptoms promptly when they do occur between appointments."

USA: American Society of Colon and Rectal Surgeons (ASCRS 2004) [23]

This recommends follow-up with routine visits, CEA, USS and colonoscopy for the first 2 years but then subsequent follow-up for life with colonoscopy for detection of metachronous tumours. There does not seem to be any elaboration at present as to precise intervals of follow-up.

Australia: Colorectal Surgical Society of Australasia (CSSA 2004) [24]

The patient website advocates an initial 2-4 week postoperative follow-up, followed by regular and frequent appointments for 5 years, and then annually thereafter. This electronic site favoured clinical history and examination along with digital rectal examination (DRE) and colonoscopy, CEA measurements and USS of the liver if suspicion arises of metastasis. The Society also recommends that a patient should be followed-up by the surgeon for as long as he/she remains fit to undergo further treatment should a new cancer develop. The conclusions are:

- "Early postoperative colonoscopy, if colonoscopy or barium enema had not been performed before the operation.
- A review at regular and frequent intervals for 5 years. These visits to be associated with digital and sigmoidoscopic examination depending on the aspects of your case.
- Colonoscopy every 3 years.
- Other tests to detect cancer according to clinical indications."

Table 4. Example of an NHS protocol for CRC follow-up: St. Mary's Hospital, London.

Time from operation date	Physical exam DRE and rigid sig	Colonoscopy	CT chest, abdomen and pelvis	Other
3 months (from operation date) or approx 6/52 from ward discharge	No	Book patient for colonoscopy for 3 months time (i.e. 6/12 postop) **ONLY IF NO pre-op full colonic evaluation was performed.** If reversal of stoma is appropriate ensure gastrografin enema is booked and complete admission request card	No	Assess wound and pain Bowel function Weight/nutrition Psychosocial issues Ensure colorectal nurse's contact details are given
6 months	Yes	Yes *only if no* full colon test pre-op See patient with results of colonoscopy	CT chest *If* lung mets excised CT Ab/Pel *If* liver mets excised Book CT chest, abdomen, pelvis for 6 months time *if* <75 yrs and/or fit for surgery	Assess bowel function Weight/nutrition Psychosocial issues **Give patient blood form for LFTs for next OPA**
12 months	Yes	Yes *only if* polyps present pre-op (then go on to follow polyp surveillance protocol) otherwise no routine colonoscopy needed	See patient with results of CT **Liver imaging and LFTs**	Assess bowel function Weight/nutrition Psychosocial issues
18 months	Yes	No	CT chest *If* lung mets excised CT Ab/Pel *If* liver mets excised Book CT for 6 months time *if* <75 yrs and fit for surgery	Assess bowel function Weight/nutrition Psychosocial issues
2 years	Yes	Complete request card to book patient for colonoscopy in 1 year (i.e. 3 years postop)	See patient with results of CT Liver imaging	Assess bowel function Weight/nutrition Psychosocial issues
3 years	Yes	**Patient has had colonoscopy** and comes to clinic for results **If colonoscopy NAD 5 yrly until 70 yrs**	No	Assess bowel function Weight/nutrition Psychosocial issues
4 years	Yes	No	No	Assess bowel function Weight/nutrition Psychosocial issues
5 years	Yes	No	No	Cease follow-up. Colorectal nurse contact no. Patient aware of what symptoms to report

Where are we going?

A multicentre, randomised, controlled trial is currently under way in the UK, comparing intensive versus no scheduled follow-up in patients who have undergone resection for CRC with curative intent. This is the FACS trial (Follow-up After Colorectal Surgery). Its primary objective is to assess overall survival and the secondary aims are to assess quality of life of the survivors, cost of NHS service and NHS cost per life years saved. The trial commenced in 2004 with 3 years for recruitment and 5 years for follow-up and seeks to recruit all patients who have undergone curative treatment for primary colorectal cancer (R0 resections, Dukes' A-C). The study requires a sample size of 4760 patients to provide adequate power to detect a 4% improvement in survival in either arm of the study. In addition to a uniform colonoscopic surveillance programme, the four arms of the study are:

- Group 1: symptomatic follow-up in primary care
- Group 2: tumour marker measurement in primary care
- Group 3: intensive hospital follow-up with CT
- Group 4: a combination of groups 2 and 3.

Its results will be eagerly awaited, especially as it is also placing emphasis on QOL and not just survival and cost issues (http://www.facs.soton.ac.uk/Information.ac.uk/Information.aspx).

Rosen et al [7] suggested that the emphasis on follow-up should be directed towards finding "the different prognostic indicators, for example genetic tumour markers, primary tumour site, tumour stage, or age of the patient at diagnosis, to determine which select group of patients will benefit most from follow-up by detecting early curable recurrent cancer" [7].

Ultimately, although CRC follow-up is important, it is more likely that screening, early detection and initial comprehensive treatment of the disease will change outcomes to a far greater extent. Follow-up of surgery with curative intent is contentious, but one could argue that if the surgery is truly curative then follow-up should only really be aimed at the detection of metachronous tumours (provided the primary did not require adjuvant therapies), which again if detected early and treated aggressively should have a very favourable outcome. Currently, there are no hard and fast rules. The evidence presented above gives a summary of proposed follow-up guidelines and is presented in Table 3, with an example of a similar guideline table already used in an NHS Trust (Table 4). The discussion above should give a flavour of the pros and cons to intensive and non-intensive follow-up with regards to which modalities should be used and which clinicians should be involved to improve efficacy and cost-effectiveness.

References

1. DeVita VT, Hellman S, Rosenberg SA, editors. *Cancer: Principles and Practice of Oncology*. 6th Edition. Lippincott, Philadelphia, 1997.
2. National Cancer Institute of Canada. Canadian Cancer Statistics 2000. National Cancer Institute of Canada, Toronto, Canada, 2000.
3. Reis LAG, Kosary CL, Hankey BF, et al. SEER Cancer Statistics Review, 1973-1996: National Cancer Institute; 1999.
4. Steele G, Jr. Follow-up plans after treatment of primary colon and rectum cancer. *World J Surg* 1991; 15: 583-8.
5. Olson RM, Perencevich NP, Malcolm AW, et al. Patterns of recurrence following curative resection of adenocarcinoma of the colon and rectum. *Cancer* 1980; 45: 2969-74.
6. Bergamaschi R, Arnaud JP. Routine compared with nonscheduled follow-up of patients with "curative" surgery for colorectal cancer. *Ann Surg Oncol* 1996; 3: 464-9.
7. Rosen M, Chan L, Beart RW, Jr., et al. Follow-up of colorectal cancer: a meta-analysis. *Dis Colon Rectum* 1998; 41: 1116-26.
8. Renehan AG, Egger M, Saunders MP, et al. Impact on survival of intensive follow-up after curative resection for colorectal cancer: systematic review and meta-analysis of randomised trials. *BMJ* 2002; 324: 813.
9. Jeffery GM, Hickey BE, Hider P. Follow-up strategies for patients treated for non-metastatic colorectal cancer. *Cochrane Database Syst Rev* 2002: CD002200.
10. Kievit J. Follow-up of patients with colorectal cancer: numbers needed to test and treat. *Eur J Cancer* 2002; 38: 986-99.

11. Bruinvels DJ, Stiggelbout AM, Kievit J, et al. Follow-up of patients with colorectal cancer. A meta-analysis. *Ann Surg* 1994; 219: 174-82.
12. Martin EW, Jr., Cooperman M, King G, et al. A retrospective and prospective study of serial CEA determinations in the early detection of recurrent colon cancer. *Am J Surg* 1979; 137: 167-9.
13. Moertel CG, Fleming TR, Macdonald JS, et al. An evaluation of the carcinoembryonic antigen (CEA) test for monitoring patients with resected colon cancer. *JAMA* 1993; 270: 943-7.
14. Putzki H, Student A, Jablonski M, et al. Comparison of the tumor markers CEA, TPA, and CA 19-9 in colorectal carcinoma. *Cancer* 1987; 59: 223-6.
15. Rosen L, Abel ME, Gordon PH, et al. Practice parameters for the detection of colorectal neoplasms - supporting documentation. The Standards Task Force. American Society of Colon and Rectal Surgeons. *Dis Colon Rectum* 1992; 35: 391-4.
16. Scalmati A, Roncucci L, Ghidini G, et al. Epithelial cell kinetics in the remaining colorectal mucosa after surgery for cancer of the large bowel. *Cancer Res* 1990; 50: 7937-41.
17. Khoury DA, Opelka FG, Beck DE, et al. Colon surveillance after colorectal cancer surgery. *Dis Colon Rectum* 1996; 39: 252-6.
18. Atkin WS, Saunders BP. Surveillance guidelines after removal of colorectal adenomatous polyps. *Gut* 2002; 51 Suppl 5: V6-9.
19. Rotondano G, Esposito P, Pellecchia L, et al. Early detection of locally recurrent rectal cancer by endosonography. *Br J Radiol* 1997; 70: 567-71.
20. Tekkis PP, Poloniecki JD, Thompson MR, et al. Operative mortality in colorectal cancer: prospective national study. *BMJ* 2003; 327: 1196-1201.
21. Scholefield JH, Steele RJ. Guidelines for follow-up after resection of colorectal cancer. *Gut* 2002; 51 Suppl 5: V3-5.
22. http://www.nice.org.uk/pdf/CSGCCfull guidance.pdf.
23. http://www.fascrs.org/displaycommon.cfm?an=1&sub articlenbr=11.
24. http://www.cssa.org.au/patientarticle.asp?ArticleNo=11.

Chapter 3

Primary prevention of colorectal cancer (diet and chemoprevention)

Patrick M Lynch JD MD, Associate Professor, University of Texas,
MD Anderson Cancer Center, Houston, Texas, USA

Marina Wallace FRCS, Consultant Colorectal Surgeon
Watford General Hospital, Watford, UK

What is the problem?

Improvements in surgical techniques have probably made as much impact as they are likely to make in achieving cures for invasive colorectal cancer and its metastases. Chemotherapy and radiation continue to yield improvements in mortality, but the benefits have been incremental and modest. Few "magic bullets" appear on the horizon. If significant progress is going to be made in achieving a reduction in colorectal cancer and cancer death, earlier diagnosis and prevention will be needed. Screening, discussed elsewhere, offers great potential for identifying early, more readily curable cancer. Some of the newer approaches to screening, including colonoscopy [1], CT colography [2], and screening for mutated DNA in the stool [3], carry potential for identifying benign adenomas, the key cancer precursor. In the case of colonoscopic polypectomy, cancer may be averted.

As promising as early diagnostic measures may be, they are relatively expensive, carry some risk, and require a level of patient willingness that has frankly not been seen in sufficient numbers as to significantly impact incidence. Fortunately, recognition of risk factors for colorectal cancer has led to several important opportunities actually to achieve primary prevention. In order to structure appropriate responses to the question of "what is the problem?" it is first necessary to stratify subjects according to risk. It is generally accepted that cancer patients at high risk of recurrence and death from metastatic disease merit more aggressive surveillance and treatment. It is also accepted that subjects at high risk of developing an index cancer (prior neoplasia, inflammatory bowel disease, positive family history) warrant more aggressive screening/surveillance measures to identify early tumours. So, it stands to reason that aggressive and potentially more expensive and risky prevention measures may be warranted for those at higher risk of developing adenomas and cancer. For each risk category, interventions that can currently be recommended clinically will be described along with those that must still be considered investigational. Interventions can broadly be grouped as dietary, including naturally occurring additives, and pharmacologic.

Where are we now?

Limitations of screening

Early detection of colorectal cancer is readily achievable through such screening measures as faecal occult blood testing (FOBT) [4, 5], sigmoidoscopy [6], and barium enema [7]. Newer techniques such as computed tomography (CT) colography and testing for mutant DNA from exfoliated epithelium in the stool may bring greater sensitivity and specificity for detection of not only early cancer, but precancerous adenomas as well, albeit at substantially greater cost. Colonoscopy, both sensitive and specific for early neoplasia, offers the additional advantage of therapeutic intervention [8]. Polypectomy of ever larger and more sessile non-invasive tumours should obviate the need for a number of surgical resections. Increasingly, colonoscopy is being offered not only to high risk groups, such as those with inflammatory bowel disease, patients with previous neoplasia, and those with a strong family history of colorectal neoplasia, but also to average risk individuals over the age of 50 [9, 10].

Unfortunately, the goal of achieving a significant reduction in colorectal cancer incidence and mortality depends on a level of public participation in screening that has simply not occurred to date [11]. Even the simplest and least expensive screening measures, such as FOBT, have not been employed by a majority of those at risk.

In addition to patient compliance, provider issues include training and performance, complications, and intervals of repeat testing [12].

So, with all deference to the key roles for surgical, radio- and chemotherapeutic treatment of established cancer, early cancer detection through screening, and prevention through endoscopic polypectomy, primary prevention may provide a key to the actual reduction of colorectal cancer incidence.

Diet as risk factor and dietary interventions

One of the earliest and still most important clues to the possibility of reducing risk of colorectal cancer was the recognition of the association between risk and diet. Specifically, variation in worldwide incidence pointed to the so-called "Western diet", high in animal fat and total calories, and low in fibre, as a factor associated with increasing risk. A compelling volume of data supports this notion and also its corollary, that reducing fat and increasing fibre ought to be associated with a decrease in risk [13, 14]. A number of excellent reviews have been written on this subject [15].

Despite the considerable body of epidemiologic data supporting a risk-reducing role for a low fat, high fibre diet, rigorous prospective, controlled intervention trials have been disappointing. Typical designs have involved subjects with a history of non-familial adenomas, treated for intervals of several years.

One important study was conducted in the early 1990s in the Southwest US [16]. Following initial assessment of a much larger group, 1429 subjects age 40-80 and with a recent history of adenoma (but not cancer or family history of colorectal cancer) were randomised (following a 6-week run-in to establish probable adherence). Subjects were randomised to a high fibre (13.5g/d) or low fibre (2g/d) diet of wheat bran-based cereal. Colonoscopy was performed on two occasions, at 1 year and 2-3 years thereafter. Perhaps not surprisingly, compliance was significantly lower in the high fibre group and decreased over time during the course of the trial. Overall rates for recurrent adenomas were 51% in the low fibre and 47% in the high fibre group, a non-significant difference. Various subset analyses also failed to show significant effects of fibre supplementation.

Published simultaneously in 2000, Schatzkin et al [17] reported results of a similar intervention. More than 2000 subjects were randomised to a high fibre, low fat diet, or to no dietary change. Specifically, the goal in the intervention group was: 20% total calories from fat; dietary fibre: 18g/1000 kcal; fruits and vegetables: 3.5 servings/1000 kcal. Information about nutritional and behavioral modification was provided in the course of intensive and prolonged counselling over the several years intervention. As measured by a food frequency questionnaire, after the 4 years of trial, those in the intervention group were able, on average, to reduce fat from 36% of total calories to 24%.

Adenoma recurrence, the primary trial endpoint, was 39.7% in the intervention group and 39.7% in the control group. Analysis of subsets, such as large or villous adenomas, or adenomas with high-grade dysplasia, also showed no intervention/control differences. Non-significant gender differences were noted, with fewer adenomas among men in the intervention group, while fewer women in the control group developed adenomas. Notably, the intervention group experienced more diagnoses of invasive colorectal cancer, 10, versus 4 in the control group, though the difference was non-significant.

A smaller study (201 subjects) from Canada, the Toronto Polyp Prevention Trial [18], showed no difference in adenoma recurrence over a 2-year interval, although an 8% reduction in fat intake and a 19g/d increase in fibre consumption was achieved in the intervention group. The larger (n=424) Australian Polyp Prevention Project [19] whose interventions included reduced dietary fat, bran fibre supplementation, and beta carotene, also failed to show a reduction in adenoma recurrence over 4 years.

It is evident that if there is a benefit from dietary manipulation in so far as colorectal neoplasia risk is concerned, it is likely to be a very modest one. Had the above trials been extended over a somewhat greater interval, it is conceivable (though unlikely) that they would have achieved a reduction in colorectal cancer, despite the absence of impact on the adenoma endpoint that was employed in each study. So, if the impact of fairly straightforward dietary intervention is really minimal or absent, have there yet been any promising chemoprevention trial data? The answer is that both in average risk and high risk groups, more aggressive pharmacologic interventions have yielded very promising results.

Non-steroidal anti-inflammatory drugs (NSAIDs)

Strong epidemiologic support for risk reduction through use of non-steroidal anti-inflammatory agents (NSAIDs) has existed for many years [20, 21]. That NSAIDs have a beneficial effect in reducing risk of colorectal neoplasia is supported by the sheer variety of retrospective, case-control investigations that have evaluated a range of agents, in varying doses and durations of use, with endpoints ranging from intermediate markers in cell cultures and animal models, to human adenomas, colorectal cancer, and mortality [15].

Most evidence points toward a mechanism of action that is predicated on the cyclo-oxygenase (COX) inhibitory effect shared by most NSAIDs [22], though there is also evidence for additional non-COX mechanisms of action [23]. Detailed biochemical characterisation of the arachidonic acid pathway has shown that certain prostaglandins are involved in mediating inflammation and neoplasia [24]. Cyclo-oxygenase exists in the key isoforms, COX-1 and COX-2, which catalyse the metabolism of arachidonic acid to downstream prostaglandins. By inhibiting cyclo-oxygenase, such prostaglandins are diminished. While COX-1 is constitutively expressed in most tissues, COX-2 is induced in the presence of inflammation and comes to be expressed in neoplastic tissues, including the colorectal mucosa.

Notwithstanding the likely primacy of cyclo-oxygenase inhibition by NSAIDs, non-COX activities are shared by NSAIDs and may be important for their anticancer effects. Upregulation of 15-lipoxygenase-1 may be important in mediating apoptosis [25]. NSAIDs also appear to activate ligands of the peroxisome proliferator-activated receptor (PPAR) [26]. Experimentally, they inhibit phosphorylation of Akt. In an elegant experiment, selective inhibitors of the COX-2 enzyme inhibited growth of cancer cell-lines that were already free of COX-2 expression, suggesting other modes of action.

In humans, chemoprevention with NSAIDs has basically proceeded along three fronts:

- Non-selective NSAIDs (mainly sulindac) in high risk groups, mainly familial adenomatous polyposis (FAP) [27-31].
- Non-selective NSAIDs (mainly aspirin) in otherwise average risk subjects with a history of non-familial adenomas [32-34].
- Development and testing of selective COX-2 inhibitors in both FAP and non-familial adenoma patients [35-40].

NSAID trials in FAP

The use of NSAIDs in FAP began in the 1980s with uncontrolled exposure of subjects to sulindac [27]. Initially encouraging results led to the conduct and publication of a series of small studies (fewer than 50 subjects) [41, 28, 30]. These generally enrolled subjects with a history of FAP and colectomy with ileorectal anastomosis (IRA), followed by recurrent adenomas in the rectal stump. The studies were short term, generally less than 1 year. The consistent finding was a 30-70% reduction in adenoma burden, compared to placebo subjects whose polyp burden remained essentially unchanged.

When follow-up was conducted following cessation of drug, adenomas recurred, though without any real evidence of rebound proliferation of polyps. Few examples exist of complete, long-term suppression of adenomas [29, 42]. Generally, clinical use of an agent such as sulindac is considered as an adjunct to regular endoscopic assessment and polyp fulguration. Of great interest and concern, long-term administration of sulindac in such FAP subjects has been associated with anecdotal reports of rectal cancer [43, 44]. Tonelli et al [45] followed 15 subjects, most of whom were started on sulindac 100mg BID at about 3 months following colectomy. Treatment continued for an average of about 4 years, with flexible sigmoidoscopy at 6-month intervals. Complete short-term regression of adenomas was observed in two patients, with flattening of polyps in most others. On long-term follow-up, virtually all had recurrent polyps, with polypectomy, often multiple, required. Three developed sessile polyps requiring surgical transanal excision. Two of these nevertheless developed recurrent adenomas requiring completion proctectomy and ileal pouch anal anastomosis (IPAA), with one of two showing invasive cancer at resection. It is likely that a given adenoma, resistant to sulindac, carries the potential for malignant transformation that will in fact eventually occur if that adenoma is not removed endoscopically or surgically. While most adenomas can be treated rather easily with such measures as snare polypectomy (including saline-assisted endoscopic mucosal resection or EMR) or thermal ablation (hot biopsy, heater probe, argon plasma coagulation, YAG laser, etc.), superficially spreading adenomas with a villous component can be difficult to remove completely by such means. Such a lesion, if present in a patient with poor follow-up or with an inattentive endoscopist, can pose a real risk of cancer. The key issue here is that chemoprevention cannot be considered a stand-alone treatment measure. Long-term, collaborative, observational studies of clinical outcomes of patients on NSAIDs are clearly warranted.

Adenoma suppression

Giardiello and colleagues at Johns Hopkins University, following their demonstration of short-term sulindac efficacy in regressing existing adenomas, undertook to study the ability of sulindac to prevent the emergence of first adenomas in young patients with FAP who were phenotypically normal [31]. A randomised, double-blind, placebo-controlled study was conducted on 41 individuals age 8-25 years who had APC mutations but were as yet described as phenotypically unaffected. They initially performed sigmoidoscopy, excluding subjects with any adenomas in the distal 20cm of colorectum that was evaluated. Such patients were thus not truly "phenotypically unaffected". Those without polyps then underwent APC testing. A great number of subjects were thus ineligible due either to presence of polyps or to non-carrier status. Eligible subjects were randomised to 75 or 150mgs (dose determined by body weight) of sulindac orally BID, or placebo for 48 months. The number and size of new colonic adenomas were scored at follow-up sigmoidoscopy. Side effects of therapy were documented.

During the 4 years of treatment, average compliance was good, exceeding 76% in the sulindac group, with mucosal prostaglandin levels lower than in the placebo group. Adenomas developed in 9 of 21 subjects (43%) in the sulindac group and 11 of 20 subjects in the placebo group (55%). There was no significant difference in the mean number of polyps between the groups (p=0.54). The authors concluded that sulindac did not prevent the emergence of first adenomas in patients with FAP. However, since there was at least a trend toward delay in polyp formation in the treated group, this small trial may have carried a type II error. That is, a larger sample might have carried the power to yield a significant difference between groups. Since examination was limited to sigmoidoscopy of the most distal 20cm of colorectum, a more sensitive measure of adenoma formation, such as full colonoscopy with the added use of dye spray for detection of microadenomas, might well have limited misclassification of subjects.

Undeterred by the essentially negative trial by Giardiello, and designed before those results were available, a multicentre trial is currently evaluating the effect of celecoxib in a larger series of APC positive, phenotype negative or minimal children. An 18-subject pilot, six subjects in three cohorts, is being treated with escalating doses approximating 200, 400, and 800mg/d, and scaled down on mg/kg basis for paediatric purposes. This part of the overall study, which has now completed enrolment, has the goals of demonstrating the safety of high dose celecoxib in children and to work out the logistics of a multicentre paediatric endoscopic/drug trial, in anticipation of a larger phase II trial. The phase II study will involve a host of US centres, St. Mark's in London, and likely additional European and world sites. Differences from the Giardiello trial will involve:

- initial APC testing to exclude non-carriers from the outset;
- use of annual, full colonoscopy with total IV anaesthesia (primary use of propofol);
- enhancement by indigo carmine dye spray (detection and modulation of micro-adenomas or aberrant crypt foci will be a secondary endpoint [46]);
- enrolment of subjects with a modest, "ablatable" adenoma burden, with analysis stratified to take into account the likely biologic difference between prevention of adenoma occurrence in those already manifesting a limited phenotype and those who are truly "pre-adenoma";
- termination of participation when adenomas develop.

Anticipated challenges include difficulty in enrolment of subjects who are in the narrow window just before polyps emerge (the Giardiello trial had many screen failures for just this reason, i.e. adenomas already present). Due to the increased sensitivity of full colonoscopy with dye spray, it is anticipated that defining and adhering to an arbitrary but reasonable adenoma burden, at baseline and as an endpoint, will be challenging.

Combination chemotherapy

One of the most important challenges in cancer treatment is drug resistance. For this reason, medical oncologists are quick to exploit multiple pathways in an effort to develop combinations of agents to overcome such single-drug resistance. That agents employed to induce regression of adenomas have met with limited success provides further testimonial to the seeming ubiquitousness of drug resistance, even at the level of very early neoplasia. While the data from non-selective NSAID and COX-2 inhibition trials in FAP (and for sporadic adenomas as well, see below) have been encouraging, "complete response" has been rare in the short term and virtually non-existent in the long term.

In an effort to improve response rates in FAP, several combination studies have been undertaken. The first of these is the so-called CAPP I trial, for Concerted Action for the Prevention of Polyposis trial, nearing completion by centres in countries of the European Union, and scattered institutions in other countries [47]. The design involves a factorial design: aspirin, 600mg/d, resistant starch in gram quantities daily, both, or neither (placebo). Preliminary data are expected very soon, as several years of follow-up are in.

At the University of Texas MD Anderson Cancer Center, along with colleagues at St. Mark's in London and at the Cleveland Clinic, the first relatively large-scale trial employing pharmacologic agents directed against specific, different pathways is currently being undertaken. The overall design and endoscopic protocol is very similar to the original celecoxib trial [38]. However, due to the efficacy of celecoxib, use of a placebo arm was not considered ethical. The control arm, therefore, is celecoxib 800mg/d in divided doses, with or without the addition of Difluoromethylornithine (DFMO) at a dose of 0.5mg/kg/d. Enrolment of the target sample of 110 subjects is about half complete at this writing. The large sample size, as FAP trials go, is due to the use of an active drug as the control arm. Even so, there continue to be major challenges to enrolment. Because FAP is a rare condition, the best source of subjects traditionally has been the families of subjects enrolled in trials or who are at least known to a Polyposis Registry. However, the need to comply with new regulatory policies on the confidentiality and privacy of family studies has made it more difficult to identify and recruit subjects from families with FAP. Because DFMO is associated with occasional, albeit reversible, ototoxicity, enrolment has been limited to subjects with normal baseline audiometry. An unusually high rate of mild hearing impairment has led to the exclusion of many subjects for this reason. This issue of hearing impairment is now being investigated in its own right.

NSAID trials for sporadic adenomas

As noted above, the body of epidemiologic support for a protective effective of NSAIDs in sporadic cancer and sporadic adenomas is extensive and largely consistent. Intuitively, one would also think that if NSAIDs have efficacy in FAP, they should work even better in subjects without a genetically programmed predisposition.

Several very important trials have been conducted and their results reported. In phase II-III trials, the impact of NSAIDs against sporadic adenomas and cancer has been positive, but not as dramatic as might have been hoped (see Hawk, 2004 [15] for an excellent review of these studies). Only one trial was conducted in previously healthy (i.e. no prior adenoma or cancer) subjects, the Physicians' Health Study. In this study of aspirin vs placebo, there was no significant reduction in colorectal cancer or adenoma incidence [48].

In three quite recent clinical trials involving patients at increased risk of colorectal neoplasia by virtue of personal history of adenomas or cancer, significant reductions in recurrent adenomas were observed among those treated with aspirin for more than a year [33, 34, 49]. Sandler et al [34] randomised more than 600 disease-free colon cancer patients to 325mg/day of aspirin or to placebo. At about 1 year of follow-up, a significantly lower proportion of treated patients were free of new adenomas. In the treated group there was also a significant prolongation in the time to development of a first adenoma. In another trial of more than 100 patients with a history of adenomas, Baron et al [33] randomised the subjects to 81 or 325mg of aspirin/day or placebo. Perhaps surprisingly, there was a 19% reduction in incidence of new adenomas in the low dose (81mg/d) aspirin group but only a 4% reduction in the high dose (325mg/d) aspirin group compared to placebo. As against the argument that small adenomas are not clinically important, the observed protection against advanced adenomas (i.e. larger, more severely dysplastic or villous) was more pronounced. They observed a 41% and 17% lower rate of advanced adenomas in the groups taking 81 or 325mg/day, as compared to placebo. Interim results from yet another phase III clinical trial of 272 previous adenoma patients have shown an advantage to use aspirin at 1 year [49]. More mature data are expected soon.

Where are we going?

Progress is clearly being made in the chemo-prevention of colorectal adenomas and cancer in conditions such as FAP. While there are no good data on the prevalence of the use of agents such as sulindac and celecoxib, it is likely to be fairly widespread (although whether such agents are being used appropriately may be less certain). Appropriate use would include usage in doses that have been effective in the published short-term trials. Appropriate use should also recognise that there are no data supporting the relaxation (lengthening) of surveillance endoscopy intervals. Such surveillance is critical. Not all patients respond to NSAID therapy. If a subject appears to be a responder, individual adenomas in the rectum or duodenum still need to be ablated, particularly if they are increasing in size. Because of reports of presumably resistant adenomas becoming malignant, any large or sessile adenoma must be completely removed. Indeed, the need to ablate large, progressively dysplastic, or numerous adenomas signals a failure of therapy and may even warrant surgical intervention.

New agents and combinations

To move beyond mere adjunctive status, future chemopreventive agents will likely need to be started early in life and continued indefinitely. They will need to address mechanisms of adenoma development in a more rigorous fashion than they have to date. They will likely have to involve combinations of agents that affect different pathways.

Very intriguing combinations of agents have been evaluated in animal studies. For example, the COX-2 inhibitor, rofecoxib (Vioxx), was given in conjunction with APC gene product replacement [23]. Min mice received rofecoxib, APC gene product, both, or neither for 2 months. All animals were placed on a high fat diet. At necropsy, intestinal tumours were counted. The APC protein evidently reached its cellular target, as DNA plasmid constructs mixed with liposomal vectors and administered by gut lavage increased the measured APC protein in the small bowel. Animals given both rofecoxib and APC protein experienced an 85% reduction in polyps, decreasing from an average of about 60 polyps/mouse in the placebo group to less than 10 in the rofecoxib/APC protein treated group. Although those mice receiving rofecoxib only or APC protein only showed a more modest reduction in polyp count, the rofecoxib effect was greater than that of the APC protein. If the underlying defect in FAP was an insufficient "dose" of endogenous APC protein, one would have expected a more dramatic effect of supplemental APC product alone. Perhaps higher levels of APC protein would have provided greater protection. Note that no toxicity was in evidence over the 2-month duration of the trial. If this is so non-toxic, then perhaps it is time to consider phase I human trials of APC protein.

The future use of COX-2 inhibitors for adenoma prevention has recently been called into question due to the withdrawal from the market of rofecoxib (Vioxx). The withdrawal was based upon reports of increased cardiovascular events in patients participating in a non-familial, sporadic adenoma recurrence trial. Similar reports in one study utilising celecoxib 400mg bd in sporadic adenoma patients suggests patient risk needs to be higher (as it is in FAP) for these agents to be recommended.

This is but one example of the type of approach that may be anticipated in the future. Scientists and clinicians will definitely benefit from co-operation in translational studies.

References

1. Lieberman DA, Weiss DG, Bond, et al. Use of colonoscopy to screen asymptomatic adults for colorectal cancer. *N Engl J Med* 2000; 343: 162-8.
2. Pickhardt PJ, Choie R, Hwang I, et al. Computed tomographic virtual colonoscopy to screen for colorectal neoplasia in adymptomatic adults. *N Engl J Med* 2003; 349: 2191-200.
3. Ahlquist DA, Skoletsky JE, Boynton KA, et al. Colorectal cancer screening by detection of altered human DNA in stool: feasibility of a mutitarget assay panel. *Gastro* 2000; 119: 1219-27.
4. Mandel JS, Bond JH, Church TR, et al. Reducing mortality from colorectal cancer by screening for fecal occult blood. *N Engl J Med* 1993; 328: 1365-71.
5. Mandel JS, Church TR, Bond JH, et al. The effect of fecal occult-blood screening on the incidence of colorectal cancer. *N Engl J Med* 2000; 343: 1603-7.
6. Selby JV, Friedman GD, Quesenberry CP, Weiss NS. Case-control study of screening sigmoidoscopy and mortality from colorectal cancer. *N Engl J Med* 1992; 326: 653-7.
7. Winawer SJ, Stewart ET, Zauber AG, et al. A comparison of colonoscopy and double-contrast barium enema for surveillance after polypectomy. *N Engl J Med* 2000; 342: 1766-72.
8. Winawer SJ, Zauber AG, Ho MN, et al. Prevention of colorectal cancer by colonoscopic polypectomy. *N Engl J Med* 1993; 329: 1977-81.
9. Winawer S, Fletcher R, Rex D, et al. Colorectal cancer screening and surveillance: clinical guidelines and rationale - update based on new evidence. *Gastro* 2003; 124: 544-60.
10. Smith RA, Cokkinides V, Eyre. American Cancer Society guidelines for the early detection of cancer. *CA Cancer J Clin* 2003; 53: 27-43.
11. Subramanian S, Klosterman M, Amonkar MM, Hunt TL. Adherence with colorectal cancer screening guidelines: a review. *Prev Med* 2004; 38: 536-50.
12. Lieberman D. Quality in colon cancer screening. *Practical Gastro* 2004; 28: 27-42.
13. Walker AR, Burkitt DP. Colonic cancer - hypotheses of causation, dietary prophylaxis, and future research. *Am J Dig Dis* 1976; 21: 910-7.
14. Wynder EL. The epidemiology of large bowel cancer. *Cancer Res* 1975; 35: 3388-94.
15. Hawk ET, Umar A, Viner JL. Colorectal cancer chemoprevention - an overview of the science. *Gastro* 2004; 126: 1423-47.
16. Alberts DS, Martinez ME, Roe DJ, et al. Lack of effect of a high-fiber cereal supplement on the recurrence of colorectal adenomas. Phoenix Colon Cancer Prevention Physicians' Network. *N Engl J Med* 2000; 342: 1156-62.
17. Schatzkin A, Lanza E, Corle D. Lack of effect of a low-fat, high-fiber diet on the recurrence of colorectal adenomas. Polyp Prevention Trial Study Group. *N Engl J Med* 2000; 342: 1149-55.

18. McKeown-Eyssen GE, Bright-See E, Bruce WR, et al. A randomized trial of a low fat high fibre diet in the recurrence of colorectal polyps. *J Clin Epidemiol* 1994; 47: 525-36.
19. MacLennan R, Macrae F, Bain C, et al. Randomized trial of intake of fat, fiber, and beta carotene to prevent colorectal adenomas: the Australian Polyp Prevention Project. *J Natl Cancer Inst* 1995; 87: 1760-6.
20. Kune GA, Kune S, Watson LF. Colorectal cancer risk, chronic illnesses, operations, and medications: case control results from the Melbourne Colorectal Cancer Study. *Ca Res* 1988; 48: 4399-04.
21. Logan RF, Little, Hawtin PG, Hardcastle JD. Effect of aspirin and non-steroidal anti-inflammatory drugs on colorectal adenomas: case control study of subjects participating in the Nottingham faecal occult blood screening programme. *BMJ* 1993; 307: 285-9.
22. Eberhart CE, Coffey RJ, Radhika A, et al. Up-regulation of cyclooxygenase 2 gene expression in human colorectal adenomas and adenocarcinomas. *Gastro* 1994; 107: 1183-8.
23. Piazza GA, Alberts DS, Hixson LJ, et al. Sulindac sulfone inhibits azoxymethane-induced colon carcinogenesis in rats without reducing prostaglandin levels. *Ca Res* 1997; 57: 2909-15.
24. Marnett LJ. Aspirin and the potential role of prostaglandins in colon cancer. *Ca Res* 1992; 52: 5575-89.
25. Shureiqi I, Chen D, Lotan R, et al. 15-lipoxygenase-1 mediates nonsteroidal anti-inflammatory drug-induced apoptosis independently of cyclooxygenase-2 in colon cancer cells. *Ca Res* 2000; 60: 6846-50.
26. Lehmann JM, Lenhard JM, Oliver BB, et al. Peroxisome proliferator-activated receptors alpha and gamma are activated by indomethacin and other non-steroidal anti-inflammatory drugs. *J Biol Chem* 1997; 272: 3406-10.
27. Waddell WR, Loughry RW. Sulindac for polyposis of the colon. *J Surg Oncol* 1983; 24: 83-7.
28. Labayle D, Fischer D, Viehl P, et al. Sulindac causes regression of rectal polyps in familial adenomatous polyposis. *Gastro* 1991; 101: 635-9.
29. Cruz CM, Hylind LM, Romans K, et al. Long-term treatment with sulindac in familial adenomatous polyposis: a prospective cohort study. *Gastro* 2002; 122(3): 641-5.
30. Giardiello, FM, Hamilton, SR, Krush, AJ, et al. Treatment of colonic and rectal adenomas with sulindac in familial adenomatous polyposis. *N Engl J Med* 1993; 1313-6.
31. Giardiello FM, Yang VW, Hylind LM, et al. Primary chemoprevention of familial adenomatous polyposis with sulindac. *N Engl J Med* 2002; 346: 1054-9.
32. Thun MJ, Namboodiri MM, Heath CW Jr. Aspirin use and reduced risk of fatal colon cancer. *N Engl J Med* 1991; 325: 1593-6.
33. Baron JA, Cole BF, Sandler RS, et al. A randomized trial of aspirin to prevent colorectal adenomas. *N Engl J Med* 2003; 348: 891-9.
34. Sandler RS, Halabi S, Baron JA, et al. A randomized trial of aspirin to prevent colorectal adenomas in patients with previous colorectal cancer. *N Engl J Med* 2003; 348: 883-90.
35. Gierse JK, Hauser SD, Creely DP, et al. Expression and selective inhibition of the constitutive and inducible forms of human cyclo-oxygenase. *Biochem J* 1995; 305: 479-84.
36. Oshima M, Dinchuk JE, Kargman SL, et al. Suppression of intestinal polyposis in Apc delta716 knockout mice by inhibition of cyclooxygenase 2 (COX-2). *Cell* 1996; 87: 803-9.
37. Kawamori T, Rao CV, Seibert K, Reddy BS. Chemopreventive activity of celecoxib, a specific cyclooxygenase-2 inhibitor, against colon carcinogenesis. *Ca Res* 1998; 58: 409-2.
38. Steinbach G, Lynch PM, Phillips RK, et al. The effect of celecoxib, a cyclooxygenase-2 inhibitor, in familial adenomatous polyposis. *N Engl J Med* 2000; 342: 1946-52.
39. Phillips RK, Wallace MH, Lynch PM, et al. A randomised, double blind, placebo controlled study of celecoxib, a selective cyclooxygenase 2 inhibitor, on duodenal polyposis in familial adenomatous polyposis. *Gut* 2002; 50: 857-60.
40. Hallak A, Alon-Baron L, Shamir R, et al. Rofecoxib reduces polyp recurrence in familial polyposis. *Dig Dis Sci* 2003; 48: 1998-2002.
41. Rigau J, Pique JM, Rubio E, et al. Effects of long-term sulindac therapy on colonic polyposis. *Ann Intern Med* 1991; 115: 952-4.
42. Winde G, Schmid KW, Schlegel W, et al. Complete reversion and prevention of rectal adenomas in colectomized patients with familial adenomatous polyposis by rectal low-dose sulindac maintenance treatment: advantages of a low-dose nonsteroidal anti-inflammatory drug regimen in reversing adenomas exceeding 33 months. *Dis Colon Rectum* 1995; 38: 813-30.
43. Niv Y, Fraser GM. Adenocarcinoma in the rectal segment in familial polyposis coli is not prevented by sulindac therapy. *Gastro* 1994; 107: 854-7.
44. Lynch HT, Thorson AG, Smyrk T. Rectal cancer after prolonged sulindac chemoprevention. *Cancer* 1995; 75: 936-8.
45. Tonelli F, Valanzano R, Messerini L, Ficari F. Long-term treatment with sulindac in familial adenomatous polyposis: is there an actual efficacy in prevention of rectal cancer? *J Surg Oncol* 2000; 74: 15-20.
46. Wallace MH, Frayling IM, Clark SK, et al. Attenuated adenomatous polyposis coli: the role of ascertainment bias through failure to dye-spray at colonoscopy. *Dis Colon Rectum* 1999; 42: 1078-80.
47. Burn J, Chapman PD, Bishop DT, et al. Diet and cancer prevention, the concerted action polyp prevention (CAPP) studies. *Proc Nutr Soc* 1998; 57: 183-6.
48. Gann PH, Manson JE, Glynn RJ, et al. Low-dose aspirin and incidence of colorectal tumors in a randomized trial. *JNCI* 1993; 85: 1220-4.
49. Benamouzig R, Deyra J, Martin A, et al. Daily soluble aspirin and prevention of colorectal adenoma recurrence: one-year results of the APACC trial. *Gastroenterology* 2003; 125: 328-36.

Chapter 4

Polyp management

Brian Saunders MD FRCP
Senior Lecturer in Endoscopy & Consultant Gastroenterologist
Wolfson Unit for Endoscopy, St. Mark's Hospital, Harrow, Middlesex, UK

Introduction

Colonoscopic polypectomy is probably the most frequently performed procedure in modern surgical practice. Prospective and case controlled studies have shown that polypectomy can prevent colorectal cancer, supplying the potential to exert a significant positive impact on population healthcare [1-8]. It is the duty of the endoscopist to ensure safe and effective practice by maximising polyp detection, removing pre-malignant lesions and organising appropriate post-procedure surveillance. This chapter provides guidance on effective, modern polyp management and gives a glimpse into the future of some of the new and emerging technologies in this rapidly evolving field of medicine.

What is the problem?

Colorectal cancer is the third most common malignancy and the second most common cause of cancer-related death in the Western world [9,10]. There is overwhelming evidence that almost all cancers develop from adenomas, whether flat or polypoid; therefore, there is a window of opportunity to find and remove adenomas before cancer develops [11,12]. Prospective and case controlled studies have shown a reduction in colorectal cancer incidence after removal of adenomas [1-8]. That said, up to 30% of the general population over the age of 50 years will have a colonic adenoma, which means therefore that not all adenomas go on to develop into cancer [13, 14, 15]. However, with an ageing population and relatively high background risk of cancer, a policy of removing all potential adenomas when detected in patients likely to benefit seems appropriate, even taking into account the small attendant risks of polypectomy. Polyps in the colon only occasionally give specific symptoms such as bleeding, change in bowel habit or mucus discharge per rectum; therefore, most are found fortuitously at diagnostic or screening investigations. Small polyps (<1cm) are less likely to contain high-grade dysplasia or early invasive malignancy, but as the polyp increases in size there is a parallel increase in risk of malignancy [16]. Polypoid, stalked lesions with an early malignant focus can usually be completely removed endoscopically without recourse to resectional surgery, and certain very early flat or sessile cancers can also be resected by using new endoscopic techniques such as endoscopic mucosal resection (EMR) [17-24]. Current evidence suggests that small left-sided metaplastic polyps carry very little risk of future malignancy; however, multiple metaplastic polyps (metaplastic polyposis) and larger right-sided metaplastic polyps (Figure 1) may herald an increased cancer risk, with some metaplastic lesions becoming serrated adenomas and then cancers along an

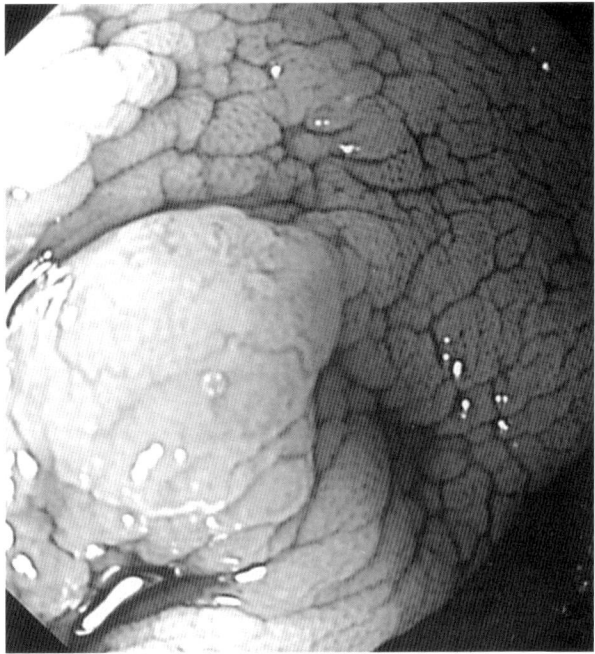

Figure 1. A large right-sided metaplastic polyp highlighted by topical indigocarmine dye. Characteristic features include minimal elevation, pale, mucinous surface and visible vessel pattern on the polyp surface.

alternative pathway of carcinogenesis [25,26]. Differentiating neoplastic from non-neoplastic polyps at the time of endoscopy is difficult and therefore all polyps are usually resected. The exception is where multiple post-inflammatory polyps are present on a background of chronic inflammatory bowel disease or multiple tiny rectal or sigmoid metaplastic polyps are present. Here several biopsies to confirm the benign diagnosis is all that is required. Polyposis syndromes such as familial adenomatous polyposis (FAP), Peutz-Jeghers syndrome and juvenile polyposis are best managed by specialised registries and are beyond the remit of this chapter. The key problems with sporadic polyp management faced by the clinician are as follows:

- What is the variation in the endoscopic appearances of neoplastic lesions?
- How can polyp detection be maximised?
- How do we differentiate between endoscopically resectable and more advanced lesions that will require surgery?
- What techniques should be used for polypectomy?
- How can we reduce complications from polypectomy?
- Which patients require endoscopic follow-up and how frequently?

Where are we now?

Overview

Patients with significant symptoms such as change in bowel habit, diarrhoea, iron deficiency anaemia and rectal bleeding all warrant colonic investigation and for the vast majority of symptom complexes colonoscopy or flexible sigmoidoscopy are the investigations of choice. Colonoscopy is more accurate than barium enema both for cancer detection and surveillance of patients with previous colonic adenomas [27-31]. Virtual colonoscopy appears to be a promising new technology and may prove to be as accurate as optical colonoscopy for detection of cancers and large polyps [32]. However, data are currently limited as to the effectiveness of this procedure. Colonoscopy remains the procedure of choice for surveillance of high risk groups, such as those with a strong family history of colorectal cancer (CRC), previous colonic neoplasia or longstanding inflammatory bowel disease. The optimal method of population screening is more controversial and colonoscopy has competition from virtual colonoscopy, flexible sigmoidoscopy, faecal occult blood testing and looking for genetic aberrations in stool, all of which have advantages and disadvantages. Regardless of which test is used for the initial screen, colonoscopy is inevitably the back-up second-line test because it allows direct visualisation, biopsy and polypectomy. Approximately 15,000,000 colonoscopies are performed each year in the USA for diagnostic or screening purposes. This unprecedented surge in demand for colonoscopy has focused professional bodies on the quality of delivered colonoscopy [33]. Key factors in determining quality include caecal intubation rates, complications, adenoma detection rates, levels of sedation used, compliance with surveillance guidelines, patient satisfaction scores and appropriate interactions with pathologists [34].

4 Polyp management

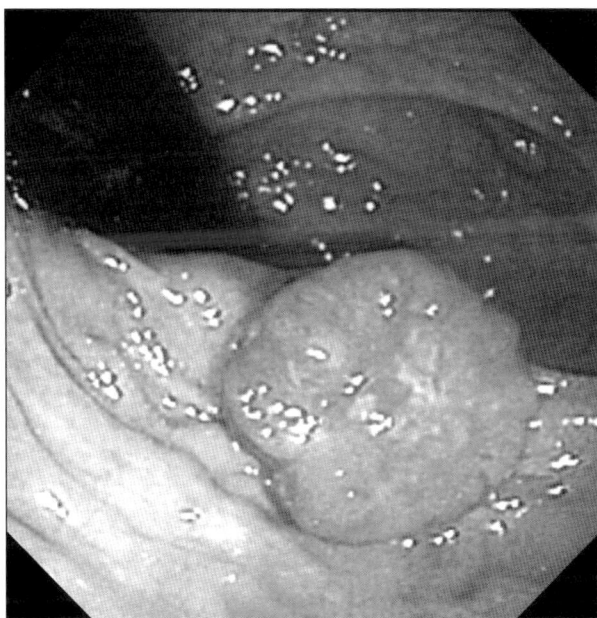

Figure 2. Early rectal cancer, best seen in retroflexion.

Examination technique

Although the major technical challenge of colonoscopy is to intubate to the caecum predictably, comfortably and safely, an accurate diagnostic assessment during the withdrawal phase of the procedure is of paramount importance. In the past, too little emphasis in colonoscopy training programmes has been apportioned to examination technique, although it has been known for some time that many polyps and even some early cancers can be missed if a meticulous approach is not adhered to [35-38]. Moreover, examination quality as determined by blinded video scoring appears to correlate with adenoma detection rates [39, 40]. A useful part of visual assessment, and some biopsies and polypectomies, can best be made during the insertion phase when the sigmoid colon is stretched out, but most diagnostic and therapeutic effort is on withdrawal. A rapid and scrupulous technique is required to scan the maximum area of the mucosa and to reduce the number of blind spots. Obsessionality is needed to aspirate all fluid or irrigate any residue that may be obscuring the surface and to look behind prominent folds or to re-scan areas that have been poorly seen. Circular muscle spasticity can significantly reduce the view, so that use of antispasmodics may improve accuracy in the hunt for small polyps. It is also inevitable that some acute bends may require more than one pass for proper inspection, and that certain flexures may be best seen after a change of position. The hepatic flexure is best seen in the left lateral position and the transverse with the patient supine. Turning the patient to the right-oblique position to examine the splenic flexure and the descending colon, but then back to left lateral for examination of the sigmoid and rectum, also improves visualisation considerably. The process of accurate colorectal examination cannot be hurried. It is impossible to examine a colon adequately on withdrawal in less than 5 minutes; to scan carefully for small polyps should take nearer 10 minutes. The technique of scope retroflexion should always be considered to maximise visualisation of the lower rectum or ascending colon, areas where small lesions are missed easily during insertion (Figure 2) [41, 42].

Flat adenomas

Traditionally, it was thought that almost all adenomas were stalked or sessile, that they projected from the bowel wall and that they were relatively easy to see at colonoscopy. The description of flat adenomas by Muto (Tokyo, Japan) in 1985 therefore caused considerable controversy, particularly when subsequent reports documented the existence of small (<1cm), flat adenocarcinomas [43-46]. Initially, Western endoscopists were sceptical, but extensive Japanese reporting has led to more detailed searches for flat lesions in the West (Figure 3) [47-54]. Prospective series have documented the prevalence of flat adenomas in Western countries to be 10-36% and small, flat cancers to constitute approximately 10% of all cancers detected at colonoscopy (Figure 4) [44, 48-50, 52-54]. These reports reflect the Japanese experience [47]. Flat adenomas can be minimally elevated (IIa), flush with the mucosa (IIb) or depressed below the level of the mucosal surface (IIc); they tend to have a more proximal distribution within the colon and histologically they are tubular adenomas. Flat adenomas with a IIb or IIc morphology only account for 10% of all flat lesions and only 2-3% of adenomas overall, but these lesions appear to have a high incidence of high-grade dysplasia or early invasive cancer, despite their small size [47]. Conversely, minimally elevated lesions (IIa) are

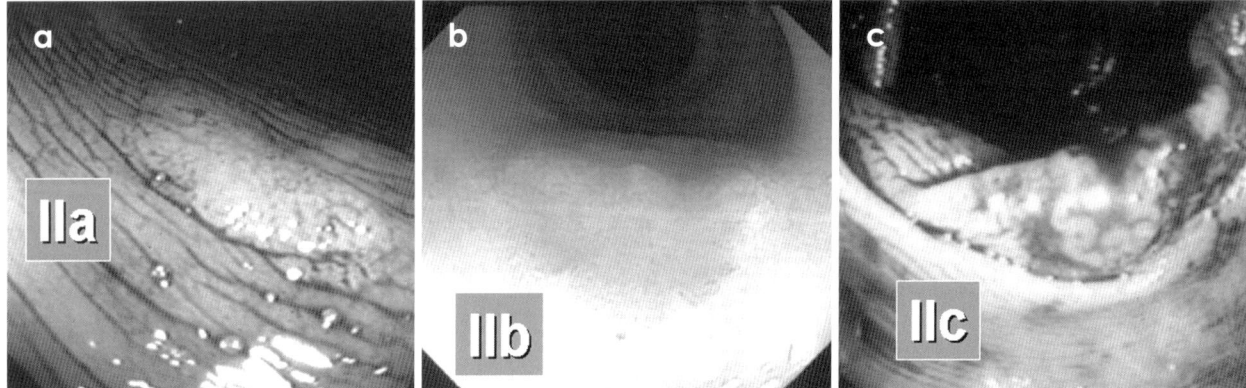

Figure 3. Flat adenomas. a) Type IIa, minimally elevated. b) Type IIb, flush with the mucosal surface. c) Type IIc, depressed below the mucosal surface. Note views augmented by the use of indigocarmine dye as a mucosal contrast.

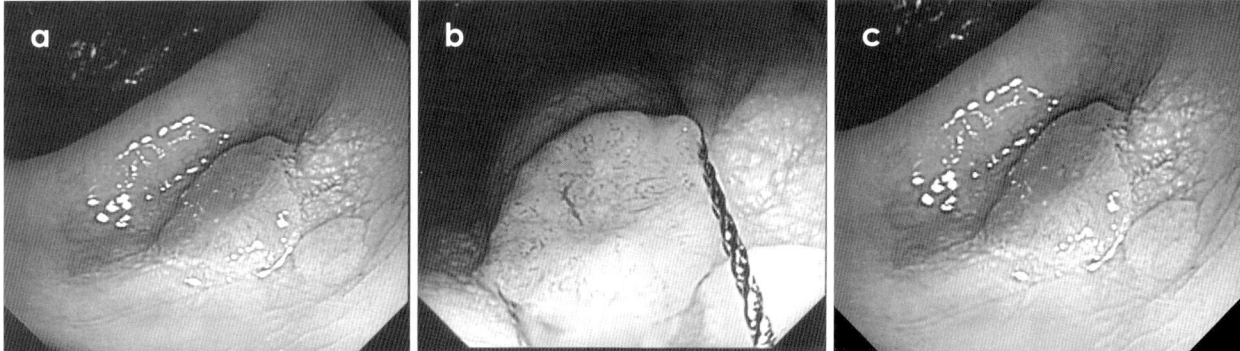

Figure 4. Examples of small, early flat cancers.

common and appear to have no increased risk of severe dysplasia or cancer and appear to grow slowly [55-57]. Research is ongoing to quantify the genetic characteristics of flat lesions. Current studies have failed to show consistent differences in the genetic make-up of flat compared to polypoid adenomas [58].

Detection of flat neoplasia at colonoscopy requires good bowel preparation and attention to careful examination technique, as emphasised above. Subtle changes in mucosal colour, loss of vessel pattern or localised disruption of a haustral fold draw attention to possible abnormalities which can be further highlighted by the use of indigocarmine dye (0.2%). Dye can be injected directly down the biopsy channel or sprayed over extensive areas using dedicated catheters. Indigocarmine is not absorbed but pools in depressions and mucosal ridges (innominate grooves). Elective pan-colonic dye spray is technically feasible and may have particular value when examining high risk groups, such as those with multiple previous adenomas, longstanding, extensive inflammatory bowel disease, and family cancer syndromes [59-65].

Polyp assessment prior to polypectomy

On detecting a colonic polyp the endoscopist must decide whether polypectomy is a safe and appropriate action. A first priority is to achieve optimal endoscopic access, orientation and visualisation. This may require a change in patient position followed by scope rotation to place the polyp opposite the instrument (biopsy) channel at 5 o'clock. Aspiration of fluid and retained stool after washing with water and use of additional anti-spasmodic (simethicone) or mucosal dye (indigocarmine 0.2%) helps the visualisation process. Provided access and visualisation are both good, almost all benign polyps can be removed endoscopically. Very large sessile lesions that extend beyond 50% of the bowel wall circumference, particularly in the thin-walled right colon, are probably best removed surgically, as are large rectal lesions abutting near or onto the dentate line which can be accessed easily via a transanal approach. Advances in endoscopic mucosal resection techniques have allowed specialist colonoscopists to treat large sessile lesions, avoiding the need for surgery in many cases; therefore, if doubt remains regarding endoscopic resectability, a second specialist endoscopic opinion should be considered before referring the patient to open or laparoscopic surgery [66-69]. Features suggesting malignant involvement which would make an attempt at endoscopic excision inappropriate include ulceration, mucosal fold deformity (in the absence of a previous polypectomy attempt) and "hard feel" to palpation with the biopsy forceps. If there is doubt regarding resectability, submucosal saline injection should be performed looking for the "non-lifting" sign of likely submucosal involvement. Lesions that fail to lift or only partially lift are likely to have deep submucosal invasion with a significant risk of already having lymph node metastases [70]. Such lesions require formal surgical resection to maximise the possibility of cure. Lesions that lift completely are safe to remove by endoscopic means and most will show no or very minimal invasion into the submucosa where the risk of lymph node involvement is extremely low [71, 72]. Alternative techniques to determine resectability, usually only available at specialist units, include magnification colonoscopy and endoscopic ultrasound [73,74]. The finding of a disrupted, (type V) pit pattern on magnification indicates malignancy, with severe disruption increasing the likelihood of lymph node metastases being present [74]. High frequency (20Mhz) endoluminal ultrasound (EUS) mini-probes can give views of the depth of submucosal involvement. Both these techniques are complementary but add little advantage over assessment of whether or not a lesion lifts with submucosal injection.

The site of any polyp that appears suspicious of malignant involvement (see above) or which is considered to be too awkward to be removed endoscopically, should be tattooed for future endoscopic or surgical recognition [75]. The optimal technique to avoid spillage of black ink in the lumen or peritoneal cavity is to first raise a submucosal bleb with saline and then inject ink directly into the large submucosal space created [76]. A single 1-2ml tattoo is sufficient in most cases but four quadrant tattoos are optimal if there is a high suspicion of malignancy and surgery appears likely (Figure 5). This approach ensures easy localisation of the polypectomy site at laparotomy, regardless of the position of the polypectomy site or the orientation of the bowel. With commercially available sterile tattoo products, complications such as abscess formation are extremely rare and the tattoo is permanent [77].

Polypectomy techniques

Small colonic polyps, less than 5mm in size, can be removed by hot biopsy, cold snare or hot snare. Hot biopsy is quick and easy to perform and almost always provides an adequate tissue specimen for histology; however, there have been some concerns recently that it is associated with an increased risk of delayed bleeding, particularly in those on aspirin, and that it may not fully remove all polyp tissue [78-81]. Good technique is essential for effective hot biopsy, in

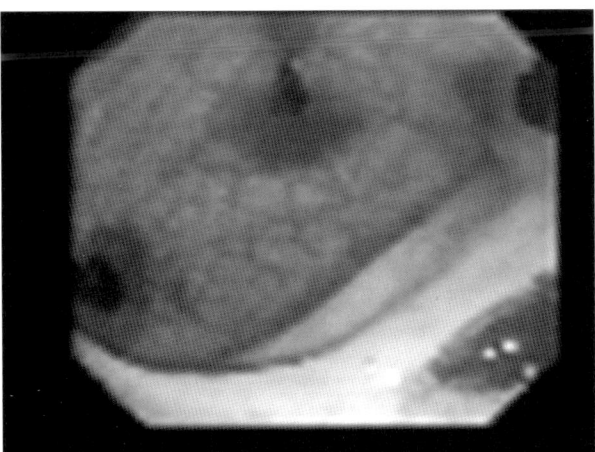

Figure 5. Four quadrant India ink tattoos.

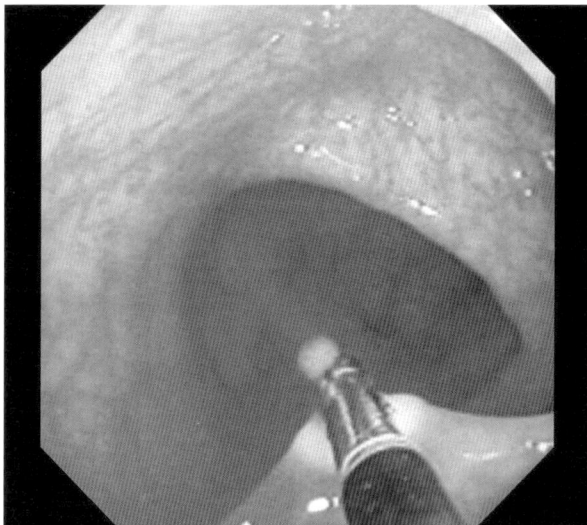

Figure 6. Hot biopsy technique. Note tenting and visible whitening at base, the so called Mt. Fuji effect.

particular ensuring adequate tenting of the mucosa to concentrate a short burst of current and heating directly below the polyp (Figure 6) [79]. Cold or hot snare of small polyps is effective, particularly with mini snares, but specimen retrieval may be more tricky with loss of the specimen in up to 30% of polyps [82]. Larger stalked polyps are usually easy to remove with conventional large or mini snares. With snare removal of stalked polyps the risk of perforation is very small; however, significant feeding blood vessels may be present within the stalk, increasing the risk of immediate or delayed bleeding. Therefore, slow transection of the stalk with low power coagulating current (15W) is recommended to allow adequate haemostasis [83]. Placing the snare approximately halfway down the stalk ensures a histologically complete excision but leaves sufficient stalk to be regrasped by the snare if there is immediate post-polypectomy bleeding. A variety of techniques and devices to avoid post-polypectomy bleeding exist, including endoclips and loops which can be placed before or after stalk transection, and pre-injection of the stalk with adrenaline, usually 1-3mls of 1/100,000 adrenaline (Figure 7) [84].

Sessile polyps larger than 1cm should generally be removed by an endoscopic mucosal resection technique. A variety of techniques for EMR have been described but all involve injection of a solution into the submucosal space to separate and lift the mucosa from the muscularis propria [85,86]. Single lesions up to approximately 2cm in diameter can be resected in one piece, but larger lesions require a piecemeal technique (Figure 8). There has been interest recently in improving the duration and quality of the mucosal "lift" by using different injection solutions. In the author's experience using dilute epinephrine provides benefits in terms of haemostasis, whilst addition of a few drops of methylene blue helps to stain the muscularis propria and submucosa defining tissue planes during resection. Hyaluronate has advantages in terms of duration and extent of mucosal lift but is currently very expensive and concerns are present that it may stimulate tumour cell proliferation at wound

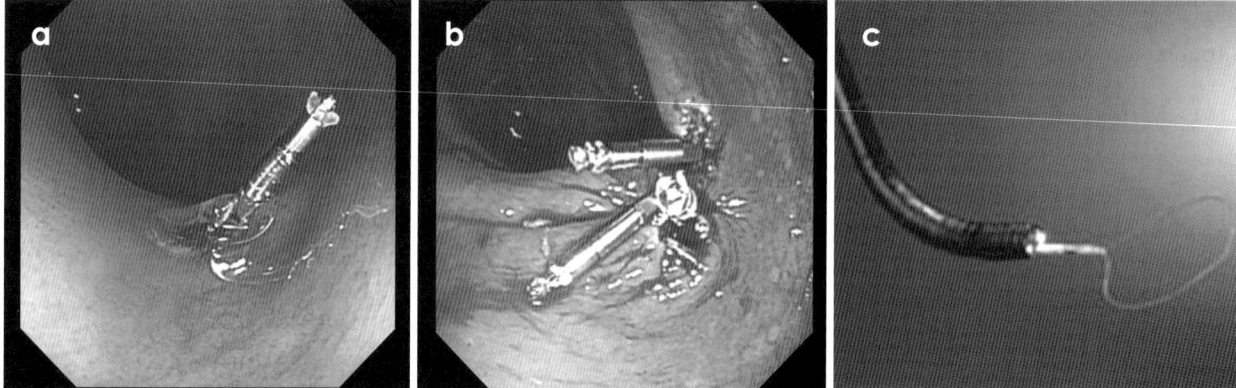

Figure 7. Endo-clips and the Endo-loop prior to deployment.

4 Polyp management

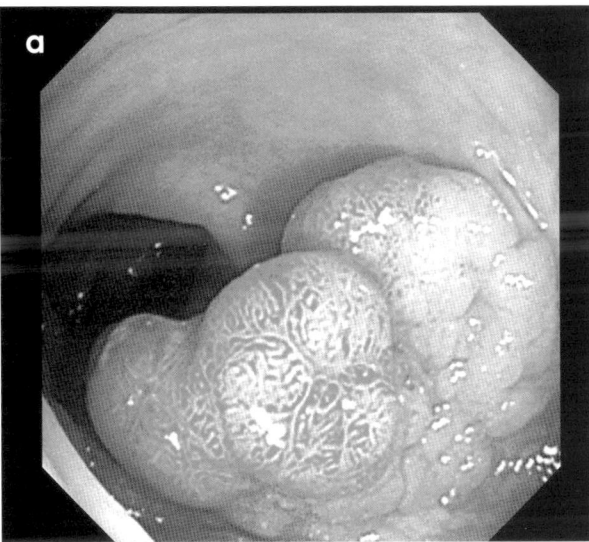 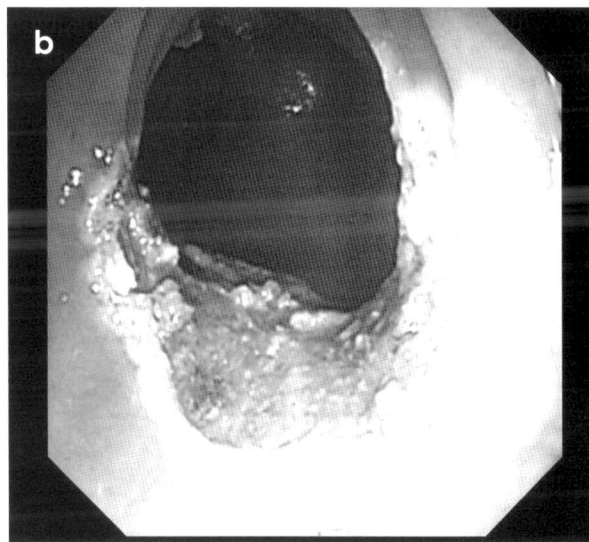

Figure 8. Piecemeal resection of large (>6cm) rectal villous adenoma.

sites [87]. Other more viscous solutions which may increase the duration of lift such as hydroxymethylcellulose, twice normal saline and 50% dextrose have also been proposed [88].

Most EMR in the colon can be achieved successfully with a standard, single-channel colonoscope and a diathermy snare. Variations on this theme include use of barbed or spiked snares to help grasp mucosa and facilitate removal of flat lesions and the use of the suction cap to perform aspiration mucosectomy. This latter technique has a high complication rate when used in the relatively thin-walled colon but may have application in the rectum, particularly for removing submucosal lesions [89]. A twin-channel colonoscope can be employed to use a "lift and cut" technique, where grasping forceps are used to retract the mucosa through the open snare. Endoscopic piecemeal resection of large lesions is a feasible and effective management, often preventing the need for surgery [90]. Piecemeal resection commits the patient to at least two endoscopies, the second 2-3 months after the initial examination to ensure complete healing of the polypectomy site. Argon plasma coagulation (APC) to treat resection margins immediately after piecemeal EMR has been shown significantly to reduce recurrence/residual neoplastic tissue [91]. APC is also the method of choice for ablation of multiple small polyps, such as those seen in the rectum of a patient with FAP post-ileorectal anastomosis.

Polyp retrieval

An attempt should be made to retrieve all polyps and the various techniques are listed below [92-95].

- Aspiration through the scope of small polyps up to 1cm in size, utilising specially designed suction traps or interrupting the suction tubing with a thin gauze swab.
- Regrasping with the snare and withdrawing the scope - taking care not to cheese-wire the polyp.
- By suctioning the polyp onto the end of the scope and withdrawing the scope maintaining suction pressure.
- Using a specific retrieval basket or the Roth retrieval net (Figure 9).
- Using tripod grasping forceps.

Treating and avoiding complications of polypectomy

The incidence of post-polypectomy bleeding is between 0.2-3%, while the other significant complications, namely post-polypectomy coagulation syndrome (full-thickness diathermy burn causing serosal irritation but without frank perforation) (0.5-1%) and perforation (0.5%) are less frequent [96-98].

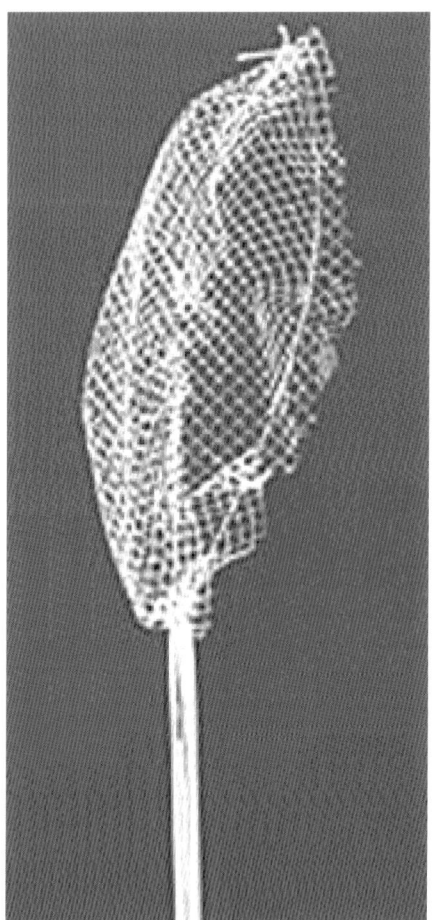

Figure 9. The Roth retrieval net.

Post-polypectomy bleeding can be characterised in different ways. It is defined as "immediate" when bleeding occurs during the procedure such that endoscopic intervention is required, or it is "delayed" if it occurs after the colonoscopy has been completed. Delayed bleeding usually starts within the first few days but has been reported as long as 30 days after polypectomy [99-101]. Immediate bleeding is usually due to inadequate coagulation of vessels in the polyp stalk or base, whereas delayed bleeding is thought to relate to detachment of the eschar several days after polypectomy when a significant submucosal vessel is exposed [102]. Therefore, the risk of bleeding either immediate or delayed is partly dependent upon the amount of tissue coagulation; too little and immediate bleeding is likely, too much and deep tissue injury with a risk of delayed bleeding may occur. The degree of tissue injury is dependent upon the power settings and duration of current application, the type of current used and most importantly the force applied to the snare during closure. For this reason endoscopists should become familiar with closing the snare themselves during application of diathermy so that they develop "feel" to guide the speed of cutting in addition to observing for "visible whitening" on the video monitor. Most colonic polypectomies can be performed using low power (15W) diathermy settings predominately set to the use of a coagulating current. Use of pure cutting current which vaporises tissue may be associated with a higher risk of immediate bleeding [103]. Coagulating current heat-seals blood vessels and is ideal for resection of large stalked polyps where centrally-located stalk vessels are often large and the risk of damage to the bowel wall, remote from the stalk, is small.

Post-polypectomy bleeding can be graded as mild, moderate or severe, depending on alterations in haemoglobin level, transfusion requirements or whether angiography or surgery become necessary. Fortunately the majority of post-polypectomy bleeds are mild and self-limiting, and therefore conservative management is usually sufficient with only a few patients with persistent bleeding requiring repeat colonoscopy or other interventions [104].

Risk factors for post-polypectomy bleeding should be anticipated and include size of polyp head or stalk, the relative experience of the endoscopist, the presence of a coagulopathy or anticoagulant medication and proximal location of the polyp in the colon [105]. There is a wide consensus and there are considerable data to assert that low-dose aspirin does not increase the risk of post-polypectomy bleeding [106,107]. However, electively stopping all antiplatelet medication, where feasible, is probably a wise precaution before attempted piecemeal excision of a large sessile polyp. Definitive data on the risk of bleeding post-polypectomy in patients taking newer anti-platelet drugs, such as clopidogrel, are not available and caution is therefore advised. Generally, warfarin should be stopped for 4 days before polypectomy and the INR checked just before the procedure. Patients with a high risk of thromboembolism (mechanical heart valves, recent vascular graft, previous endocarditis) should be covered with heparin which is stopped a few hours before the procedure [108].

In order to avoid the more severe consequences of bleeding, several novel approaches have been developed to encourage haemostasis after removal of high risk polyps or in patients more likely to bleed. These include mechanical devices, such as endo-loops and clips, adjunctive thermal modalities, such as APC, the heater probe and hot biopsy forceps, and the use of injection therapy with saline or hypertonic saline mixed with epinephrine [109-111]. Sclerosants are generally no longer used because of the perceived increased risk of perforation.

Perforation is a less frequent complication than bleeding (0.05-1% of polypectomies) and can also be delayed in presentation, hence patients undergoing colonoscopy should be warned to report immediately any severe abdominal pain or fever [112]. Localised pain, fever and leucocytosis are characteristic features of post-polypectomy syndrome, where there is localised peritonitis from a full thickness burn but no frank perforation [113]. With all significant complications the immediate principle of management is to hospitalise the patient with close observation of vital signs. Post-polypectomy syndrome and some small perforations can be managed conservatively with bed rest, fluids and broad spectrum antibiotics, whilst frank perforations will usually require immediate repair with open or laparoscopic surgery [112, 114]. Perforation is more likely in the thin-walled right colon, and here diathermy should be kept to a minimum and for larger sessile lesions a submucosal injection technique is mandatory to reduce heat damage to the muscle layer [115]. Marking the snare handle to avoid capture of excessively large volumes of tissue and being responsive to patient discomfort (indicating serosal irritation) are also important safety tips.

Surveillance post-polypectomy

Data on appropriate colonoscopic surveillance intervals post-polypectomy are limited. Where large sessile lesions have been removed piecemeal, a check of the polypectomy site should occur 2-3 months later to ensure complete healing with no residual polyp [116]. Tiny areas of recurrence in the polypectomy scar are best seen with the application of indigocarmine (0.2%) dye which should be used routinely. If a recurrent or residual polyp is present this is treated aggressively with a snare or APC and a further 2-3 month check organised. Occasionally recurrence may be seen late and therefore a second check at 1 year is recommended, even if the scar appears completely healed at 3 months. Post-polypectomy surveillance studies concur that the greatest risk factor for future development of advanced adenomas is multiplicity of adenomas at the baseline examination. High-grade dysplasia in an adenoma and size >1cm are also risk factors [117]. The British Society of Gastroenterology has recently produced guidelines for colonoscopic surveillance post-polypectomy where three groups are recognised [116]. High risk patients are those with five or more adenomas who are recommended to undergo initial surveillance at 1 year. Intermediate risk patients are those with three to four small polyps or an adenoma that is >1cm in size, and low risk are those with one or two small adenomas. There is little evidence that patients found to have one or two small adenomas (<1cm) (i.e. low risk) have any increased cancer risk compared to the general average risk population. However, given that currently no bowel screening is available in the UK, it is reasonable to offer a further examination in 5 years. All screening intervals must take into account age, comorbidity and associated risk factors such as family history. Patient risk is dependent on current colonoscopic findings which means that patients can move from low to high risk and vice versa. Thus someone with five adenomas at an initial colonoscopy who is high risk (1 year follow-up) would become low risk if they subsequently, at the 1 year follow-up only had one or two small adenomas. They would then be moved to 5-yearly follow-up but might become high risk again if at the next colonoscopy (undertaken 5 years later), they had five adenomas.

Where are we going?

There has been an unprecedented increase in demand for colonoscopy and this seems likely to continue for the foreseeable future. Colonoscopy is the primary screening modality already in the USA and with improved resources and colonoscopic training other countries may follow suit [118, 119]. In the future some diagnostic and perhaps screening colonoscopy will be done by virtual colonoscopy but optical colonoscopy will remain the preferred diagnostic

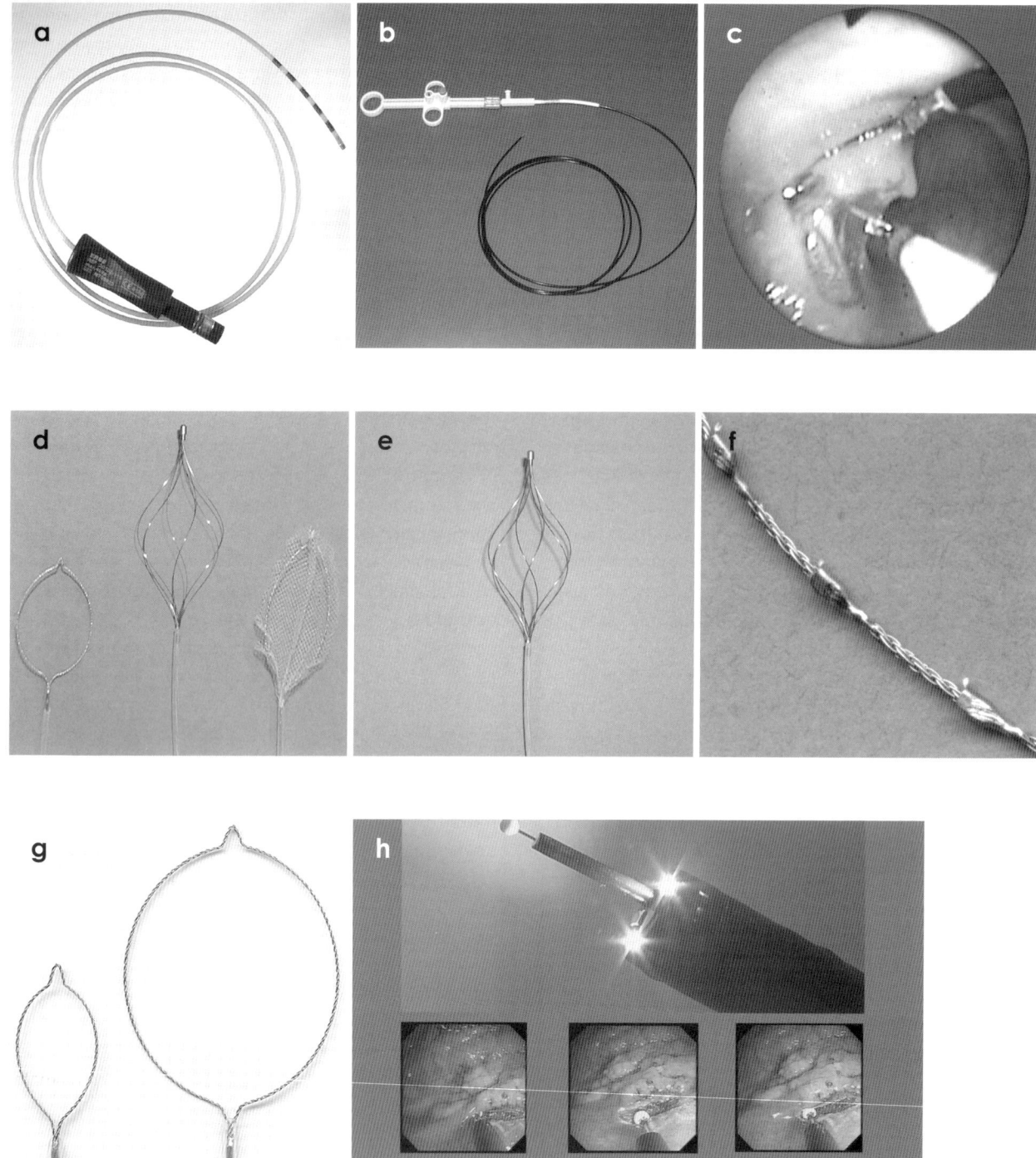

Figure 10. Existing through-the-scope diathermy devices, scissors and knives. a) APC catheter. b) Full snare device. c) Endoscopic scissors. d) Snares and baskets. e) New memory metal basket. f) Barbed snare. g) Snares. h) I-T knife.

modality for surveillance of high risk patients. Quality issues around colonoscopy performance are becoming increasingly important and it seems likely that in the future all procedures will be recorded electronically for audit, accreditation and review purposes. Those individual colonoscopists not complying with quality indicators may be required to retrain and stop performing screening procedures!

Adenoma detection at colonoscopy is likely to become easier with the advent of new optical technologies such as tissue autofluorescence [120-124]. Autofluorescence or tissue spectroscopy works by interrogating the mucosal surface with light of a known, narrow wavelength and capturing the reflective light pattern. Different types of mucosa have different reflective "tissue signatures" which can be relayed onto a monitor as colour changes allowing immediate recognition of dysplastic areas. A video colonoscope which combines all the functionality of a conventional scope with an autofluorescence system is undergoing evaluation. Another way of improving the view is to increase the standard field of view (140 degrees) with a wide-angled lens or even by incorporating simultaneous forward and backward viewing video camera systems [125]. Having detected lesions there is a very real prospect in the near future of being able to obtain highly accurate *in vivo* histology to guide endoscopic or surgical therapy. Promising techniques include magnification and confocal laser microscopy [126-128]. The latter can actually image below the mucosal surface, providing cross-sectional images very similar to those obtained using standard haematoxilyn and eosin staining and light microscopy. Preliminary data suggest very high positive and negative predictive values for determining neoplastic from non-neoplastic lesions [127].

Once abnormalities are detected the potential for endoscopic surgery is immense [129]. *En bloc* resection of large lesions is clearly advantageous and ideally would also include a margin of normal mucosa to aid interpretation of completeness of excision [130]. Possible methods of *en bloc* endoscopic resection include circumferential incision with special diathermy knives followed by a large snare resection or submucosal dissection using endoscopic scissors or diathermy devices [131]. Sessile lesions invariably lie over contoured haustral folds and a dissection technique whereby the submucosal plane is established and developed in a controlled way is likely to be the safest and most effective approach. Establishing the submucosal plane is relatively easy using existing diathermy knives (needle-knife, "hooking knife" or "triangle-tipped knife") but optimal dissection devices (scissors/knives) have yet to be developed (Figure 10). To enable accurate and quick dissection of the submucosal plane, traction on the mucosa above the line of dissection is usually necessary and this could be achieved by utilising a twin channel instrument with grasping forceps or creating an accessory channel with tubing attached externally onto the colonoscope. An alternative would be to use two ultra-thin endoscopes in parallel, possibly inserted via channels in an overtube [131]. In the future, purpose designed colonoscopes with multiple therapeutic channels will be available, the so-called "operating colonoscope". This instrument will need to maintain the flexibility of a conventional colonoscope with the therapeutic ability of current Trans-Endoscopic Microsurgery (TEMS) Units. Ultimately, there is the prospect for full thickness excision of early cancers [132]. To enable this, new accessory devices to allow cutting, haemostasis and tissue apposition would be needed. If these major engineering challenges can be overcome then endoscopic surgery from within, combined initially with laparoscopic assistance, will become the ultimate and perhaps preferred method of minimally invasive surgery [133].

References

1. Winawer SJ, Stewart ET, Zauber AG, Bond JH, Ansel H, Waye JD. A comparison of colonoscopy and double-contrast barium enema for surveillance after polypectomy. *N Engl J Med* 2000; 342: 1766-72.
2. Thiis-Evensen E, Hoff GS, Sauar J, Langmark F, Majak BM, Vatn MH. Population-based surveillance by colonoscopy: effect on the incidence of colorectal cancer. Telemark Polyp Study I. *Scand J Gastroenterol* 1999; 34(4): 414-20.
3. Zheng S, Liu XY, Ding KF, Wang LB, Qiu PL, Ding XF, Shen YZ, Shen GF, Sun QR, Li WD, Dong Q, Zhang SZ. Reduction of the incidence and mortality of rectal cancer by polypectomy: a prospective cohort study in Haining County. *World J Gastroenterol* 2002; 8(3): 488-92.
4. Muller AD, Sonnenberg A. Prevention of colorectal cancer by flexible endoscopy and polypectomy. A case-control study of 32,702 veterans. *Ann Intern Med* 1995; 123(12): 904-10.
5. Meagher AP, Stuart M. Does colonoscopic polypectomy reduce the incidence of colorectal carcinoma? *ANZ J Surg* 1994; 64(6): 400-4.
6. Atkin WS, Morson BC, Cuzick J. Long-term risk of colorectal cancer after excision of rectosigmoid adenomas. *N Engl J Med* 1992; 326(10): 658-62.
7. Jorgensen OD, Kronborg O, Fenger C. The Funen Adenoma Follow-up Study. Incidence and death from colorectal carcinoma in an adenoma surveillance program. *Scand J Gastroenterol* 1993; 28(10): 869-74.
8. Citarda F, Tomaselli G, Capocaccia R, Barcherini S, Crespi M; Italian Multicentre Study Group. Efficacy in standard clinical practice of colonoscopic polypectomy in reducing colorectal cancer incidence. *Gut* 2001; 48(6): 812-5.
9. Parkin DM. International variation. *Oncogene* 2004; 23(38): 6329-40.
10. Jemal A, Clegg LX, Ward E, Ries LA, Wu X, Jamison PM, Wingo PA, Howe HL, Anderson RN, Edwards BK. Annual report to the nation on the status of cancer, 1975-2001, with a special feature regarding survival. *Cancer* 2004; 101(1): 3-27.
11. Fearon ER, Vogelstein B. A genetic model for colorectal tumorigenesis. *Cell* 1990; 61(5): 759-67.
12. Yamaji Y, Mitsushima T, Ikuma H, Watabe H, Okamoto M, Kawabe T, Wada R, Doi H, Omata M. Incidence and recurrence rates of colorectal adenomas estimated by annually repeated colonoscopies on asymptomatic Japanese. *Gut* 2004; 53(4): 568-72.
13. Sandler RS, Halabi S, Baron JA, Budinger S, Paskett E, Keresztes R, Petrelli N, Pipas JM, Karp DD, Loprinzi CL, Steinbach G, Schilsky R. A randomized trial of aspirin to prevent colorectal adenomas in patients with previous colorectal cancer. *N Engl J Med* 2003; 348(10): 883-90.
14. Lieberman DA, Weiss DG, Bond JH, Ahnen DJ, Garewal H, Chejfec G. Use of colonoscopy to screen asymptomatic adults for colorectal cancer. Veterans Affairs Cooperative Study Group 380. *N Engl J Med* 2000; 343(3): 162-8.
15. Rembacken BJ, Fujii T, Cairns A, Dixon MF, Yoshida S, Chalmers DM, Axon AT. Flat and depressed colonic neoplasms: a prospective study of 1000 colonoscopies in the UK. *Lancet* 2000; 355(9211): 1211-4.
16. Gschwantler M, Kriwanek S, Langner E, Goritzer B, Schrutka-Kolbl C, Brownstone E, Feichtinger H, Weiss W. High-grade dysplasia and invasive carcinoma in colorectal adenomas: a multivariate analysis of the impact of adenoma and patient characteristics. *Eur J Gastroenterol Hepatol* 2002; 14(2): 183-8.
17. Masaki T, Muto T. Predictive value of histology at the invasive margin in the prognosis of early invasive colorectal carcinoma. *J Gastroenterol* 2000; 35(3): 195-200.
18. Williams CB, Saunders BP, Talbot IC. Endoscopic management of polypoid early colon cancer. *World J Surg* 2000; 24(9): 1047-51.
19. Netzer P, Forster C, Biral R, Ruchti C, Neuweiler J, Stauffer E, Schonegg R, Maurer C, Husler J, Halter F, Schmassmann A. Risk factor assessment of endoscopically removed malignant colorectal polyps. *Gut* 1998; 43(5): 669-74.
20. Netzer P, Binek J, Hammer B, Lange J, Schmassmann A. Significance of histologic criteria for the management of patients with malignant colorectal polyps and polypectomy. *Scand J Gastroenterol* 1997; 32(9): 910-6.
21. Kikuchi R, Takano M, Takagi K, Fujimoto N, Nozaki R, Fujiyoshi T, Uchida Y. Management of early invasive colorectal cancer. Risk of recurrence and clinical guidelines. *Dis Colon Rectum* 1995; 38(12): 1286-95.
22. Cooper HS, Deppisch LM, Gourley WK, Kahn EI, Lev R, Manley PN, Pascal RR, Qizilbash AH, Rickert RR, Silverman JF, et al. Endoscopically removed malignant colorectal polyps: clinicopathologic correlations. *Gastroenterology* 1995; 108(6): 1657-65.
23. Chantereau MJ, Faivre J, Boutron MC, Piard F, Arveux P, Bedenne L, Hillon P. Epidemiology, management, and prognosis of malignant large bowel polyps within a defined population. *Gut* 1992; 33(2): 259-63.
24. Geraghty JM, Williams CB, Talbot IC. Malignant colorectal polyps: venous invasion and successful treatment by endoscopic polypectomy. *Gut* 1991; 32(7): 774-8.
25. Baker K, Zhang Y, Jin C, Jass JR. Proximal versus distal hyperplastic polyps of the colorectum: different lesions or a biological spectrum? *J Clin Pathol* 2004; 57(10): 1089-93.
26. Jass JR. Hyperplastic polyps and colorectal cancer: is there a link? *Clin Gastroenterol Hepatol* 2004; 2(1): 1-8.
27. Rex DK, Rahmani EY, Haseman JH, Lemmel GT, Kaster S, Buckley JS. Relative sensitivity of colonoscopy and barium enema for detection of colorectal cancer in clinical practice. *Gastroenterology* 1997; 112(1): 17-23.
28. Winawer SJ, Stewart ET, Zauber AG, Bond JH, Ansel H, Waye JD, Hall D, Hamlin JA, Schapiro M, O'Brien MJ, Sternberg SS, Gottlieb LS. A comparison of colonoscopy and double-contrast barium enema for surveillance after polypectomy. National Polyp Study Work Group. *N Engl J Med* 2000; 342(24): 1766-72.
29. Smith GA, O'Dwyer PJ. Sensitivity of double contrast barium enema and colonoscopy for the detection of colorectal neoplasms. *Surg Endosc* 2001; 15(7): 649-52.
30. de Zwart IM, Griffioen G, Shaw MP, Lamers CB, de Roos A. Barium enema and endoscopy for the detection of colorectal neoplasia: sensitivity, specificity complications and its determinants. *Clin Radiol* 2001; 56(5): 401-9.
31. Rex DK, Mark D, Clarke B, Lappas JC, Lehman GA. Flexible sigmoidoscopy plus air-contrast barium enema versus colonoscopy for evaluation of symptomatic patients without evidence of bleeding. *Gastrointest Endosc* 1995; 42(2): 132-8.
32. Pickhardt PJ, Choi JR, Hwang I, Butler JA, Puckett ML, Hildebrandt HA, Wong RK, Nugent PA, Mysliwiec PA,

Schindler WR. Computed tomographic virtual colonoscopy to screen for colorectal neoplasia in asymptomatic adults. *N Engl J Med* 2003; 349(23): 2191-200. Epub 2003 Dec 01.
33. Rex DK. Colonoscopy turning the focus on quality. *Dig Liver Dis* 2002; 34(12): 831-2.
34. Rex DK, Bond JH, Winawer S, Levin TR, Burt RW, Johnson DA, Kirk LM, Litlin S, Lieberman DA, Waye JD, Church J, Marshall JB, Riddell RH; U.S. Multi-Society Task Force on Colorectal Cancer. Quality in the technical performance of colonoscopy and the continuous quality improvement process for colonoscopy: recommendations of the U.S. Multi-Society Task Force on Colorectal Cancer. *Am J Gastroenterol* 2002; 97(6): 1296-308.
35. Rex DK, Cutler CS, Lemmel GT, Rahmani EY, Clark DW, Helper DJ, et al. Colonoscopic miss rates of adenomas determined by back-to-back colonoscopies. *Gastroenterology* 1997; 112: 24-8.
36. Bretthauer M, Skovlund E, Grotmol T, Thiis-Evensen E, Gondal G, Huppertz-Hauss G, Efskind P, Hofstad B, Thorp Holmsen S, Eide TJ, Hoff G. Inter-endoscopist variation in polyp and neoplasia pick-up rates in flexible sigmoidoscopy screening for colorectal cancer. *Scand J Gastroenterol* 2003; 38(12): 1268-74.
37. Hixson LJ, Fennerty MB, Sampliner RE, et al. Prospective blinded trial of the colonoscopic miss-rate of large colorectal polyps. *Gastrointest Endosc* 1991; 37: 125-7.
38. Hosokawa O, Shirasaki S, Kaizaki Y, Hayashi H, Douden K, Hattori M. Invasive colorectal cancer detected up to 3 years after a colonoscopy negative for cancer. *Endoscopy* 2003; 35(6): 506-10.
39. Rex DK. Colonoscopic withdrawal technique is associated with adenoma miss rates. *Gastrointest Endosc* 2000; 51(1): 33-6
40. Atkin W, Rogers P, Cardwell C, Cook C, Cuzick J, Wardle J, Edwards R. Wide variation in adenoma detection rates at screening flexible sigmoidoscopy. *Gastroenterology* 2004; 126(5): 1247-56.
41. Rex DK. Accessing proximal aspects of folds and flexures during colonoscopy: impact of a pediatric colonoscope with a short bending section. *Am J Gastroenterol* 2003; 98(7): 1504-7.
42. Harrison M, Singh N, Rex DK. Impact of proximal colon retroflexion on adenoma miss rates. *Am J Gastroenterol* 2004; 99(3): 519-22.
43. Muto T, Kamiya J, Sawada T, Konishi F, Sugihara K, Kubota Y, Adachi M, Agawa S, Saito Y, Morioka Y, et al. Small "flat adenoma" of the large bowel with special reference to its clinicopathologic features. *Dis Colon Rectum* 1985; 28(11): 847-51.
44. Suzuki N, Talbot IC, Saunders BP. The prevalence of small, flat colorectal cancers in a western population. *Colorectal Dis* 2004; 6(1): 15-20.
45. Balachandar G, Trowers EA. Early colorectal cancer in a flat adenoma. *J Natl Med Assoc* 1999; 91(11): 631-2.
46. Trecca A, Fujii T, Kato S, Hasebe T, Tajiri H, Yoshida S. Small advanced colorectal adenocarcinomas: report on three cases. *Endoscopy* 1998; 30(5): 493-5.
47. Kudo S, Kashida H, Tamura T, Kogure E, Imai Y, Yamano H, Hart AR. Colonoscopic diagnosis and management of nonpolypoid early colorectal cancer. *World J Surg* 2000; 24(9): 1081-90.
48. Rembacken BJ, Fujii T, Cairns A, Dixon MF, Yoshida S, Chalmers DM, Axon AT. Flat and depressed colonic neoplasms: a prospective study of 1000 colonoscopies in the UK. *Lancet* 2000; 355(9211): 1211-4.
49. Diebold MD, Samalin E, Merle C, Bouche O, Higuero T, Jolly D, Ramaholimihaso F, Renard P, Yaziji N, Thiefin G, Cadiot G. Colonic flat neoplasia: frequency and concordance between endoscopic appearance and histological diagnosis in a French prospective series. *Am J Gastroenterol* 2004; 99(9): 1795-800.
50. Tsuda S, Veress B, Toth E, Fork FT. Flat and depressed colorectal tumours in a southern Swedish population: a prospective chromoendoscopic and histopathological study. *Gut* 2002; 51(4): 550-5.
51. Hart AR, Kudo S, Mackay EH, Mayberry JF, Atkin WS. Flat adenomas exist in asymptomatic people: important implications for colorectal cancer screening programmes. *Gut* 1998; 43(2): 229-31.
52. Jaramillo E, Watanabe M, Slezak P, Rubio C. Flat neoplastic lesions of the colon and rectum detected by high-resolution video endoscopy and chromoscopy. *Gastrointest Endosc* 1995; 42(2): 114-22.
53. Hurlstone DP, Brown S, Cross SS. The role of flat and depressed colorectal lesions in colorectal carcinogenesis: new insights from clinicopathological findings in high-magnification chromoscopic colonoscopy. *Histopathology* 2003; 43(5): 413-26.
54. Saitoh Y, Waxman I, West AB, Popnikolov NK, Gatalica Z, Watari J, Obara T, Kohgo Y, Pasricha PJ. Prevalence and distinctive biologic features of flat colorectal adenomas in a North American population. *Gastroenterology* 2001; 120(7): 1657-65.
55. Rozen P, Brazowski E. Flat colorectal neoplasia: identification, pathogenesis and clinical significance. *Dig Liver Dis* 2003; 35(3): 135-7.
56. O'brien MJ, Winawer SJ, Zauber AG, Bushey MT, Sternberg SS, Gottlieb LS, Bond JH, Waye JD, Schapiro M; National Polyp Study Workgroup. Flat adenomas in the National Polyp Study: is there increased risk for high-grade dysplasia initially or during surveillance? *Clin Gastroenterol Hepatol* 2004; 2(10): 905-11.
57. Kaneko K, Kurahashi T, Makino R, Konishi K, Mitamura K. Growth patterns of superficially elevated neoplasia in the large intestine. *Gastrointest Endosc* 2000; 51(4 Pt 1): 443-50.
58. Jass JR. Histopathology of early colorectal cancer. *World J Surg* 2000; 24(9): 1016-21.
59. Lee JH, Kim JW, Cho YK, Sohn CI, Jeon WK, Kim BI, Cho EY. Detection of colorectal adenomas by routine chromoendoscopy with indigocarmine. *Am J Gastroenterol* 2003; 98(6): 1284-8.
60. Hurlstone DP, Cross SS, Slater R, Sanders DS, Brown S. Detecting diminutive colorectal lesions at colonoscopy: a randomised controlled trial of pan-colonic versus targeted chromoscopy. *Gut* 2004; 53(3): 376-80.
61. Kiesslich R, von Bergh M, Hahn M, Hermann G, Jung M. Chromoendoscopy with indigocarmine improves the detection of adenomatous and nonadenomatous lesions in the colon. *Endoscopy* 2001; 33(12): 1001-6.
62 Hurlstone DP, Fujii T, Lobo AJ. Early detection of colorectal cancer using high-magnification chromoscopic colonoscopy. *Br J Surg* 2002; 89(3): 272-82.
63. Brooker JC, Saunders BP, Shah SG, Thapar CJ, Thomas HJ, Atkin WS, Cardwell CR, Williams CB. Total colonic dye-spray increases the detection of diminutive adenomas during routine

colonoscopy: a randomized controlled trial. *Gastrointest Endosc* 2002; 56(3): 333-8.
64. Kiesslich R, Fritsch J, Holtmann M, Koehler HH, Stolte M, Kanzler S, Nafe B, Jung M, Galle PR, Neurath MF. Methylene blue-aided chromoendoscopy for the detection of intraepithelial neoplasia and colon cancer in ulcerative colitis. *Gastroenterology* 2003; 124(4): 880-8.
65. Rutter MD, Saunders BP, Schofield G, Forbes A, Price AB, Talbot IC. Pancolonic indigo carmine dye spraying for the detection of dysplasia in ulcerative colitis. *Gut* 2004; 53(2): 256-60.
66. Brooker JC, Saunders BP, Shah SG, Williams CB. Endoscopic resection of large sessile colonic polyps by specialist and non-specialist endoscopists. *Br J Surg* 2002; 89(8): 1020-4.
67. Iishi H, Tatsuta M, Iseki K, Narahara H, Uedo N, Sakai N, Ishikawa H, Otani T, Ishiguro S. Endoscopic piecemeal resection with submucosal saline injection of large sessile colorectal polyps. *Gastrointest Endosc* 2000; 51(6): 697-700.
68. Church JM. Experience in the endoscopic management of large colonic polyps. *ANZ J Surg* 2003; 73(12): 988-95.
69. Binmoeller KF, Bohnacker S, Seifert H, Thonke F, Valdeyar H, Soehendra N. Endoscopic snare excision of "giant" colorectal polyps. *Gastrointest Endosc* 1996; 43(3): 183-8.
70. Kato H, Haga S, Endo S, Hashimoto M, Katsube T, Oi I, Aiba M, Kajiwara T. Lifting of lesions during endoscopic mucosal resection (EMR) of early colorectal cancer: implications for the assessment of resectability. *Endoscopy* 2001; 33(7): 568-73.
71. Nascimbeni R, Burgart LJ, Nivatvongs S, Larson DR. Risk of lymph node metastasis in T1 carcinoma of the colon and rectum. *Dis Colon Rectum* 2002; 45(2): 200-6.
72. Kikuchi R, Takano M, Takagi K, Fujimoto N, Nozaki R, Fujiyoshi T, Uchida Y. Management of early invasive colorectal cancer. Risk of recurrence and clinical guidelines. *Dis Colon Rectum* 1995; 38(12): 1286-95.
73. Togashi K, Konishi F, Ishizuka T, Sato T, Senba S, Kanazawa K. Efficacy of magnifying endoscopy in the differential diagnosis of neoplastic and non-neoplastic polyps of the large bowel. *Dis Colon Rectum* 1999; 42(12): 1602-8.
74. Matsumoto T, Hizawa K, Esaki M, Kurahara K, Mizuno M, Hirakawa K, Yao T, Iida M. Comparison of EUS and magnifying colonoscopy for assessment of small colorectal cancers. *Gastrointest Endosc* 2002; 56(3): 354-60.
75. Hancock JH, Talbot RW. Accuracy of colonoscopy in localisation of colorectal cancer. *Int J Colorectal Dis* 1995; 10(3): 140-1.
76. Sawaki A, Nakamura T, Suzuki T, Hara K, Kato T, Kato T, Hirai T, Kanemitsu Y, Okubo K, Tanaka K, Moriyama I, Kawai H, Katsurahara M, Matsumoto K, Yamao K. A two-step method for marking polypectomy sites in the colon and rectum. *Gastrointest Endosc* 2003; 57(6): 735-7.
77. Price N, Gottfried MR, Clary E, Lawson DC, Baillie J, Mergener K, Westcott C, Eubanks S, Pappas TN. Safety and efficacy of India ink and indocyanine green as colonic tattooing agents. *Gastrointest Endosc* 2000; 51(4 Pt 1): 438-42.
78. Weston AP, Campbell DR. Diminutive colonic polyps: histopathology, spatial distribution, concomitant significant lesions, and treatment complications. *Am J Gastroenterol* 1995; 90(1): 24-8.
79. Williams CB. Small polyps: the virtues and the dangers of hot biopsy. *Gastrointest Endosc* 1991; 37(3): 394-5.
80. Dyer WS, Quigley EM, Noel SM, Camacho KE, Manela F, Zetterman RK. Major colonic hemorrhage following electrocoagulating (hot) biopsy of diminutive colonic polyps: relationship to colonic location and low-dose aspirin therapy. *Gastrointest Endosc* 1991; 37(3): 361-4.
81. Monkemuller KE, Fry LC, Jones BH, Wells C, Mikolaenko I, Eloubeidi M. Histological quality of polyps resected using the cold versus hot biopsy technique. *Endoscopy* 2004; 36(5): 432-6.
82. McAfee JH, Katon RM. Tiny snares prove safe and effective for removal of diminutive colorectal polyps. *Gastrointest Endosc* 1994; 40(3): 301-3.
83. Fraser C, Saunders B. Preventing postpolypectomy bleeding: obligatory and optional steps. *Endoscopy* 2004; 36(10): 898-900.
84. Dobrowolski S, Dobosz M, Babicki A, Dymecki D, Hac S. Prophylactic submucosal saline-adrenaline injection in colonoscopic polypectomy: prospective randomized study. *Surg Endosc* 2004; 18(6): 990-3. Epub 2004 Apr 27.
85. Hawes RH. Perspectives in endoscopic mucosal resection. *Gastrointest Endosc Clin N Am* 2001; 11(3): 549-52.
86. Waye JD. Endoscopic mucosal resection of colon polyps. *Gastrointest Endosc Clin N Am* 2001; 11(3): 537-48.
87. Matsui Y, Inomata M, Izumi K, Sonoda K, Shiraishi N, Kitano S. Hyaluronic acid stimulates tumor-cell proliferation at wound sites. *Gastrointest Endosc* 2004; 60(4): 539-43.
88. Fujishiro M, Yahagi N, Kashimura K, Mizushima Y, Oka M, Enomoto S, Kakushima N, Kobayashi K, Hashimoto T, Iguchi M, Shimizu Y, Ichinose M, Omata M. Comparison of various submucosal injection solutions for maintaining mucosal elevation during endoscopic mucosal resection. *Endoscopy* 2004; 36(7): 579-83.
89. Nagai T, Torishima R, Nakashima H, Ookawara H, Uchida A, Kai S, Sato R, Murakami K, Fujioka T. Saline-assisted endoscopic resection of rectal carcinoids: cap aspiration method versus simple snare resection. *Endoscopy* 2004; 36(3): 202-5.
90. Conio M, Repici A, Demarquay JF, Blanchi S, Dumas R, Filiberti R. EMR of large sessile colorectal polyps. *Gastrointest Endosc* 2004; 60(2): 234-41.
91. Brooker JC, Saunders BP, Shah SG, Thapar CJ, Suzuki N, Williams CB. Treatment with argon plasma coagulation reduces recurrence after piecemeal resection of large sessile colonic polyps: a randomized trial and recommendations. *Gastrointest Endosc* 2002; 55(3): 371-5.
92. Miller K, Waye JD. Polyp retrieval after colonoscopic polypectomy: use of the Roth Retrieval Net. *Gastrointest Endosc* 2001; 54(4): 505-7. PMID: 11577319 [PubMed - indexed for MEDLINE].
93. Khanduja KS, Pons R. Efficient technique for retrieving small polyps from the colon and rectum following snare polypectomy. *Dis Colon Rectum* 1994; 37(2): 190.
94. Waye JD, Lewis BS, Atchison MA, Talbott M. The lost polyp: a guide to retrieval during colonoscopy. *Int J Colorectal Dis* 1988; 3(4): 229-31.
95. Webb WA, McDaniel L, Jones L. Experience with 1000 colonoscopic polypectomies. *Ann Surg* 1985; 201(5): 626-32.
96. Cappell MS, Abdullah M. Management of gastrointestinal bleeding induced by gastrointestinal endoscopy. *Gastroenterol Clin North Am* 2000; 29(1): 125-67, vi-vii.

97. Waye JD, Kahn O, Auerbach ME. Complications of colonoscopy and flexible sigmoidoscopy. *Gastrointest Endosc Clin N Am* 1996; 6(2): 343-77.
98. Vernava AM, III, Longo WE. Complications of endoscopic polypectomy. *Surg Oncol Clin N Am* 1996; 5(3): 663-73.
99. Rex DK, Lewis BS, Waye JD. Colonoscopy and endoscopic therapy for delayed post-polypectomy hemorrhage. *Gastrointest Endosc* 1992; 38(2): 127-29.
100. Rosen L, et al. Hemorrhage following colonoscopic polypectomy. *Dis Colon Rectum* 1993; 36(12): 1126-31.
101. Singaram C, Torbey CF, Jacoby RF. Delayed postpolypectomy bleeding. *Am J Gastroenterol* 1995; 90(1): 146-47.
102. Van Gossum A, et al. Colonoscopic snare polypectomy: analysis of 1485 resections comparing two types of current. *Gastrointest Endosc* 1992; 38(4): 472-75.
103. Parra-Blanco A, Kaminaga N, Kojima T, Endo Y, Tajiri A, Fujita R. Colonoscopic polypectomy with cutting current: is it safe? *Gastrointest Endosc* 2000; 51(6): 676-81.
104. Gibbs DH, et al. Postpolypectomy colonic hemorrhage. *Dis Colon Rectum* 1996; 39(7): 806-10.
105. Cappell MS, Abdullah M. Management of gastrointestinal bleeding induced by gastrointestinal endoscopy. *Gastroenterol Clin North Am* 2000; 29(1): 125-vii.
106. Yousfi M, Gostout CJ, Baron TH, Hernandez JL, Keate R, Fleischer DE, Sorbi D. Postpolypectomy lower gastrointestinal bleeding: potential role of aspirin. *Am J Gastroenterol* 2004; 99(9): 1785-9.
107. Hui AJ, Wong RM, Ching JY, Hung LC, Chung SC, Sung JJ. Risk of colonoscopic polypectomy bleeding with anticoagulants and antiplatelet agents: analysis of 1657 cases. *Gastrointest Endosc* 2004; 59(1): 44-8.
108. Timothy SK, Hicks TC, Opelka FG, Timmcke AE, Beck DE. Colonoscopy in the patient requiring anticoagulation. *Dis Colon Rectum* 2001; 44(12): 1845-8; discussion, 1848-9.
109. Dobrowolski S, et al. Prophylactic submucosal saline-adrenaline injection in colonoscopic polypectomy: prospective randomized study. *Surg Endosc* 2004; 18(6): 990-3.
110. Fraser C, Saunders B. Preventing postpolypectomy bleeding: obligatory and optional steps. *Endoscopy* 2004; 36(10): 898-900.
111. Parra-Blanco A, Kaminaga N, Kojima T, Endo Y, Uragami N, Okawa N, Hattori T, Takahashi H, Fujita R. Hemoclipping for postpolypectomy and postbiopsy colonic bleeding. *Gastrointest Endosc* 2000; 51(1): 37-41.
112. Cobb WS, Heniford BT, Sigmon LB, Hasan R, Simms C, Kercher KW, Matthews BD. Colonoscopic perforations: incidence, management, and outcomes. *Am Surg* 2004; 70(9): 750-7; discussion 757-8.
113. Church JM. Avoiding surgery in patients with colorectal polyps. *Dis Colon Rectum* 2003; 46(11): 1513-6.
114. Ker TS, Wasserberg N, Beart RW Jr. Colonoscopic perforation and bleeding of the colon can be treated safely without surgery. *Am Surg* 2004; 70(10): 922-4.
115. Conio M, Repici A, Demarquay JF, Blanchi S, Dumas R, Filiberti R. EMR of large sessile colorectal polyps. *Gastrointest Endosc* 2004; 60(2): 234-41
116. Atkin WS, Saunders BP; British Society for Gastroenterology; Association of Coloproctology for Great Britain and Ireland. Surveillance guidelines after removal of colorectal adenomatous polyps. *Gut* 2002; 51 Suppl 5: V6-9.
117. Rex DK. Postpolypectomy and post-cancer resection surveillance. *Rev Gastroenterol Disord* 2003; 3(4): 202-9.
118. Rex DK; ACG Board of Trustees. American College of Gastroenterology action plan for colorectal cancer prevention. *Am J Gastroenterol* 2004; 99(4): 574-7.
119. Rex DK, Johnson DA, Lieberman DA, Burt RW, Sonnenberg A. Colorectal cancer prevention 2000: screening recommendations of the American College of Gastroenterology. American College of Gastroenterology. *Am J Gastroenterol* 2000; 95(4): 868-77.
120. Kelly K, Alencar H, Funovics M, Mahmood U, Weissleder R. Detection of invasive colon cancer using a novel, targeted, library-derived fluorescent peptide. *Cancer Res* 2004; 64(17): 6247-51.
121. Gono K, Obi T, Yamaguchi M, Ohyama N, Machida H, Sano Y, Yoshida S, Hamamoto Y, Endo T. Appearance of enhanced tissue features in narrow-band endoscopic imaging. *J Biomed Opt* 2004; 9(3): 568-77.
123. Mayinger B, Jordan M, Horner P, Gerlach C, Muehldorfer S, Bittorf BR, Matzel KE, Hohenberger W, Hahn EG, Guenther K. Endoscopic light-induced autofluorescence spectroscopy for the diagnosis of colorectal cancer and adenoma. *J Photochem Photobiol B* 2003; 70(1): 13-20.
124. Mycek MA, Schomacker KT, Nishioka NS. Colonic polyp differentiation using time-resolved autofluorescence spectroscopy. *Gastrointest Endosc* 1998; 48(4): 390-4.
125. Rex DK, Chadalawada V, Helper DJ. Wide angle colonoscopy with a prototype instrument: impact on miss rates and efficiency as determined by back-to-back colonoscopies. *Am J Gastroenterol* 2003; 98(9): 2000-5.
126. Fleischer DE. Chromoendoscopy and magnification endoscopy in the colon. *Gastrointest Endosc* 1999; 49(3 Pt 2): S45-9.
127. Kiesslich R, Burg J, Vieth M, Gnaendiger J, Enders M, Delaney P, Polglase A, McLaren W, Janell D, Thomas S, Nafe B, Galle PR, Neurath MF. Confocal laser endoscopy for diagnosing intraepithelial neoplasias and colorectal cancer *in vivo*. *Gastroenterology* 2004; 127(3): 706-13.
128. Kiesslich R, Jung M, DiSario JA, Galle PR, Neurath MF. Perspectives of chromo and magnifying endoscopy: how, how much, when, and whom should we stain? *J Clin Gastroenterol* 2004; 38(1): 7-13.
129. Hawes RH. Perspectives in endoscopic mucosal resection. *Gastrointest Endosc Clin N Am* 2001; 11(3): 549-52.
130. Yamamoto H, Koiwai H, Yube T, Isoda N, Sato Y, Sekine Y, Higashizawa T, Utsunomiya K, Ido K, Sugano K. A successful single-step endoscopic resection of a 40 millimeter flat-elevated tumor in the rectum: endoscopic mucosal resection using sodium hyaluronate. *Gastrointest Endosc* 1999; 50(5): 701-4.
131. Brooker JC, Saunders BP, Suzuki N, Sibbons P. Twin-endoscope scissors resection (T-ESR): a new minimally invasive technique for performing colonic mucosectomy. *Surg Endosc* 2001; 15(12): 1463-6.
132. Rajan E, Gostout CJ, Burgart LJ, Leontovich ON, Knipschiel MA, Herman LJ, Norton ID. First endoluminal system for transmural resection of colorectal tissue with a prototype full-thickness resection device in a porcine model. *Gastrointest Endosc* 2002; 55(7): 915-20.
133. Franklin ME Jr, Diaz-E JA, Abrego D, Parra-Davila E, Glass JL. Laparoscopic-assisted colonoscopic polypectomy: the Texas Endosurgery Institute experience. *Dis Colon Rectum* 2000; 43(9): 1246-9.

Chapter 5

Endoscopy training: state of the art

Siwan Thomas-Gibson BSc MRCP, Research Fellow, Gastroenterology
Margaret Vance RGNDip MSc, Nurse Consultant, Gastroenterology
St. Mark's Hospital, Harrow, Middlesex, UK

What is the problem?

Endoscopy services and training are in the process of undergoing major change in the UK. This has been driven by several factors. Colorectal cancer is the second most common cause of cancer death in the UK after lung cancer, with more than 34,000 new cases diagnosed in the UK each year and around 16,000 deaths. The survival rates in the UK are amongst the lowest in Europe and almost 20% lower than in the USA. Poor survival rates in the UK correlate with the advanced stage at which most colorectal cancers are diagnosed. In 2000, the National Health Service (NHS) cancer plan was published to provide a national strategy to reform the way cancer services are delivered with the focus being prevention, early detection and treatment of cancers and a specific aim of reducing the mortality rate of cancer by 20% in people under 75 by 2010 [1]. The cancer plan was formulated in response to findings of the Calman-Hine report [2], which highlighted variations in cancer treatments across the UK. To coincide with the cancer plan the "two-week standard" was rolled out nationally. This target guaranteed that any patient with suspected colorectal cancer (amongst others) had to be seen by a specialist within 2 weeks of the general practitioner (GP) referal. This emphasis on early detection highlighted the importance of diagnostic services, including endoscopy, in the detection, staging and treatment of disease.

In 2002, the Secretary of State for Health publicly supported the development and implementation of a national screening programme for colorectal cancer by 2007 [3]. This will lead to an increase in the demand for endoscopic services to assist with the detection and treatment of colorectal neoplasia. This is in the context of an already over-stretched NHS where there is a recognised lack of medical manpower to provide endoscopy services for patients [4]. Endoscopy services have, until recently, been under resourced with no national strategy for service development and training. The introduction of the NHS plan and the development of targets for both suspected cancer referrals and waiting times for endoscopic procedures has led to close examination of endoscopy services in the UK. The demand for endoscopic procedures has been steadily rising, with a 66% increase in colonoscopy activity in the UK between 1996 and 2001. This demand will increase with the introduction of colorectal cancer screening. To assist the implementation of the NHS cancer plan and to prepare for colorectal cancer screening, the National Endoscopy Project was set up by the NHS

Modernisation agency to redesign endoscopy services, increase the number of endoscopists and tackle variation in existing approaches to their training [3].

Major changes in the working lives of doctors have also had an increasing impact on all areas of training in clinical medicine, including endoscopy. The introduction of the European Working Time Directive changed British Law in 1998 and, as a result, soon no doctor will be able to work more than 48 hours per week. In addition, in 1993 the Calman report proposed reforms of the registrar training grades (the specialty training years in which endoscopic skills are learned) to bring medical training into line with the European Union [5]. The Royal Colleges recognise that this will have substantial implications for the training of specialists of the future. It has been calculated that a trainee surgeon will now work a total of 6000 hours between becoming a senior house officer and gaining a consultant post. This compares with a total of 30,000 hours before these two major changes [6]. Many aspects of training and assessment will have to be reviewed in order to preserve the safety of patients whilst accommodating these changes. This may require fundamental changes in approach to training by experienced surgeons and physicians [7]. Endoscopy is no exception, particularly in the light of a recent major UK study which showed evidence of low colonoscopy completion rates and inadequate training [8]. This prospective study by the British Society of Gastroenterology (BSG) reported wide variation in the standard of colonoscopy training. Only 17% of trainees had received supervised training for their first 100 colonoscopies and only 39% of clinicians had attended an endoscopy training course. Variable standards of procedure performance were also reported, with an adjusted caecal intubation rate of just 57% when recognised landmarks were used to identify the caecum. This figure falls well below the recommended caecal intubation rate of at least 90%. In a large UK-based multicentre study on screening flexible sigmoidoscopy, adenoma detection rates were found to be highly variable, with a two-fold difference between some endoscopists [9]. It has been proposed that differences in the endoscopist's technique are responsible for this, which is perhaps hardly surprising as there are no standardised training methods in endoscopy and no accreditation process. There is concern about the quality of training elsewhere across Europe and the rest of the world [10-12]. A common theme is that there is no uniform, clear structure to training or assessment of competence.

These major influences - increasing demands on diagnostic endoscopy services, concern over the quality of existing services, the likely introduction of colorectal cancer screening and a reduction in hours spent in training - have driven major change in endoscopy training in the UK.

Where are we now?

As a result of these problems and issues the way in which clinical skills such as flexible sigmoidoscopy and colonoscopy are taught has recently been scrutinised by the professional bodies which oversee endoscopy training. As well as a general trend towards providing more structure in day-to-day teaching, in the UK there has been a considerable drive to produce high quality, intensive endoscopy training courses. This is coupled with rapidly developing technology, which is having a direct impact on how training is delivered.

The Joint Advisory Group (JAG) on Gastro-intestinal Endoscopy is a professional group representing the Royal Colleges of Physicians, Surgeons, Radiologists and General Practitioners in the UK. The JAG has published guidelines on the training, appraisal and assessment of trainees in gastrointestinal endoscopy. It is recognised that endoscopy training should be of a high standard within the unit in which an individual is working but that this should be complemented by periods of more intensive training in the format of approved courses. Much work has gone into developing these courses and trainees must complete them in order to gain their certificate of completion of specialist training. Training units should undertake at least 300 colonoscopies annually and an individual trainee should have experience of at least 100 per annum [13]. For surgeons and physicians in the UK this equates to an experience of at least 500 cases by the time specialty training has been completed.

Training methods

The focus on postgraduate medical education and skills training has precipitated a more formalised approach to endoscopy training. The reduction in hours a doctor is allowed to work means there are fewer hours in which training can be delivered and received. In addition, there is far closer scrutiny of the quality and quantity of training each trainee receives. It is increasingly being recognised that practitioners with expertise in a particular clinical skill are not necessarily skilled as teachers, and therefore attention is also being paid to training the trainers so that their knowledge and skills can be more effectively passed on to their trainees.

A more formalised structure to the method of training will enhance the traditional apprenticeship approach. Medical education literature describes the four domains involved in acquiring a clinical skill: knowledge, skill, attitude and social behaviour [14]. Modern endoscopic training should incorporate teaching in all of these domains. Peyton describes a stepwise approach to teaching surgical procedures in which a trainee progresses through a hierarchy of skills from being a novice to mastering the technique. There has been an attempt to rationalise the approach to teaching flexible sigmoidoscopy and colonoscopy in this way, reinforced with the advent of JAG courses [13]. Procedures are taught with a trainee building their skills from observing and describing what the trainer is doing to being able to demonstrate that they *know what to do* next and then *know how to do* it before they go onto the stage of *showing how to do* it.

Endoscopy is suited well to this method of teaching. Flexible sigmoidoscopy and colonoscopy procedures can be broken down into several steps. Each step of the procedure can be followed in this four-stage process and then the entire procedure built up from the individual steps as they are mastered. The focus of training progresses from one stage to another once the trainee has demonstrated their ability. The trainer may perform the procedure up to the point where the trainee is learning a new stage where the teaching for that case will take place. This method makes clinical teaching more feasible with less frustration and delay than if an inadequately prepared trainee tries to take on an entire case. It allows the trainer to set clear objectives for the teaching session and will more likely result in the trainee having a feeling of accomplishment instead of failure. This is an important motivator in all adult learners. Variations in this approach may be carried out for novices or for procedures which have to be taught but do not present themselves clinically very often. Here the trainer may perform more of the procedure. Another key feature of training, which is often neglected but is encouraged in this method of endoscopy teaching, is feedback. Feedback is immediate information, requiring little preparation and highly desired by the medical learner. This aspect of training, often a scarce occurrence, can be highly formative in the development of skills. It is non-judgemental and should not be confused with evaluation. Giving good feedback is an essential part of all training and is of particular relevance in clinical skills such as endoscopy [15].

Training aids

Advances in technology have brought exciting new developments to the field of endoscopy training. Two of the most significant of these have been the very recent advances in computer simulation and the development of a 3-D endoscope imaging system.

Simulators

The use of simulators in clinical teaching is attractive as they provide the opportunity for a trainee to gain skill whilst avoiding putting patients at risk. Other advantages of simulators are shown in Table 1. In procedures such as colonoscopy, which in addition is often performed with minimal sedation, this has long been seen as an attractive teaching option. The concept of simulation in endoscopy has been around at least since 1972. Flat-board static models were used to teach the "macromanoeuvres" involved in colonoscopy but these were largely used in specialist training centres and required constant trainer supervision. Modern static rubber simulators, such as the Koken model (Koken Ltd, Japan), are useful, particularly in teaching novices the basic skills required for steering the endoscope using a one-handed technique. More sophisticated models, such

Table 1. Advantages of training using simulators.

- Does patients no harm
- Allows trainee "permission to fail" in a safe learning environment
- Multiple variations of procedures
- Multiple repetitions possible
- Immediate feedback trains out error
- Unlimited training time adds convenience
- Less support from trainer required
- Training may be standardised
- External stress factors may be controlled for

as the Erlanger Endo-trainer, which was originally developed as an upper gastrointestinal model [16], now has a colonic version. This utilises porcine colon and has the advantage of providing real tissue feel. These models allow safe, stepwise teaching on simple therapeutic manoeuvres, such as colonic polypectomy, control of haemorrhage, foreign body retrieval and colonic dilatation. Multicentre studies are currently underway to evaluate rates of improvement and to establish the learning curves achieved with the Erlanger system.

The first endoscopic computer simulators were developed in the late 1980s but with significant limitations imposed by the processing speed of computers at that time [17]. A long history of success in simulation for training in the aviation industry, however, is often cited as the drive for continued interest in development of medical simulation, and the new millennium saw the introduction of computerised endoscopy simulators capable of simulating both flexible sigmoidoscopy and colonoscopy. Evidence in support of endoscopic computer simulators is beginning to emerge. Currently, two systems are commercially available, the Simbionix GI-Mentor (Israel) and the AccuTouch (Immersion Medical, Gaithersburg, USA) (Figure 1). An Olympus system is in the final stages of development. These simulators all work on a similar basis. A specialised colonoscope that functions as a normal endoscope is inserted into a computer-based model. The colonic lumen is displayed on a video screen, as in reality. Real time images are displayed as progress is made through the virtual colon. Several flexible sigmoidoscopy and colonoscopy cases of different complexity are available. The Simbionix system has a "game" module designed to enhance particular dexterity skills. Both systems have a "virtual trainer" that can give the trainee advice during the case. The trainee can administer drugs and perform some ancillary manoeuvres during the procedure. Basic therapeutic skills such as hot biopsy and snare polypectomy are simulated and although not entirely realistic they do allow stepwise teaching of a complex, multi-stage procedure associated with considerable risk, particularly when being performed by the novice in a real patient. Performance parameters are automatically displayed at the end of each case and stored on the computer's database. Aabakken was one of the first to report on the ease of use and realism of the Simbionix system for colonoscopy [18]. Feedback from its use by 33 endoscopists suggested it had a reasonable level of realism (face validity) and unsurprisingly, it was felt that it was most useful during early stages of training. Most respondents felt it was less difficult than real life colonoscopy and one concern is that a computer simulator which is too easy may give the trainee false confidence resulting in complications when they encounter the complexity of

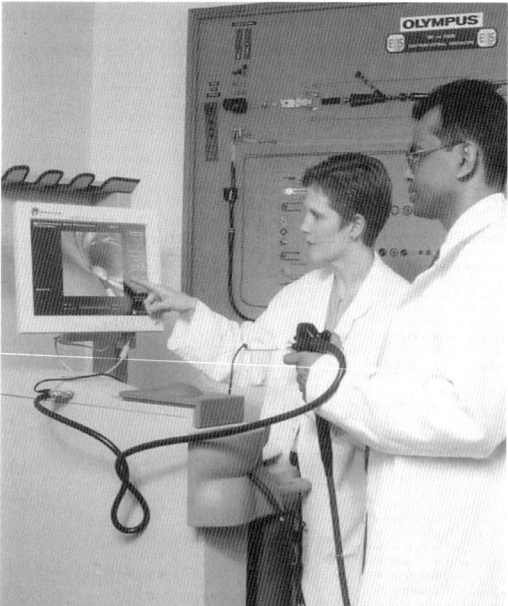

Figure 1. Computer simulators have the ability to teach basic hand skills required for colonoscopy.

a real colon. Several groups have demonstrated that these simulators can differentiate between experts and novices (the construct validity) based on some of the performance criteria measured [19-21]; however, not all performance criteria that should differentiate between individuals of different expertise do so. Sedlack has shown that intensive, structured use of a computer-based colonoscopy simulator at the start of colonoscopy training has an advantage over traditional patient-based initial training. Trainees who had used the simulator demonstrated a higher degree of competency during the early stages of their patient-based practice. But these advantages were negligible after 30 patient-based procedures [22]. This raises the possibility that early training with computer-based simulators may accelerate the learning curve; with further improvements in software these effects may be seen for a longer time period.

One group has described preliminary work using a computer simulator together with simulated patients (actors) to teach and assess the other skill domains important in endoscopy, such as interaction with the patient and communication skills. In Kneebone's small study [23], novice nurse endoscopists underwent computer-based simulator training in the presence of a simulated patient with the aim of integrating the different learning domains.

Further studies into the transferability of skills on the simulator to skills in human subjects are in progress. Firm, conclusive evidence for the effectiveness of computer simulators in endoscopy training may be difficult to achieve but they are likely to be used as an adjunct to traditional teaching methods which have the ability to teach basic skills whilst avoiding the risks associated with exposing real patients to complete novices. By definition, simulators are not "the real thing" and functional fidelity, that is how the user feels when involved with the simulator, requires immersive behaviour and if this can be achieved, value may be added to the training process.

The 3-dimensional endoscope imaging system

The 3-D endoscope imaging system or Scope Guide produced by Olympus has been a major innovation in training and practising colonoscopy. This non-radiographical technique for picturing the colonoscope in real time was designed initially to aid insertion through difficult colons where recurrent looping hindered progress. Although its use has not been widely taken up yet, the major teaching units in the UK are utilising it routinely in their training programme and, where available, regularly in day-to-day practice. The system was initially described in 1993 [24,25]. Its validation and practicality has been demonstrated [26] but it has taken a decade to produce the commercial version. The 3-D endoscope imaging system comprises a low-voltage magnetic field sequentially produced by a series of several electromagnetic generator coils positioned about 10cm apart within a specifically designed colonoscope. Each magnetic pulse is detected by a series of sensor coils in a receiving plate placed alongside the patient. From the electronic signal produced, the precise position and orientation in three dimensions is calculated. Computer software draws a smooth line between the calculated points, generating a graphical image of the colonoscope shaft within the patient. The imager view is updated every 0.2 seconds, making the image virtually real-time. The 3-D imaging system can accurately determine the position of the colonoscope; it can detect and observe loop formation and straightening; and accurate tip location can allow localisation of pathological findings [27,28]. The entire system is easily set-up, unobtrusive and mobile (Figure 2). With trainees and experienced endoscopists, this system speeds up intubation time and reduces the number of attempts at loop straightening. Colonoscopy completion rates have also been shown to improve significantly in trainees [29].

This system has also demonstrated that during standard practice even very experienced endoscopists do not always correctly interpret loop formation and that ancillary manoeuvres such as abdominal pressure and patient position change are often ineffective [30]. It seems likely that utilising this technology will speed up a trainee's ability to correctly interpret and manage loop formation during colonoscopy. There is already some evidence that this system enhances the acquisition of colonoscopy skills in trainees [31]. Further work needs to be done to demonstrate real benefits in the leaning curve; however, even sceptics admit that the system certainly has the ability to make teaching more enjoyable and

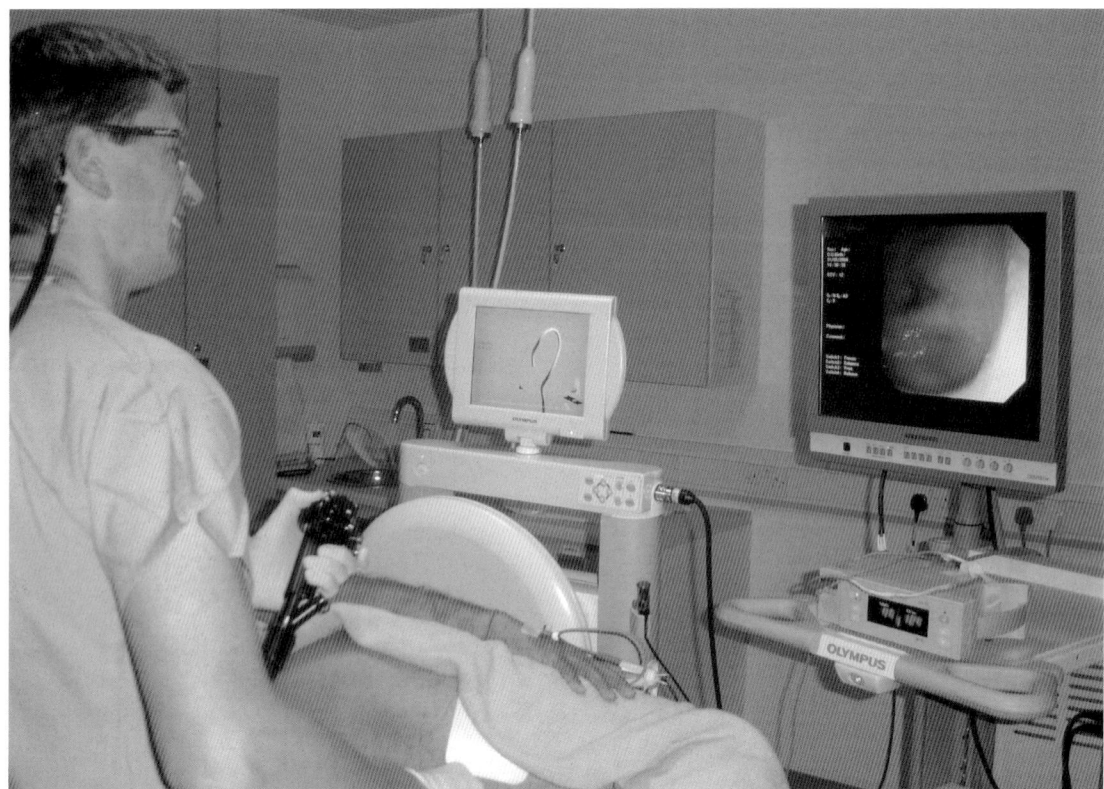

Figure 2. The 3-dimensional endoscope imaging system (the screen on the left) enables the endoscopist to observe and manage colonoscope looping within the patient.

interactive for all those involved [32]. Its application as it stands also has the ability to assist in difficult clinical procedures, outwith training, thereby benefiting and educating experienced endoscopists as well [29].

Where are we going?

Tackling the problems in endoscopy training requires a multi-faceted approach:

- Managing clinical demand.
- Expansion of the available workforce.
- Optimising endoscopy training.
- Ensuring competency in practising endoscopists and accreditation.

Managing clinical demand

Managing clinical demand is beyond the scope of this chapter; however, an improvement in general training should result in an improvement in referral patterns leading to a reduction in procedures being performed inappropriately - for example, by adherence to guidelines for surveillance intervals. The introduction of a colorectal cancer screening programme will necessitate careful planning for increased demand on stretched services.

Workforce expansion

Workforce expansion is already in place for medical and nursing staff; however, the expansion will undoubtedly need to continue as the changes in working hours are introduced. Training resources should be directed towards those who have a committed interest in performing endoscopic procedures long term.

Specific training for screening endoscopists should be built into screening programmes rather than assuming existing staff will shoulder the burden.

Although endoscopists, whether nurses or doctors, are judged to the same standards of clinical practice, training programmes in the UK have recognised that the different educational background of nurses means that they require in depth theory and knowledge in order to undertake this role [33,34].

Optimising training

The JAG has developed a series of courses in endoscopy designed to teach a uniform training approach. Core information relevant to clinical endoscopy is taught on the course supported by key literature as background reading. Individual trainers in teaching centres are encouraged to attend train-the-trainer courses to ensure that in addition, a safe approach is adopted at the local level [13]. These courses are now mandatory for all personnel training in endoscopic procedures. The courses routinely utilise the 3-D endoscope imager. Some training courses incorporate teaching on the simulator, in particular the courses for novice nurse endoscopists. The success of these courses in raising standards remains to be proven, but preliminary unpublished data are encouraging. (See Table 2 for a list of training centres.)

Table 2. National and regional endoscopy training centres in England.

Useful contacts: JAG website - www.thejag.org.uk

Training centres	Centre lead
Royal Liverpool Hospital	Professor Anthony Morris
St. George's Hospital	Mr Roger Leicester
St. Mark's Hospital	Dr Brian Saunders
Gloucestershire Hospital	Dr John Anderson
Hull Hospital	Dr Graeme Duthie
Norfolk and Norwich Hospital	Dr Richard Tighe
Sheffield Hospital	Dr Stuart Riley
South Tees Hospitals	Professor Mike Bramble
South Devon Trust (Torbay)	Dr Robin Teague
Royal Wolverhampton Hospital	Dr Edwin Swarbrick

Ensuring competency

One important area of ongoing and future development in flexible sigmoidoscopy and colonoscopy is the development of objective, validated performance assessments. Performance assessment is an essential part of any learning process and, whereas day-to-day feedback is non-judgemental, some form of regular assessment that does evaluate competence is helpful in judging whether training interventions are having their desired effect and to guide further training. Accreditation in endoscopic procedures, like many other fields of medicine, is likely to become mandatory in the UK in the near future. How exactly this will be done is uncertain. Performance assessments need to incorporate all domains of the skill: knowledge, skills, attitudes and social behaviour. These very different aspects require different assessment methods. To date in the UK and in many other countries, competency assessments have been largely unstructured and subjective. In the UK and other countries such as Australia, physicians have no formal test of endoscopic knowledge; it is assumed that working within the discipline for several years is sufficient to gain essential knowledge. Surgeons in the UK however, do have formal examinations but endoscopy is not a specific focus of these. Nurse training programmes in the UK do include formal knowledge-based assessments [23, 33]. In some countries such as Brazil and the USA, endoscopic knowledge is tested in an end of training examination in gastroenterology.

There is good evidence that testing knowledge *per se* and even some aspects of interpretation and application are best assessed by multiple choice question (MCQ) techniques [7]. Work on knowledge assessment of flexible sigmoidoscopy and colonoscopy is being done in the UK and is likely to become part of the accreditation process [35].

To date, the skill of performing the procedure has been recorded in a numbers-based logbook but in reality these are completed by the trainees themselves and are open to inaccuracy and subjective bias. Recording caecal intubation rates may be of some use and can be done easily using the Cusum method, which readily provides a visual record of the learning curve [36, 37]. The caecal intubation rate, however, only gives a narrow view of competence.

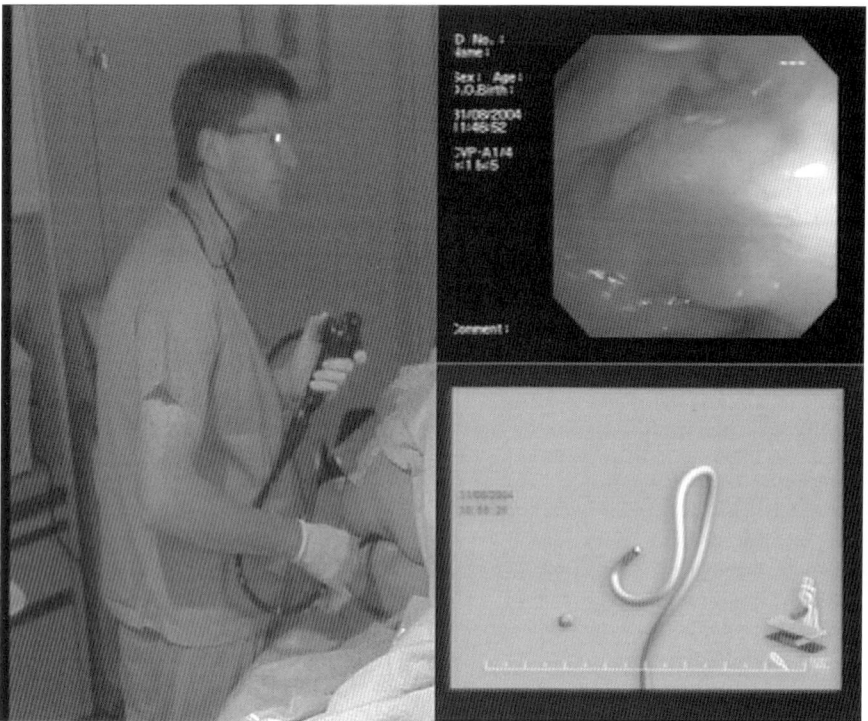

Figure 3. The tri-split view showing the endoscopist handling the endoscope, the endoscopic mucosal view and the 3-D imager view simultaneously.

New methods to assess hand skills are being investigated. Simulators have the potential to fulfil this role, at least in part. One supposed advantage of a simulator is that standardised cases could be used to assess competence at different levels [38]. In other branches of clinical medicine, such as anaesthetics and laparoscopic surgery, the use of simulators in the assessment of clinical skills has been described [39, 40]. Exciting literature from the field of neurosurgery raises the possibility that actual patient data could be fed into a simulator so that an endoscopist could be assessed on a virtually real colonoscopy generated from true patient data [41].

Video assessment of clinical skills is not a new concept [42], but its use in endoscopic practice is hampered by the complexity of the hand skills involved. A method of assessment using a tri-split image of the endoscopist's hands, the endoscopic mucosal view and the view of the magnetic endoscope imager has potential as an objective assessment tool for the hand skills necessary in colonoscopy (Figure 3) [43]. Some work has been done looking at performance assessment of extubation technique in screening flexible sigmoidoscopy and colonoscopy, using solely the endoscopic views recorded on video tape [44, 45].

In the UK, the JAG has introduced structured score sheets to be completed by trainees with their trainers for every single endoscopy case performed until they are judged competent. These Direct Observation of Procedure or Skill (D.O.P.S) forms aim to encompass evaluation of most domains of the endoscopic skill and are to be completed at the time of the procedure [46]. It is proposed that the introduction of other forms of assessment such as 360 degree appraisal will complement these.

It seems likely that adding structure to and formalising traditional methods of teaching and assessment will continue to be the cornerstone of training in flexible sigmoidoscopy and colonoscopy. But the advent of exciting new technological developments will undoubtedly serve as adjuncts to the process. Embracing new technology is viewed with suspicion by many and too easily welcomed by some. A balanced approach requiring a reasonable level of evidence should ensure an improvement in the provision of endoscopic services.

References

1. HMSO. The NHS Cancer Plan; 2000.
2. Calman KHD. A Policy Framework for Commissioning Cancer Services, 1995.
3. HMSO. Department of Health Modernisation Agency Meeting The Challenges, 2004.
4. Barrison IG, Bramble MG, Wilkinson M, et al. Provision of Endoscopy Related Services in District General Hospitals. British Society of Gastroenterology Working Party Report, 2001.
5. Calman KC, Department of Health WGoSMT. Hospital doctors: training for the future. Report of the working group on specialist medical training [Calman Report]. Heywood: Health Publications Unit, 1993.
6. Chikwe J, de Souza AC, Pepper JR. No time to train the surgeons. *BMJ* 2004; 328(7437): 418-9.
7. Rowley DI. The surgeon's job: how should we assess the trainee? *J Roy Soc Med* 2004; 97(8): 363-5.
8. Bowles CJ, Leicester R, Romaya C, et al. A prospective study of colonoscopy practice in the UK today: are we adequately prepared for national colorectal cancer screening tomorrow? *Gut* 2004; 53(2): 277-83.
9. Atkin W, Rogers P, Cardwell C, et al. Wide variation in adenoma detection rates at screening flexible sigmoidoscopy. *Gastroenterology* 2004; 126(5): 1247-56.
10. Bisschops R, Wilmer A, Tack J. A survey on gastroenterology training in Europe. *Gut* 2002; 50(5): 724-9.
11. Lal SK, Barrison A, Heeren T. A national survey of flexible sigmoidoscopy training in primary care graduate and postgraduate education programs. *Am J Gastroenterol* 2004; 99(5): 830-6.
12. Wilkins T, Jester D, Kenrick J, et al. The current state of colonoscopy training in family medicine residency programs. *Fam Med* 2004; 36(6): 407-11.
13. Teague R, Soehendra N, Carr-Locke D, et al. Setting standards for colonoscopic teaching and training. *J Gastroenterol Hepatol* 2002; 17 Suppl: S50-S53.
14. Peyton JWR. *Teaching and Learning in Medical Practice*. First Edition. Manticore, 1998.
15. Wood BP. Feedback: a key feature of medical training. *Radiology* 2000; 215(1): 17-9.
16. Neumann M, Hochberger J, Felzmann T, et al. Part 1. The Erlanger endo-trainer. *Endoscopy* 2001; 33(10): 887-90.
17. Williams CB, Baillie J, Gillies DF, et al. Teaching gastrointestinal endoscopy by computer simulation: a prototype for colonoscopy and ERCP. *Gastrointest Endosc* 1990; 36(1): 49-54.
18. Aabakken L, Adamsen S, Kruse A. Performance of a colonoscopy simulator: experience from a hands-on endoscopy course. *Endoscopy* 2000; 32(11): 911-3.
19. Ferlitsch A, Glauninger P, Gupper A, et al. Evaluation of a virtual endoscopy simulator for training in gastrointestinal endoscopy. *Endoscopy* 2002; 34(9): 698-702.
20. Sedlack RE, Kolars JC. Validation of a computer-based colonoscopy simulator. *Gastrointest Endosc* 2003; 57(2): 214-8.
21. Datta V, Mandalia M, Mackay S, et al. The PreOp flexible sigmoidoscopy trainer. Validation and early evaluation of a virtual reality based system. *Surg Endosc* 2002; 16(10): 1459-63.
22. Sedlack RE, Kolars JC. Computer simulator training enhances the competency of gastroenterology fellows at colonoscopy: results of a pilot study. *Am J Gastroenterol* 2004; 99(1): 33-7.
23. Kneebone RL, Nestel D, Moorthy K, et al. Learning the skills of flexible sigmoidoscopy - the wider perspective. *Med Educ* 2003; 37 Suppl 1: 50-8.
24. Bladen JS, Anderson AP, Bell GD, et al. Non-radiological technique for three-dimensional imaging of endoscopes. *Lancet* 1993; 341(8847): 719-22.
25. Williams C, Guy C, Gillies D, et al. Electronic three-dimensional imaging of intestinal endoscopy. *Lancet* 1993; 341(8847): 724-5.
26. Saunders BP, Bell GD, Williams CB, et al. First clinical results with a real time, electronic imager as an aid to colonoscopy. *Gut* 1995; 36(6): 913-7.
27. Wehrmann K, Fruhmorgen P. Evaluation of a new three-dimensional magnetic imaging system for use during colonoscopy. *Endoscopy* 2002; 34(11): 905-8.
28. Shah SG, Pearson HJ, Moss S, et al. Magnetic endoscope imaging: a new technique for localizing colonic lesions. *Endoscopy* 2002; 34(11): 900-4.
29. Shah SG, Brooker JC, Williams CB, et al. Effect of magnetic endoscope imaging on colonoscopy performance: a randomised controlled trial. *Lancet* 2000; 356(9243): 1718-22.
30. Shah SG, Saunders BP, Brooker JC, et al. Magnetic imaging of colonoscopy: an audit of looping, accuracy and ancillary maneuvers. *Gastrointest Endosc* 2000; 52(1): 1-8.
31. Shah SG, Thomas-Gibson S, Lockett M, et al. Effect of real-time magnetic endoscope imaging on the teaching and acquisition of colonoscopy skills: results from a single trainee. *Endoscopy* 2003; 35(5): 421-5.
32. Waye JD. Imaging of the colonoscope: magnetic, fluoroscopic, or neither? *Gastrointest Endosc* 2000; 52(1): 131-3.
33. Duthie GS, Drew PJ, Hughes MA, et al. A UK training programme for nurse practitioner flexible sigmoidoscopy and a prospective evaluation of the practice of the first UK trained nurse flexible sigmoidoscopist. *Gut* 1998; 43(5): 711-4.
34. *The Nurse Endoscopist*. British Society of Gastroenterology, London, 1994.
35. Thomas-Gibson S, Rutter MD, Suzuki N, et al. The development of a multiple choice question paper for training and assessment in colonoscopy. *Gut* 2003; 52[S1]: A74.
36. Bolsin S, Colson M. The use of the Cusum technique in the assessment of trainee competence in new procedures. *Int J Qual Health Care* 2000; 12(5): 433-8.
37. Parry BR, Williams SM. Competency and the colonoscopist: a learning curve. *ANZ J Surg* 1991; 61(6): 419-22.
38. Sedlack RE, Kolars JC. Colonoscopy curriculum development and performance-based assessment criteria on a computer-based endoscopy simulator. *Acad Med* 2002; 77(7): 750-1.

39. Schwid HA, O'Donnell D. Anesthesiologists' management of simulated critical incidents. *Anesthesiology* 1992; 76(4): 495-501.
40. Taffinder N, Smith S, Jansen J, *et al*. Objective measurement of surgical dexterity - validation of the Imperial College Surgical Assessment Device (ICSAD). *Minimally Invasive Therapy and Allied Techniques* 1998; 7 (suppl 1): 11.
41. Radetzky A, Nurnberger A. Visualization and simulation techniques for surgical simulators using actual patient's data. *Artif Intell Med* 2002; 26(3): 255-79.
42. Stranc MF, McDiarmid JG, Stranc LC. Video assessment of surgical technique. *Br J Plast Surg* 1991; 44(1): 65-8.
43. Shah SG, Thomas-Gibson S, Brooker JC, *et al*. Use of video and magnetic endoscope imaging for rating competence at colonoscopy: validation of a measurement tool. *Gastrointest Endosc* 2002; 56(4): 568-73.
44. Rex DK. Colonoscopic withdrawal technique is associated with adenoma miss rates. *Gastrointest Endosc* 2000; 51(1): 33-6.
45. Thomas-Gibson S, Swain D, Schofield G, *et al*. Quality of performance at screening flexible sigmoidoscopy correlates with adenoma detection rates. *Gut* 2004; 53: A8.
46. Joint Advisory Group on Gastrointestinal Endoscopy. Guidelines for the training, appraisal and assessment of trainees in gastrointestinal endoscopy, 2004.

Chapter 6

The evaluation of rectal cancer

Kirsten M Boyle MB ChB MRCS, Clinical Research Fellow, Colorectal Surgery
Dermot Burke PhD FRCS, Senior Lecturer in Surgery and Consultant Surgeon
The General Infirmary at Leeds, Leeds, UK

What is the problem?

The aim of pre-operative evaluation of rectal cancer is to assess the stage and potential resectability of the tumour. This allows the selection of patients for adjuvant therapy and permits the optimum choice of surgical procedure, with a view to minimising local recurrence and improving outcome. The value of pre-operative radiological evaluation has been measured by comparing the predicted tumour stage on imaging and the corresponding final pathological stage, which is still considered the gold standard. The major disadvantage of pathological staging is that it is available to the treating clinicians only after surgery.

There is growing evidence that adjuvant therapy is more effective if given pre-operatively than postoperatively [1,2,3]. Localised disease, and by this we mean tumour confined within the limits of the mesorectal fascia, is potentially curable with surgery alone, avoiding unnecessary and potentially harmful pre-operative therapy. Where the tumour approaches the mesorectal fascia ("threatened margin"), pre-operative therapy is used in order to induce tumour regression from the anticipated surgical resection margin and improve the likelihood of a negative margin. For patients with locally advanced and initially unresectable disease, detailed spatial depiction of the tumour allows radiotherapy regimens to be tailored. After therapy, repeat evaluation permits a review of whether the tumour has undergone sufficient shrinkage to allow potentially curative surgery.

Where are we now?

Clinical examination remains of prime importance in the evaluation of rectal cancer. An impression of the macroscopic appearance of most low and mid rectal tumours may be gained in the outpatient clinic. Proctoscopy gives useful visual information on tumour height, circumferential location, size and whether it is flat or pedunculated, with a broad base or a narrow stalk. A formal rectal examination under general anaesthetic allows for a more thorough assessment, in particular of mobility. However, the subjective assessment of tumour mobility is prone to error; peritumoural inflammation may make a superficial tumour appear tethered to underlying structures. Clinical examination also gives no information on nodal metastases.

Histological confirmation of malignancy is essential prior to the commencement of potentially radical therapy, and biopsy findings may influence the treatment pathway. The finding of poor differentiation in a biopsy specimen may increase the radicality of overall treatment, either by the addition or prolongation of radiotherapy or chemotherapy, or by extending surgical resection (for example anterior resection [AR] to abdominoperineal excision of the rectum [APE]). In the case of very low lesions, it is important to differentiate squamous cell tumours of the anus that are invading cranially from low rectal adenocarcinomas extending caudally.

Radiological staging has assumed primacy in the evaluation of primary rectal cancer, and is the main subject of this chapter. Computed tomography (CT) was the first imaging modality that was able to give useful information on the local invasion of rectal cancer and on distant metastases. The use of endorectal ultrasound (EUS) in the pre-operative staging of rectal cancer was first described by Hildebrandt and Feifel in 1985 [4]. EUS quickly realised its potential and became the gold standard in the 1990s. Around the same time magnetic resonance imaging (MRI) and positron emission tomography (PET) techniques were being developed. Early reports of MR imaging of the pelvis showed its great potential in visualising soft tissues [5], in particular the rectum and perirectal tissues [6]. At present, MRI is rapidly overtaking both CT and EUS to become the prime imaging modality for the local staging of rectal cancer. PET has no role in the routine staging of primary rectal cancer at this time.

Specific issues in evaluation

Assessment of invasion through rectal wall (T staging)

Table 1 summarises reported accuracy rates, along with overstaging and understaging, of EUS, CT and MRI in the assessment of tumour invasion through the rectal wall [7-26]. A recent meta-analysis of 78 studies

Table 1. T staging: overstaging, understaging and accuracy rates of surface MRI, endorectal MRI, CT and EUS.

	Overstaged	Understaged	Accuracy
Surface MRI	0-18%	0-22%	61-100%
Endorectal MRI	11-33%	0-25%	42-84%
CT	8-17%	8-36%	56-85%
EUS	10-29%	4-13%	59-81%

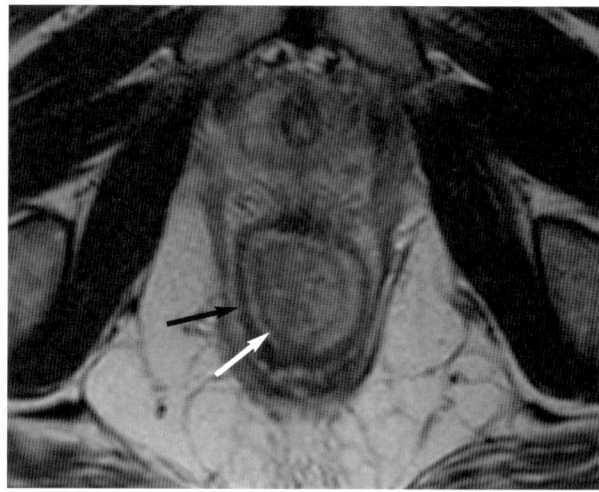

Figure 1. 1.5T high resolution axial MR image showing the layers of the rectal wall. The low signal muscularis propria (black arrow) and the equally low signal mucosa (white arrow) are visible. This image is at the level of the low rectum.

performed between 1980 and 1998 found that CT had an accuracy of 73% for T staging compared with 87% for EUS, 82% for surface MRI and 84% for endorectal MRI [27].

MRI is gaining acceptance as the primary modality for the local evaluation of rectal cancer. Rapid technical advances in surface coil MRI, including fast-spin echo, phased-array coils and breathhold techniques, have improved image quality and dramatically shortened examination time. Modern scanners using field strengths of 1.5 Tesla provide high-resolution thin section images in any chosen plane (Figure 1) covering the entire mesorectum and immediate locoregional structures. All tumours, including bulky obstructing lesions, can be assessed. Intravenous gadolinium chelates such as gadolinium-DTPA (Magnevist®) can improve contrast enhancement in the rectal wall [28-30]. Improved lesional display can be obtained by producing double-contrast MR images of the rectum after the instillation of agents such as superparamagnetic iron oxide particles and barium sulphate preparations [28, 31]. These two techniques are not part of standard imaging protocols for the staging of rectal carcinoma.

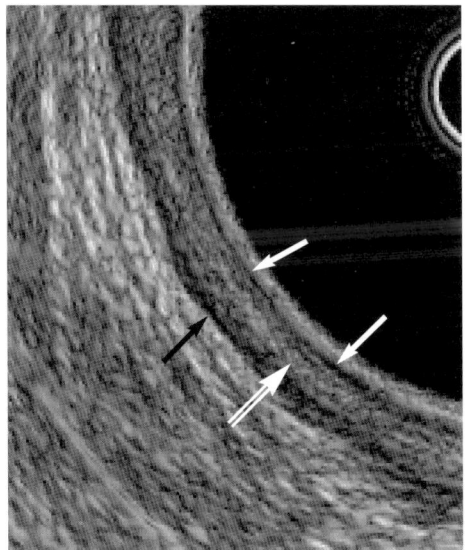

Figure 2. EUS image of the normal rectal wall. The muscularis mucosae and muscularis propria (black arrow) are hypoechoic. The mucosa (white arrows) and submucosa (empty arrow) are echogenic. The fifth layer is the echogenic perirectal fat.

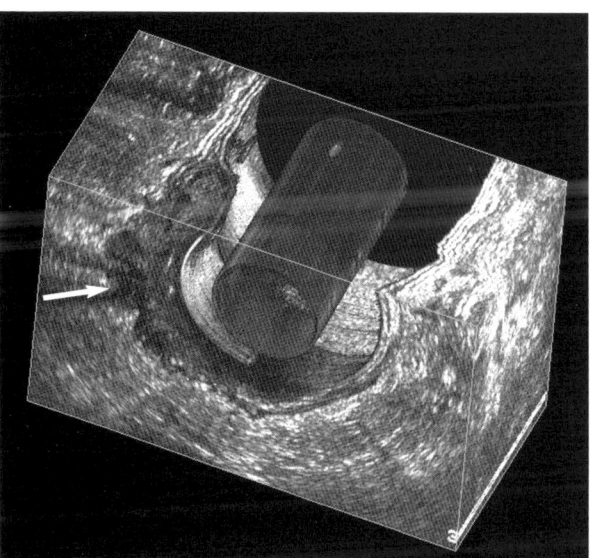

Figure 3. 3D EUS reconstruction showing a T3 tumour (arrowed).

In units without access to MR, for patients with pacemakers or large metallic implants who cannot safely enter the MR environment and for patients with severe claustrophobia, EUS and CT will be the main modes of assessment of local invasion. EUS is particularly useful in the assessment of rectal wall invasion in early superficial tumours, but is much less accurate in advanced tumours [14]. Due to its low spatial resolution, CT is more useful at assessing T stage in those tumours which are locally advanced compared with superficial tumours [10]. Early studies with conventional CT focused on locally advanced rectal cancer with good results [32, 33], but later studies on less advanced tumours were more disappointing [6, 34-36]. Accuracy rates are improving with the arrival of new technologies such as multislice CT [37].

Early tumours confined to the rectal wall

EUS is currently considered the gold standard technique for the pre-operative visualisation of tumour infiltration through the rectal wall. EUS is more accurate in the assessment of depth of invasion of early rectal tumours when compared with CT and surface MRI [26], and is particularly useful if local excision is being considered. Five layers of the rectal wall can be seen (Figure 2). Tumours appear hypoechoic (Figure 3), and may be surrounded by a layer of hypoechoic inflammatory tissue reaction and oedema [38]. EUS has the advantage of being more readily available than CT and MRI, is much less expensive and requires no contrast agents. However, the large, rigid EUS probe is unable to examine bulky, stricturing and upper rectal tumours [39]. It can also prove difficult to obtain adequate images of villous or pedunculated tumours [40]. In addition, EUS is highly operator-dependent and there is a significant learning curve [14, 41-44]. Currently, the technique is largely confined to specialised units.

Endorectal MR has a similar accuracy to EUS in the assessment of T stage in early tumours. The technique has not gained widespread acceptance as it has the same limitations as EUS [25, 45], with up to 40% insertion failure rate [39]. It is also a less widely available technique.

One problem with local excision is that it is impossible to assess nodal involvement or

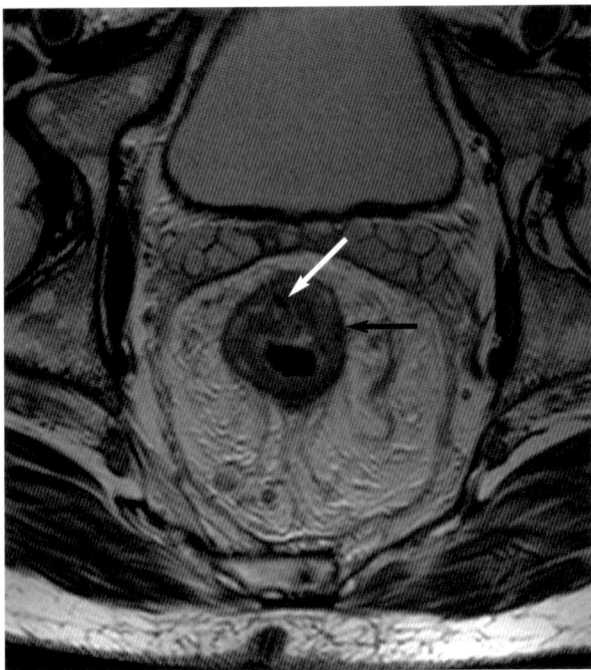

Figure 4. 1.5T high-resolution axial MR image showing T2 tumour (white arrow). The tumour is confined within the low signal muscularis propria (black arrow).

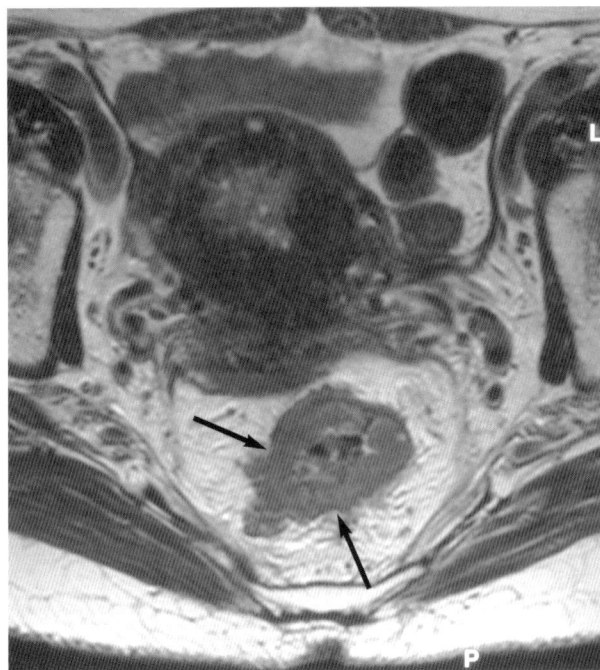

Figure 5. 1.5T high-resolution axial MR image showing a T3 tumour. The pushing tumour margin has breached the muscularis propria between 6 and 9 o'clock (between arrows) and approaches the mesorectal fascia.

extramural tumour deposits at pathological analysis, and staging therefore may be inaccurate. MRI or CT should be performed pre-operatively in addition to EUS if local excision is to be considered, as the discovery of perirectal lymphadenopathy or extramural tumour deposits will require formal excision of the rectum in order to achieve complete tumour clearance.

Tumour penetration through rectal wall and into mesorectal fat

The differentiation between T2 and early T3 tumours can be difficult, but in both cases the risk of surgical failure due to circumferential resection margin (CRM) involvement is low, and in the absence of perirectal lymphadenopathy pre-operative therapy is not usually required (Figures 4 and 5). For tumours that have definitely breached the rectal wall, it is essential to obtain precise spatial information on the anatomical location of the tumour, in terms of height and circumferential location, in order to assess the need for pre-operative therapy and plan the optimum surgical approach. T3 tumours that invade a short distance into mesorectal fat have lower local recurrence rates and improved survival in comparison with those that invade further [46-50], leading to the concept of "good" and "bad" T3 tumours. The thickness of mesorectal fat varies around the circumference of the mesorectum and with height from the anal verge, being thinnest anteriorly and tapering towards the anal canal, and so a tumour with even a few millimetres of invasion into perirectal fat may quickly reach the mesorectal fascia placing the surgical resection margin at risk.

At the present time, surface coil MRI is the most useful modality in the assessment of depth of invasion through mesorectal fat. A T2-weighted fast-spin echo non-high resolution sagittal sequence is initially performed, and from this are planned the high-resolution axial sequences. It is important to obtain the axial images in a plane orthogonal to the tumour and to encompass the entire mesorectal package, as images in an oblique plane may lead to overestimation of depth of invasion. The MR diagnosis of a T3 lesion is based on the presence of tumour signal extending into the perirectal fat with a broad-based nodular or bulging configuration in continuity with the intramural portion of the tumour. In the past, irregularity of the outer border of the muscularis propria was used to define a T3 tumour [11]. It is now apparent that the outer coat of the muscularis propria often has an irregular appearance in the absence of tumour, mainly due to penetrating perirectal vessels which can lead to interpretative difficulty [12]. Kim et al reported an accuracy of 87% in the staging of T3 tumours [19]. Using a 1.5T surface coil, Brown et al in 1999 correctly predicted the histopathological stage in all of 25 consecutive patients with T2, T3 and T4 tumours [12]. Beets-Tan reported accuracy rates of 83% and 95% respectively for two observers in predicting T3 tumours [8].

Peritumoural fibrosis can complicate pre-operative staging. Tumour tissue has a high signal intensity on T2-weighted images, in contrast to the low signal intensity of fibrosis [51]. Some malignant tumours provoke a desmoplastic reaction [40] which can result in finger-like spiky protuberances extending from the rectal wall. This appearance contrasts with the more broad-based pushing appearance of tumour extension. Radiotherapy-induced fibrosis may contain residual viable tumour cells, and there is an argument for complete resection of all tissues that contained tumour prior to radiotherapy. Peritumoural tissue reaction is also a cause of overstaging at EUS [38, 52].

MRI can also identify vascular and lymphatic invasion (Figure 6). In a recent study by Brown et al, extramural venous invasion was defined as "serpiginous extension of tumour signal within a vascular structure", and tumour involvement of vessels greater than 3mm in diameter was correctly identified in 15 of 18 patients, although smaller vessels were not visible [53].

The MERCURY study (Magnetic Resonance Imaging and Rectal Cancer European Equivalence Study) is a prospective study involving a large number of UK and European centres that was designed to establish an accurate pre-operative staging process for the treatment of rectal cancer through the application of MRI, surgery and pathological audit. Encouraging preliminary results were made available in the summer of 2004.

CT has inherently lower soft tissue contrast resolution than MRI and is currently less accurate. EUS and endorectal MRI have a limited field of view and are therefore unable to assess reliably the true extent of mesorectal invasion.

Mesorectal fascia

When the technique of mesorectal excision is followed, the mesorectal fascia is the anticipated surgical resection margin. On pathological examination of the surgical specimen, involvement of the CRM has been shown to be an independent prognostic factor of increased local recurrence and poorer survival [54-59]. The early identification on imaging of potential breach of the mesorectal fascia by tumour allows optimisation of pre-operative therapy.

The earliest report on the identification of the mesorectal fascia on CT dates from 1983 [60]. Currently, surface MRI with phased-array coils is the only imaging modality that can visualise the fascia with any degree of accuracy. The fascia is identified on axial images as a fine linear structure enveloping the

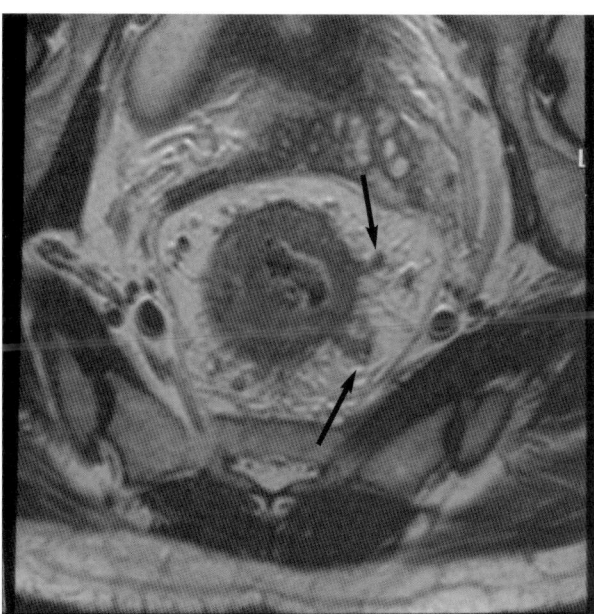

Figure 6. 1.5T high-resolution axial MR image showing extramural vascular invasion (arrowed). Note the tubular nature of the finger-like projections with the same signal intensity as the tumour in the rectal wall.

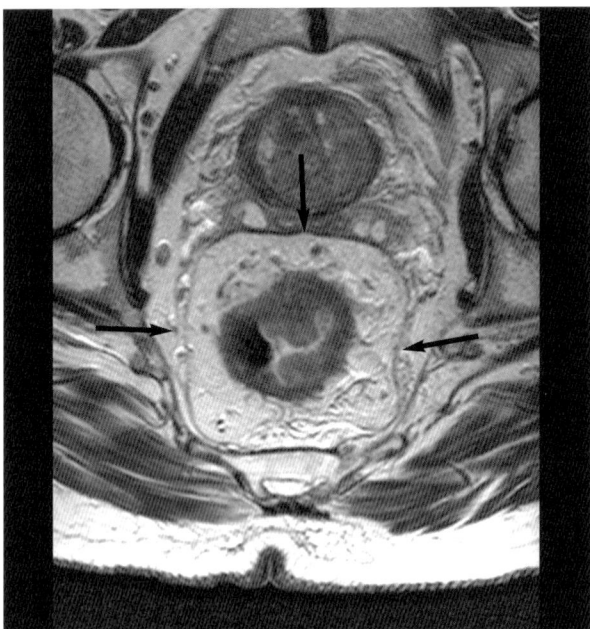

Figure 7. 1.5T high-resolution axial MR image orthogonal to the rectal wall. The mesorectal fascia (arrowed) is hypointense on T2-weighted images.

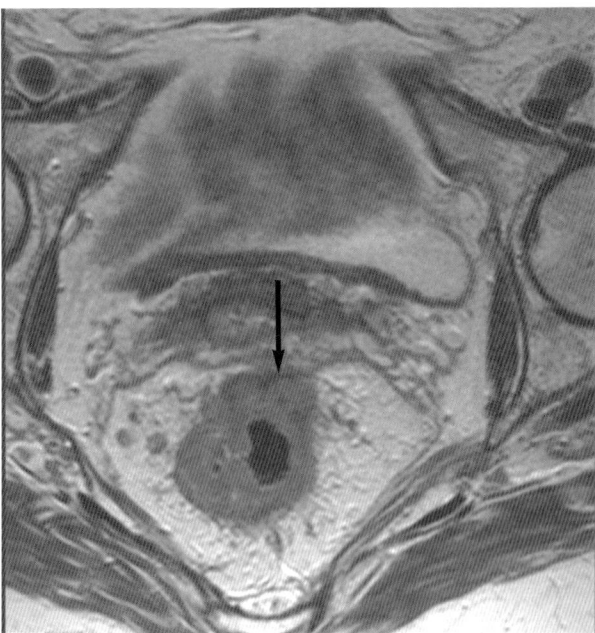

Figure 8. 1.5T high-resolution axial MR image showing transmural tumour extension reaching the mesorectal fascia anteriorly (arrowed).

mesorectum, hypointense on T2-weighted images (Figures 7 and 8) [8]. The fascia cannot reliably be seen using EUS or endorectal coil MRI due to the small field of view [25, 61].

Several studies have been published recently on the prediction of mesorectal fascial involvement using MRI [8, 62-64]. Beets-Tan et al claimed that a tumour-free resection margin of at least 1mm can be accurately predicted when the measured distance on MRI is at least 5mm [8]. Blomqvist et al reported that MRI could predict a tumour-free resection margin with an accuracy of 81% (sensitivity 88%, specificity 78%) [62]. Bissett et al were able to predict tumour penetration through the mesorectal fascia with an accuracy of 95% (sensitivity 67%, specificity 100%) [63]. In a cohort of 99 patients and using a 1.5T system with high-resolution images, Martling et al predicted a positive margin with 80% accuracy; 50 of 56 patients (89.3%) with a negative CRM were correctly identified as such by MRI. In addition, patients who were predicted to have a positive margin on MRI had a significantly higher local recurrence rate compared with patients who were predicted negative [64].

Locally advanced tumours

Locally advanced tumours that have crossed the mesorectal fascia to invade adjacent viscera require pre-operative chemoradiotherapy in order to attempt tumour shrinkage (Figure 9). Reassessment after therapy will allow a decision as to whether potentially curative surgery is possible. With precise knowledge of tumour invasion into adjacent structures, a detailed plan can be made for operations that may involve en bloc resections, pelvic exenteration or distal sacrectomy.

Beets-Tan et al compared CT and high-resolution phased-array MRI in the assessment of invasion into surrounding viscera in locally advanced and recurrent rectal cancer. MRI had a sensitivity of 97% and specificity of 98% in the detection of invasion compared with 70% and 85% respectively for CT, resulting in an accuracy of 80% for MRI and only 19% for CT [51]. In a previous study, T4 tumours were identified with 100% accuracy by two independent observers [8]. Kim et al showed that MRI and EUS had 100% accuracy in the detection of posterior vaginal wall invasion compared with only 28.5% for CT [18]. Bony invasion is better seen with MRI than CT [65].

6 The evaluation of rectal cancer

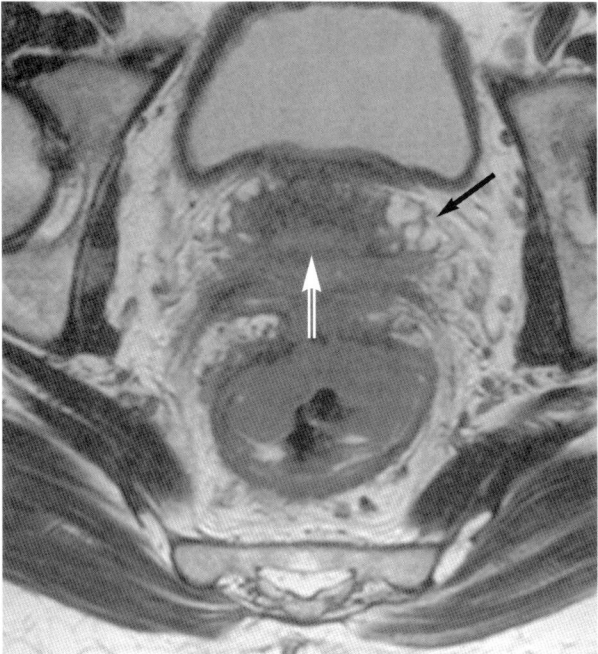

Figure 9. 1.5T high-resolution axial MR image showing direct tumour invasion (white arrow) into seminal vesicles. Residual normal seminal vesicle is shown by the black arrow.

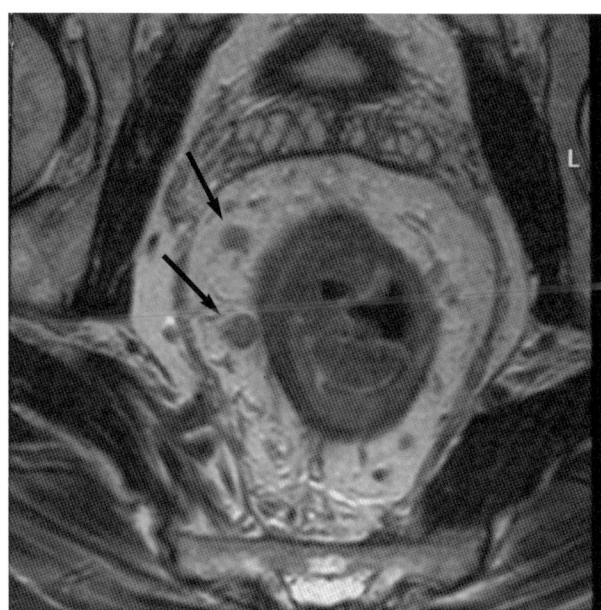

Figure 10. 1.5T high-resolution axial MR image showing perirectal lymph nodes (arrowed) within the mesorectal envelope.

Nodal staging

No imaging modality is currently able to identify which nodes are involved by tumour. Nodal staging has traditionally relied on size criteria (Figure 10). However, nodal enlargement does not indicate tumour involvement, and lymph nodes that are infiltrated by tumour are not always enlarged. Table 2 summarises reported nodal staging accuracy, sensitivity and specificity rates for MRI (surface and endorectal) and EUS. With improved resolution of all imaging modalities, morphologic criteria have proved more useful than size. Beynon reported as early as 1989 that lymph nodes potentially involved by tumour can be identified on EUS as circular or oval structures with an irregular border and echogenicity similar to that of the primary tumour [66]. These features have recently been shown to remain of prognostic value using high-resolution MRI by Brown et al [67]. On EUS, lymph nodes are hyperechoic, and as a result are not always seen in the echogenic perirectal fat [65]. The field of view of EUS with a 7.5 MHz transducer is approximately 5cm [11], and so only nodes close to the rectal wall may be visualised with any certainty. For routine rectal staging MR, lymph nodes are easily recognised on the T2-weighted sequences [65]. The identification of lateral pelvic sidewall nodes is important as they may signify locally advanced disease (Figure 11). Extended pelvic lymphadenectomy is not routine in the West, and radiotherapy fields are tailored to cover potentially involved nodes. In two recent studies by Kim et al, accuracy rates of only 12.5% and 29% were obtained in the identification of lateral pelvic nodes on CT and MRI respectively [18, 19].

Table 2. N staging: sensitivity, specificity and accuracy rates of surface MRI, endorectal MRI and EUS.

	Sensitivity	Specificity	Accuracy
Surface MRI	66-85%	41-51%	55-63%
Endorectal MRI	78-81%	41-66%	63-73%
EUS	33-92%	54-82%	59-81%

Low tumours

MRI can obtain detailed images of the peri-anal structures [68]. Sequences in the coronal plane are particularly useful to detect infiltration of the levator ani and the anal sphincter complex [29, 69]. Coronal images

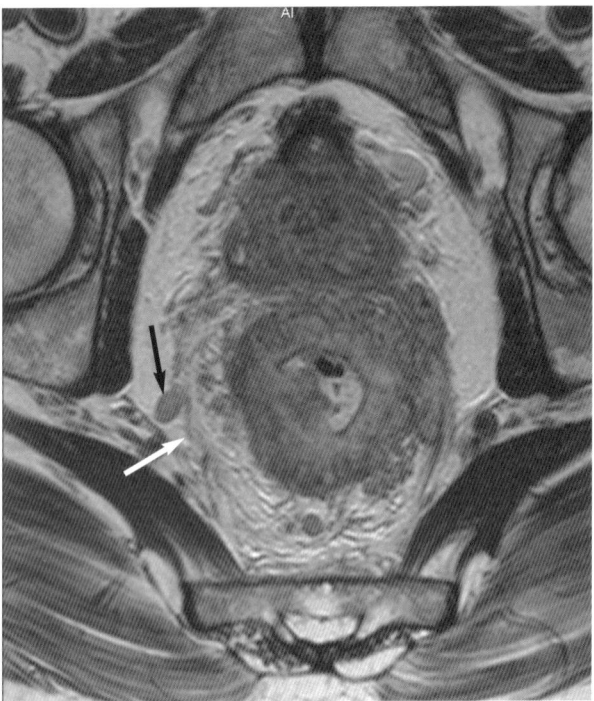

Figure 11. 1.5T high-resolution axial MR image showing a lymph node (black arrow) outside the mesorectal fascia (white arrow). Note the extensive mesorectal fascial compromise anterolaterally and the pathological prostate.

are routinely obtained as part of the staging protocol of low tumours. Although EUS is useful in the assessment of rectal wall invasion, problems with image interpretation can occur in tumours close to the anal verge as it is difficult to position the probe at 90° to the tumour [17, 40, 70].

Distant metastases

Cross-sectional imaging of the thorax and abdomen is essential to identify distant metastases (Figures 12 and 13). CT is the main imaging modality used to identify distant metastases in the liver, lungs and brain, and can identify enlarged and potentially involved locoregional and distant lymph nodes. Advances in techniques for hepatic and pulmonary resection mean that an increasing number of distant metastases are suitable for potentially curative metastasectomy (Figure 14).

CT can also detect extracolonic pathology such as adrenal masses and abdominal aortic aneurysms [71]. MRI is particularly useful in characterising equivocal liver lesions identified on CT. PET may be useful to evaluate indeterminate or "nuisance" lesions detected on CT or MRI (Figure 15) and to ensure that apparently resectable hepatic and pulmonary metastases are indeed isolated [72]. PET has been shown to detect hepatic metastases with up to 100% sensitivity [73-75]. A recent meta-analysis showed that

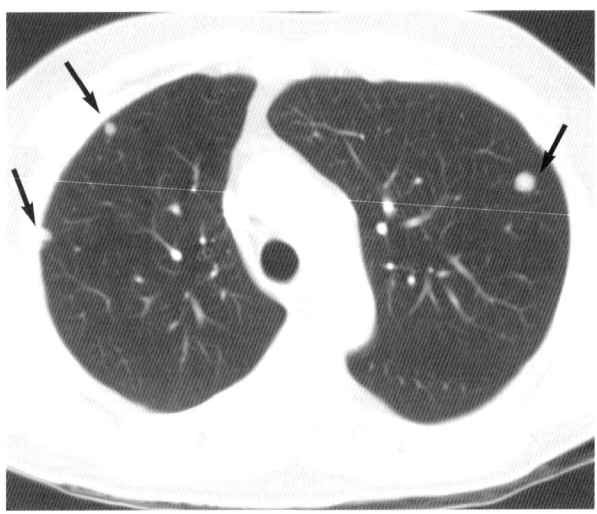

Figure 12. CT showing multiple pulmonary metastases (arrowed).

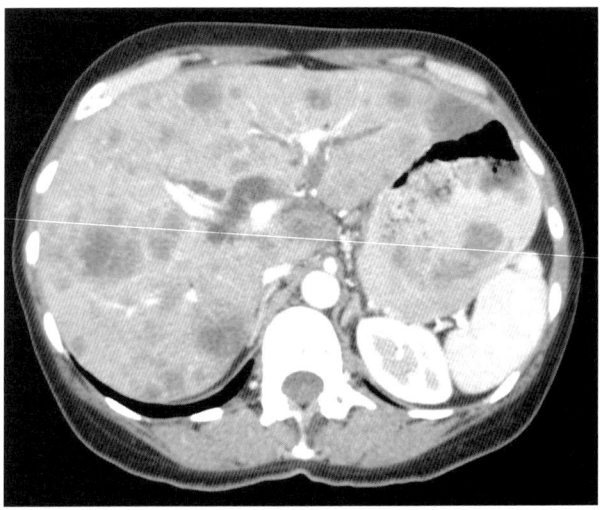

Figure 13. CT showing disseminated liver metastases.

6 The evaluation of rectal cancer

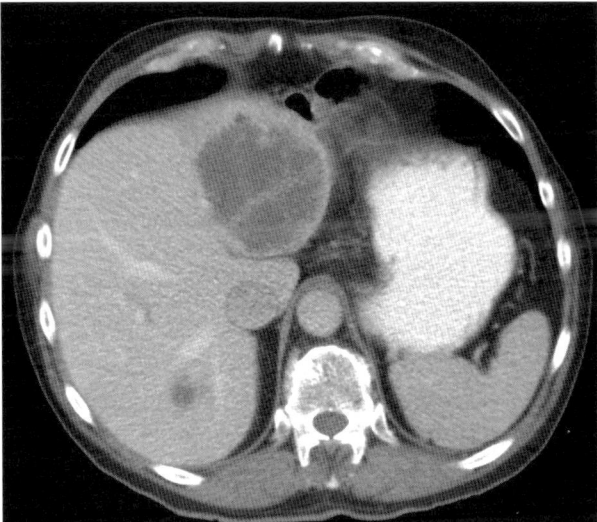

Figure 14. CT showing potentially resectable liver metastases.

PET had higher sensitivity and specificity than CT in the detection of metastases from recurrent colorectal cancer at a number of sites [76].

Assessment of the obstructing tumour

Patients who present acutely with an obstructing rectal tumour require assessment prior to urgent surgery. A water-soluble contrast or barium enema study is required in order to diagnose complete obstruction. A defunctioning stoma may be essential prior to formal staging imaging. It is impossible to pass EUS and endorectal MRI probes through stenosing tumours, and so local staging will require CT or MRI depending on availability. The presence of unresectable distant metastases will change the chosen surgical procedure and a defunctioning stoma, Hartmann's procedure or colonic stenting may be sufficient to palliate symptoms without more radical operative measures.

Response to therapy

After long-course radiotherapy, structural change may take several days or weeks to occur, whereas tumour metabolism may be affected much sooner [77]. There is an assumption that all tumours will respond to radiotherapy and chemotherapy to some degree. In approximately 50% percent of patients, the tumour fails to respond or even enlarges during pre-operative

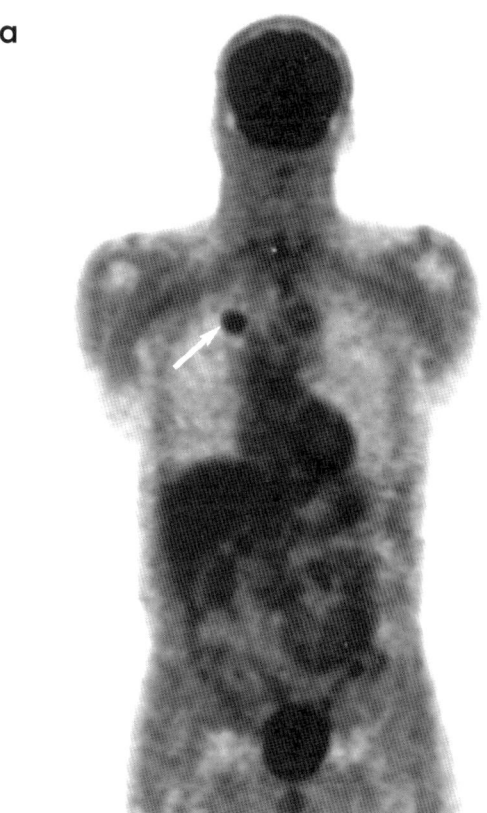

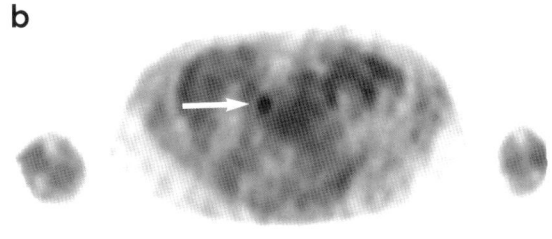

Figure 15. a) Coronal and b) axial PET scans showing solitary right upper lobe lung metastasis (arrowed).

chemoradiotherapy. If non-responders could be identified early on serial imaging, pre-operative therapy could be altered or even discontinued in favour of immediate surgery, and the side effects of ineffective therapy could be avoided.

There are a number of pitfalls when using non-functional imaging modalities such as CT and MRI to assess response to therapy. One might think that downsizing of the primary tumour might be obvious on high-resolution MR images. However, it is difficult on static imaging to differentiate intrinsic tumour-associated fibrosis from post-radiotherapy fibrosis. Apparent shrinkage of the tumour with peritumoural fibrosis may lead to a false sense of security and surgery may not be as radical as was previously anticipated or planned. Downstaging is more difficult to predict clearly. Disappearance of all previously visualised nodes on imaging after therapy may be a favourable observation, although it is impossible to say that no residual viable tumour cells remain. "Softer" observations, such as a reduction in nodal size and change in signal characteristics during therapy, may also be reported. It is possible for the dedicated pathologist to dissect out all nodes from the mesorectum and map the nodes for direct comparison with pre-operative imaging. EUS is not reliable in the assessment of downstaging after radiotherapy [78].

Where are we going?

Rapid technological advances in imaging modalities hold great promise in the assessment of local invasion, nodal involvement, distant metastases and response to pre-operative therapy.

Local tumour staging

Several new endoluminal ultrasound techniques have been developed. 3D endorectal ultrasound allows a better understanding of the objective size of the tumour and the spatial relationship between the tumour and the surrounding structures (Figure 2), leading to improved diagnostic confidence [79]. Miniprobes, with a diameter as small as 6 French gauge, can be passed down the instrument channel of flexible endoscopes and allow 360° ultrasonographic imaging of colorectal tumours during routine colonoscopy [80]. Hamada et al reported accuracy rates for depth of invasion and nodal status of 82% and 87% respectively [81]. Hünerbein et al reported a similar experience [82]. Miniprobes may also prove of value in the imaging of stenosing rectal tumours that do not allow passage of the standard EUS probe.

MRI techniques are still evolving, and scanners with larger magnets and improved contrast resolution will become available. 3.0T scanners are now in preliminary use [83]. Tumour-targeted MR contrast agents, such as polyethylene glycol (PEG)-coated liposomes, are being developed [84]. It is also possible to load the liposomes with traditional contrast agents such as gadolinium.

Multislice spiral CT will undoubtedly improve the quality of local and distant staging as it can produce thin section images over large anatomical areas. CT is unlikely to be able to replace MRI in the assessment of local tumour invasion in the pelvis, although it will prove useful in patients who are unable to undergo MRI. CT colonography, also known as virtual colonoscopy, is an emerging CT-based 3D reconstruction imaging technique that results in detailed views of the entire colonic lumen. Novel techniques such as MR spectroscopy and refraction contrast X-ray imaging are being evaluated [85, 86].

Functional imaging

Functional imaging is a current "hot topic" in clinical research. It has the potential to provide information on the biological behaviour of a tumour and to complement conventional anatomical imaging. In addition to the diagnosis of tumour tissue (primary tumour, involved lymph nodes or distant metastases), functional imaging will also prove invaluable in the assessment of response to therapy. Several imaging modalities are able to assess *in vivo* biological behaviour, including MRI and PET. New techniques using radioactive labelled tracers, fluorescence probes and compounds targeted at specific tumour antigens will emerge as our knowledge of tumour biology improves.

Functional MRI (fMRI) has been used to measure blood flow and assess changes in tumour microcirculation during pre-operative therapy [85, 87, 88]. Capillary permeability measured using dynamic contrast-enhanced MRI has been shown to be associated with tumour response to chemo-radiotherapy [89]. Diffusion-weighted MRI and dynamic contrast-enhanced CT have been reported to be of potential use in the assessment of tumour response to therapy [90, 91]. Dynamic CT has been used in the assessment of response of colorectal hepatic metastases.

18F-FDG PET has the potential to be a very useful tool in the assessment of response to pre-operative chemoradiotherapy [92]. There have been a few preliminary studies into the response to therapy in rectal cancer and colorectal liver metastases [93,94,95]. Currently, the spatial resolution of PET is considerably lower than that of other cross-sectional imaging modalities and malignant lesions below 0.5-1.0cm may not be detected [96]. The new generation of PET scanners that combine CT or MRI and enable the integration of anatomical and functional imaging are likely to become routine in the pre-operative staging of rectal cancer [97].

A number of emerging technical developments will enhance endorectal ultrasound. Doppler ultrasonography may allow a quantitative assessment of tumour blood flow using contrast agents such as microbubbles [98]. The "perfusion index" measured using Doppler ultrasound was correlated with overall survival in a series of 120 patients with colorectal cancer [99]. Elastography is a novel technique that uses ultrasound-based technology to detect shear waves, and calculate the relative shear stiffness of the tissues of interest. Preliminary work has been performed in a variety of settings [100-103].

Lymph node detection

The major downfall with all current staging imaging modalities is the lack of ability to detect involved lymph nodes. It is in the accurate identification of pathological lymph nodes that progress is most needed. Lymph node-specific contrast agents are in development. Ultrasmall superparamagnetic iron oxide (USPIO) nanocolloid particles have been shown in a limited number of phase III trials to differentiate between normal and metastatic lymph nodes on MRI [104,105,106]. Cross-linked iron oxides, so-called second generation superparamagnetic compounds, have dendritic arms that allow complexing of targeting molecules such as antibodies or fluorescent tags [107]. Microbubbles are a new lymph node contrast agent that vibrate in response to sound waves and can therefore be made to oscillate in the ultrasound field [108]. PET may offer advantages over CT and MRI in the detection of involved lymph nodes. Accumulation of FDG in nodes is independent of size, and the high biological contrast between tumour and non-tumour tissue may assist in the detection of involved nodes in difficult anatomical areas such as the pelvic sidewall [109].

Summary

The pre-operative staging of rectal cancer is key for the identification of patients at high risk of local recurrence in order to plan the optimal multidisciplinary treatment. High-resolution phased-array MRI is the most useful imaging modality for local staging. If an early tumour is identified, EUS is most accurate in assessing the degree of tumour invasion through the rectal wall. Endorectal MRI is as accurate as EUS, but is more expensive and now rarely used in clinical practice. CT of the chest and abdomen is mandatory in order to exclude metastatic disease. New developments in imaging technology such as PET and functional MRI promise improved results in the future.

Acknowledgements

The authors would like to thank Dr. Alan Chalmers and Dr. Brendan Carey for kindly providing the radiological images.

References

1. Improved survival with preoperative radiotherapy in resectable rectal cancer. Swedish Rectal Cancer Trial. *N Engl J Med* 1997; 336: 980-7.
2. Kapiteijn E, Marijnen CA, Nagtegaal ID, *et al*. Preoperative radiotherapy combined with total mesorectal excision for resectable rectal cancer. *N Engl J Med* 2001; 345: 638-46.
3. Pahlman L, Glimelius B. Pre-operative and post-operative radiotherapy and rectal cancer. *World J Surg* 1992; 16: 858-65.
4. Hildebrandt U, Feifel G. Preoperative staging of rectal cancer by intrarectal ultrasound. *Dis Colon Rectum* 1985; 28: 42-6.
5. Bryan PJ, Butler HE, Lisborg PH. Magnetic resonance imaging of the pelvis. *Radiol Clin North Am* 1984; 22: 897-915.

6. Butch RJ, Stark DD, Wittenberg J, et al. Staging rectal cancer by MR and CT. *Am J Roentgenol* 1986; 146: 1155-60.
7. Akasu T, Sugihara K, Moriya Y, Fujita S. Limitations and pitfalls of transrectal ultrasonography for staging of rectal cancer. *Dis Colon Rectum* 1997; 40: S10-S15.
8. Beets-Tan RG, Beets GL, Vliegen RF et al. Accuracy of magnetic resonance imaging in prediction of tumour-free resection margin in rectal cancer surgery. *Lancet* 2001; 357: 497-504.
9. Akasu T, Kondo H, Moriya Y et al. Endorectal ultrasonography and treatment of early stage rectal cancer. *World J Surg* 2000; 24: 1061-8.
10. Barbaro B, Valentini V, Manfredi R. Combined modality staging of high risk rectal cancer. *Rays* 1995; 20: 165-81.
11. Blomqvist L, Machado M, Rubio C, et al. Rectal tumour staging: MR imaging using pelvic phased-array and endorectal coils vs endoscopic ultrasonography. *Eur Radiol* 2000; 10: 653-60.
12. Brown G, Richards CJ, Newcombe RG, et al. Rectal carcinoma: thin-section MR imaging for staging in 28 patients. *Radiology* 1999; 211: 215-22.
13. Fuchsjager MH, Maier AG, Schima W, et al. Comparison of transrectal sonography and double-contrast MR imaging when staging rectal cancer. *Am J Roentgenol* 2003; 181: 421-7.
14. Garcia-Aguilar J, Pollack J, Lee SH, et al. Accuracy of endorectal ultrasonography in preoperative staging of rectal tumors. *Dis Colon Rectum* 2002; 45: 10-5.
15. Gualdi GF, Casciani E, Guadalaxara A, d'Orta C, Polettini E, Pappalardo G. Local staging of rectal cancer with transrectal ultrasound and endorectal magnetic resonance imaging: comparison with histologic findings. *Dis Colon Rectum* 2000; 43: 338-45.
16. Heriot AG, Grundy A, Kumar D. Preoperative staging of rectal carcinoma. *Br J Surg* 1999; 86: 17-28.
17. Herzog U, von Flue M, Tondelli P, Schuppisser JP. How accurate is endorectal ultrasound in the preoperative staging of rectal cancer? *Dis Colon Rectum* 1993; 36: 127-34.
18. Kim NK, Kim MJ, Yun SH, Sohn SK, Min JS. Comparative study of transrectal ultrasonography, pelvic computerized tomography, and magnetic resonance imaging in preoperative staging of rectal cancer. *Dis Colon Rectum* 1999; 42: 770-5.
19. Kim NK, Kim MJ, Park JK, Park SI, Min JS. Preoperative staging of rectal cancer with MRI: accuracy and clinical usefulness. *Ann Surg Oncol* 2000; 7: 732-7.
20. Lindmark G, Elvin A, Pahlman L, Glimelius B. The value of endosonography in preoperative staging of rectal cancer. *Int J Colorectal Dis* 1992; 7: 162-6.
21. Maldjian C, Smith R, Kilger A, Schnall M, Ginsberg G, Kochman M. Endorectal surface coil MR imaging as a staging technique for rectal carcinoma: a comparison study to rectal endosonography. *Abdom Imaging* 2000; 25: 75-80.
22. Mathur P, Smith JJ, Ramsey C, et al. Comparison of CT and MRI in the pre-operative staging of rectal adenocarcinoma and prediction of circumferential resection margin involvement by MRI. *Colorectal Dis* 2003; 5: 396-401.
23. Osti MF, Padovan FS, Pirolli C, et al. Comparison between transrectal ultrasonography and computed tomography with rectal inflation of gas in preoperative staging of lower rectal cancer. *Eur Radiol* 1997; 7: 26-30.
24. Sailer M, Leppert R, Kraemer M, Fuchs KH, Thiede A. The value of endorectal ultrasound in the assessment of adenomas, T1- and T2-carcinomas. *Int J Colorectal Dis* 1997; 12: 214-9.
25. Schnall MD, Furth EE, Rosato EF, Kressel HY. Rectal tumor stage: correlation of endorectal MR imaging and pathologic findings. *Radiology* 1994; 190: 709-14.
26. Starck M, Bohe M, Simanaitis M, Valentin L. Rectal endosonography can distinguish benign rectal lesions from invasive early rectal cancers. *Colorectal Dis* 2003; 5: 246-50.
27. Kwok H, Bissett IP, Hill GL. Preoperative staging of rectal cancer. *Int J Colorectal Dis* 2000; 15: 9-20.
28. Maier AG, Kersting-Sommerhoff B, Reeders JW, et al. Staging of rectal cancer by double-contrast MR imaging using the rectally administered superparamagnetic iron oxide contrast agent ferristene and IV gadodiamide injection: results of a multicenter phase II trial. *J Magn Reson Imaging* 2000; 12: 651-60.
29. Urban M, Rosen HR, Holbling N, et al. MR imaging for the preoperative planning of sphincter-saving surgery for tumors of the lower third of the rectum: use of intravenous and endorectal contrast materials. *Radiology* 2000; 214: 503-8.
30. Schiedler J, Reiser MF. MRI of the female and male pelvis: current and future applications of contrast enhancement. *Eur J Radiol* 2000; 34: 220-8.
31. Wallengren NO, Holtås S, Andrén-Sandberg Å, Jonsson E, McGill S. Rectal carcinoma: double-contrast MR imaging for preoperative staging. *Radiology* 2000; 215: 108-14.
32. Thoeni RF, Moss AA, Schnyder P. Detection and staging of primary rectal and rectosigmoid cancer by computed tomography. *Radiology* 1981; 141: 135-8.
33. Zaunbauer W, Haertel M, Fuchs WA. Computed tomography in carcinoma of the rectum. *Gastrointest Radiol* 1981; 6: 79-84.
34. Holdsworth PJ, Johnston D, Chalmers AG, et al. Endoluminal ultrasound and computed tomography in the staging of rectal cancer. *Br J Surg* 1988; 75: 1019-22.
35. Rifkin MD, Ehrlich SM, Marks G. Staging of rectal carcinoma: prospective comparison of endorectal US and CT. *Radiology* 1989; 170: 319-22.
36. Hodgman CG, Maccarty RL, Wolff BG, et al. Preoperative staging of rectal carainoma by computed tomography and 0.15T magnetic resonance imaging. Preliminary report. *Dis Colon Rectum* 1986; 29: 446-50.
37. Chiesura-Corona M, Muzzio PC, Giust G, Zuliani M, Pucciarelli S, Toppan P. Rectal cancer: CT local staging with histopathologic correlation. *Abdom Imaging* 2001; 26: 134-8.
38. Maier AG, Barton PP, Neuhold NR, Herbst F, Teleky BK, Lechner GL. Peritumoral tissue reaction at transrectal US as a possible cause of overstaging in rectal cancer: histopathologic correlation. *Radiology* 1997; 203: 785-9.
39. Beets-Tan RG. MRI in rectal cancer: the T stage and circumferential resection margin. *Colorectal Dis* 2003; 5: 392-5.
40. Kruskal JB, Kane RA, Sentovich SM, Longmaid HE. Pitfalls and sources of error in staging rectal cancer with endorectal US. *Radiographics* 1997; 17: 609-26.
41. Orrom WJ, Wong WD, Rothenberger DA, Jensen LL, Goldberg SM. Endorectal ultrasound in the preoperative staging of rectal tumors. A learning experience. *Dis Colon Rectum* 1990; 33: 654-9.

42. Solomon MJ, McLeod RS. Endoluminal transrectal ultrasonography: accuracy, reliability, and validity. *Dis Colon Rectum* 1993; 36: 200-5.
43. Solomon MJ, McLeod RS, Cohen EK, Simons ME, Wilson S. Reliability and validity studies of endoluminal ultrasonography for anorectal disorders. *Dis Colon Rectum* 1994; 37: 546-51.
44. Gold DM, Halligan S, Kmiot WA, Bartram CI. Intraobserver and interobserver agreement in anal endosonography. *Br J Surg* 1999; 86: 371-5.
45. Drew PJ, Farouk R, Turnbull LW, Ward SC, Hartley JE, Monson JR. Preoperative magnetic resonance staging of rectal cancer with an endorectal coil and dynamic gadolinium enhancement. *Br J Surg* 1999; 86: 250-4.
46. Mann B. Prognostic relevant factors within pT3 rectal carcinomas: depth of invasion or circumferential resection margins? *Int J Colorectal Dis* 2003; 18: 493-4.
47. Picon AI, Moore HG, Sternberg SS, et al. Prognostic significance of depth of gross or microscopic perirectal fat invasion in T3 N0 M0 rectal cancers following sharp mesorectal excision and no adjuvant therapy. *Int J Colorectal Dis* 2003; 18: 487-92.
48. Willett CG, Badizadegan K, Ancukiewicz M, Shellito PC. Prognostic factors in stage T3N0 rectal cancer: do all patients require postoperative pelvic irradiation and chemotherapy? *Dis Colon Rectum* 1999; 42: 167-73.
49. Merkel S, Mansmann U, Siassi M, Papadopoulos T, Hohenberger W, Hermanek P. The prognostic inhomogeneity in pT3 rectal carcinomas. *Int J Colorectal Dis* 2001; 16: 298-304.
50. Cawthorn SJ, Parums DV, Gibbs NM, et al. Extent of mesorectal spread and involvement of lateral resection margin as prognostic factors after surgery for rectal cancer. *Lancet* 1990; 335: 1055-9.
51. Beets-Tan RG, Beets GL, Borstlap AC, et al. Preoperative assessment of local tumor extent in advanced rectal cancer: CT or high-resolution MRI? *Abdom Imaging* 2000; 25: 533-41.
52. Hulsmans FJ, Tio TL, Fockens P, Bosma A, Tytgat GN. Assessment of tumor infiltration depth in rectal cancer with transrectal sonography: caution is necessary. *Radiology* 1994; 190: 715-20.
53. Brown G, Radcliffe AG, Newcombe RG, Dallimore NS, Bourne MW, Williams GT. Preoperative assessment of prognostic factors in rectal cancer using high-resolution magnetic resonance imaging. *Br J Surg* 2003; 90: 355-64.
54. Quirke P, Dixon MF. The prediction of local recurrence in rectal adenocarcinoma by histopathological examination. *Int J Colorectal Dis* 1988; 3: 127-31.
55. Nagtegaal ID, Marijnen CA, Kranenbarg EK, Van De Velde CJ, van Krieken JH. Circumferential margin involvement is still an important predictor of local recurrence in rectal carcinoma: not one millimeter but two millimeters is the limit. *Am J Surg Pathol* 2002; 26: 350-7.
56. Wibe A, Rendedal PR, Svensson E, et al. Prognostic significance of the circumferential resection margin following total mesorectal excision for rectal cancer. *Br J Surg* 2002; 89: 327-34.
57. Birbeck KF, Macklin CP, Tiffin NJ, et al. Rates of circumferential resection margin involvement vary between surgeons and predict outcomes in rectal cancer surgery. *Ann Surg* 2002; 235: 449-57.
58. Adam IJ, Mohamdee MO, Martin IG, et al. Role of circumferential margin involvement in the local recurrence of rectal cancer. *Lancet* 1994; 344: 707-11.
59. Haas-Kock DF, Baeten CG, Jager JJ, et al. Prognostic significance of radial margins of clearance in rectal cancer. *Br J Surg* 1996; 83: 781-5.
60. Grabbe E, Lierse W, Winkler R. The perirectal fascia: morphology and use in staging of rectal carcinoma. *Radiology* 1983; 149: 241-6.
61. De Souza NM, Hall AS, Puni R, Gilderdale DJ, Young IR, Kmiot WA. High resolution magnetic resonance imaging of the anal sphincter using a dedicated endoanal coil. *Dis Colon Rectum* 1996; 39: 926-34.
62. Blomqvist L, Rubio C, Holm T, Machado M, Hindmarsh T. Rectal adenocarcinoma: assessment of tumour involvement of the lateral resection margin by MRI of resected specimen. *Br J Radiol* 1999; 72: 18-23.
63. Bissett IP, Fernando CC, Hough DM, et al. Identification of the fascia propria by magnetic resonance imaging and its relevance to preoperative assessment of rectal cancer. *Dis Colon Rectum* 2001; 44: 259-65.
64. Martling A, Holm T, Bremmer S, Lindholm J, Cedermark B, Blomqvist L. Prognostic value of preoperative magnetic resonance imaging of the pelvis in rectal cancer. *Br J Surg* 2003; 90: 1422-8.
65. Thoeni RF. Colorectal cancer. Radiologic staging. *Radiol Clin North Am* 1997; 35: 457-85.
66. Beynon J, Mortensen NJ, Foy DM, Channer JL, Rigby H, Virjee J. Preoperative assessment of mesorectal lymph node involvement in rectal cancer. *Br J Surg* 1989; 76: 276-9.
67. Brown G, Richards CJ, Bourne MW, et al. Morphologic predictors of lymph node status in rectal cancer with use of high-spatial-resolution MR imaging with histopathologic comparison. *Radiology* 2003; 227: 371-7.
68. Morren GL, Beets-Tan RG, van Engelshoven JM. Anatomy of the anal canal and perianal structures as defined by phased-array magnetic resonance imaging. *Br J Surg* 2001; 88: 1506-12.
69. Holzer B, Urban M, Holbling N, et al. Magnetic resonance imaging predicts sphincter invasion of low rectal cancer and influences selection of operation. *Surgery* 2003; 133: 656-61.
70. Goh V, Halligan S, Bartram CI. Local radiological staging of rectal cancer. *Clin Radiol* 2004; 59: 215-26.
71. Ng CS, Doyle TC, Courtney HM, Campbell GA, Freeman AH, Dixon AK. Extracolonic findings in patients undergoing abdomino-pelvic CT for suspected colorectal carcinoma in the frail and disabled patient. *Clin Radiol* 2004; 59: 421-30.
72. Rohren EM, Turkington TG, Coleman RE. Clinical applications of PET in oncology. *Radiology* 2004; 231: 305-32.
73. Topal B, Flamen P, Aerts R, et al. Clinical value of whole-body emission tomography in potentially curable colorectal liver metastases. *Eur J Surg Oncol* 2001; 27: 175-9.
74. Boykin KN, Zibari GB, Lilien DL, McMillan RW, Aultman DF, McDonald JC. The use of FDG-positron emission tomography for the evaluation of colorectal metastases. *Am Surg* 1999; 65: 1183-5.

75. Vitola JV, Delbeke D, Sandler MP, et al. Positron emission tomography to stage suspected metastatic colorectal carcinoma to the liver. *Am J Surg* 1996; 171: 21-6.
76. Huebner RH, Park KC, Shepherd JE, et al. A meta-analysis of the literature for whole-body FDG PET detection of recurrent colorectal cancer. *J Nucl Med* 2000; 41: 1177-89.
77. van der Hiel B, Pauwels EK, Stokkel MP. Positron emission tomography with 2-[18F]-fluoro-2-deoxy-D-glucose in oncology. Part IIIa: Therapy response monitoring in breast cancer, lymphoma and gliomas. *J Cancer Res Clin Oncol* 2001; 127: 269-77.
78. Lindmark GE, Kraaz WG, Elvin PA, Glimelius BL. Rectal cancer: evaluation of staging with endosonography. *Radiology* 1997; 204: 533-8.
79. Hunerbein M, Schlag PM. Three-dimensional endosonography for staging of rectal cancer. *Ann Surg* 1997; 225: 432-8.
80. Hunerbein M. Endorectal ultrasound in rectal cancer. *Colorectal Dis* 2003; 5: 402-5.
81. Hamada S, Akahoshi K, Chijiiwa Y, Sasaki I, Nawata H. Preoperative staging of colorectal cancer by a 15 MHz ultrasound miniprobe. *Surgery* 1998; 123: 264-9.
82. Hünerbein M, Totkas S, Ghadimi BM, Schlag PM. Preoperative evaluation of colorectal neoplasms by colonoscopic miniprobe ultrasonography. *Ann Surg* 2000; 232: 46-50.
83. De Bazelaire CMJ, Duhamel GD, Rofsky NM, Alsop DC. MR imaging relaxation times of abdominal and pelvic tissues measured *in vivo* at 3.0 T: preliminary results. *Radiology* 2004; 230: 652-9.
84. Luciani A, Olivier JC, Clement O, et al. Glucose-receptor MR imaging of tumors: study in mice with PEGlycated paramagnetic niosomes. *Radiology* 2004; 231: 135-42.
85. Dzik-Jurasz A. The development and application of functional nuclear magnetic resonance to *in vivo* therapeutic anticancer research. *Br J Radiol* 2004; 77: 296-307.
86. Lewis RA, Hall CJ, Hufton AP, et al. X-ray refraction effects: application to the imaging of biological tissues. *Br J Radiol* 2003; 76: 301-8.
87. DeVries AF, Griebel J, Kremser C, et al. Tumor microcirculation evaluated by dynamic magnetic resonance imaging predicts therapy outcome for primary rectal cancer. *Cancer Res* 2001; 61: 2513-6.
88. De Vries A, Griebel J, Kremser C, et al. Monitoring of tumour microcirculation during fractionated radiation therapy in patients with rectal carcinoma: preliminary results and implications for therapy. *Radiology* 2000; 217: 385-91.
89. George ML, Dzik-Jurasz AS, Padhani AR, et al. Non-invasive methods of assessing angiogenesis and their value in predicting response to treatment in colorectal cancer. *Br J Surg* 2001; 88: 1628-36.
90. Dzik-Jurasz A, Domenig C, George M, et al. Diffusion MRI for prediction of response of rectal cancer to chemoradiation. *Lancet* 2002; 360: 307-8.
91. Harvey C, Morgan J, Blomley M, Dooher A, de Souza N, Dawson P. Tumor responses to radiation therapy: use of dynamic contrast material-enhanced CT to monitor functional and anatomical indices. *Acad Radiol* 2002; 9 Suppl 1: S215-S219.
92. Calvo FA, Domper M, Matute R, et al. 18FDG-positron emission tomography staging and restaging in rectal cancer treated with preoperative chemoradiation. *Int J Radiat Oncol Biol Phys* 2004; 58: 528-35.
93. Findlay M, Young H, Cunningham D, et al. Noninvasive monitoring of tumor metabolism using fluorodeoxyglucose and positron emission tomography in colorectal cancer liver metastases: correlation with tumor response to fluorouracil. *J Clin Oncol* 1996; 14: 700-8.
94. Young H, Baum R, Cremerius U, et al. Measurement of clinical and subclinical tumour response using [18F]-fluorodeoxyglucose and positron emission tomography: review and 1999 EORTC recommendations. European Organization for Research and Treatment of Cancer (EORTC) PET Study Group. *Eur J Cancer* 1999; 35: 1773-82.
95. Guillem JG, Puig-La Calle J, Jr., Akhurst T, et al. Prospective assessment of primary rectal cancer response to preoperative radiation and chemotherapy using 18-fluorodeoxyglucose positron emission tomography. *Dis Colon Rectum* 2000; 43: 18-24.
96. Tutt AN, Plunkett TA, Barrington SF, Leslie MD. The role of positron emission tomography in the management of colorectal cancer. *Colorectal Dis* 2004; 6: 2-9.
97. Townsend DW, Beyer T. A combined PET/CT scanner: the path to true image fusion. *Br J Radiol* 2002; 75: S24-S30.
98. Takeuchi N, Ohmori K, Kondo I, et al. Interaction with leukocytes: phospholipid-stabilized versus albumin-shell microbubbles. *Radiology* 2004; 230: 735-42.
99. Leen E, Goldberg JA, Angerson WJ, McArdle CS. Potential role of doppler perfusion index in selection of patients with colorectal cancer for adjuvant therapy. *Lancet* 2000; 355: 34-7.
100. Bercoff J, Chaffai S, Tanter M, et al. *In vivo* breast tumor detection using transient elastography. *Ultrasound Med Biol* 2003; 29: 1387-96.
101. Cochlin DL, Ganatra RH, Griffiths DF. Elastography in the detection of prostatic cancer. *Clin Radiol* 2002; 57: 1014-20.
102. Varghese T, Zagzebski JA, Rahko P, Breburda CS. Ultrasonic imaging of myocardial strain using cardiac elastography. *Ultrason Imaging* 2003; 25: 1-16.
103. Varghese T, Zagzebski JA, Lee FT, Jr. Elastographic imaging of thermal lesions in the liver *in vivo* following radiofrequency ablation: preliminary results. *Ultrasound Med Biol* 2002; 28: 1467-73.
104. Koh D-W, Brown G, Temple L, et al. Rectal cancer: mesoretal lymph nodes at MR imaging with USPIO versus histopathologic findings - initial observations. *Radiology* 2004; 231: 91-9.
105. Harisinghani MG, Saini S, Slater GJ, Schnall MD, Rifkin MD. MR imaging of pelvic lymph nodes in primary pelvic carcinoma with ultrasmall superparamagnetic iron oxide (Combidex): preliminary observations. *J Magn Reson Imaging* 1997; 7: 161-3.
106. Vassallo P, Matei C, Heston WD, McLachlan SJ, Koutcher JA, Castellino RA. AMI-227-enhanced MR lymphography: usefulness for differentiating reactive from tumor-bearing lymph nodes. *Radiology* 1994; 193: 501-6.
107. Thrall JH. Nanotechnology and medicine. *Radiology* 2004; 230: 315-8.
108. Rubin JM. Do microbubbles react differently with leukocytes? *Radiology* 2004; 230: 604-5.
109. Schwaiger M. Functional imaging for assessment of therapy. *Br J Radiol* 2002; 75: S67-S73.

Chapter 7

Invasive palliative therapies for colorectal cancer

Rakesh Bhardwaj FRCS FRCS (Ed), Specialist Registrar
Michael C Parker BSc MS FRCS FRCS (Ed), Consultant Surgeon
Darent Valley Hospital, Dartford, Kent, UK

What is the problem?

The World Health Organisation defines palliative care as an approach that improves the quality of life of patients and their families facing a life-threatening illness through the prevention and relief of suffering by means of early identification, impeccable assessment and with treatment of pain and other problems - physical, psychosocial and spiritual.

The ACPGBI Colorectal Cancer Study (2004) showed that the frequency of Dukes' "D" tumours in patients having surgery from April 2001 to March 2002 had fallen from 16.5% a year earlier to 8% [1]. The authors suggested this represented either a fall in the number of cases presenting with metastatic disease or a change in clinical practice, possibly due to increased use of colonic stents or palliative chemotherapy. The earlier ACPGBI Colorectal Cancer Study (2002) showed that all palliative surgical procedures had a significantly higher mortality rate [2]. Surgery in those with advanced colorectal malignancy may be considered inappropriate, as this group of patients is often frail with poor optimisation of operative risk factors in the emergency setting. Palliation of colorectal cancer often presents a difficult multidisciplinary challenge.

Strategies that can be deemed as invasive therapies to palliate colorectal carcinoma aim to prevent or resolve symptoms and signs of colonic obstruction and symptoms from the tumour bulk, which include pain, bleeding and change in bowel habit. The determination of the site of the colorectal malignancy requiring palliation is crucial as this reflects which therapeutic modality is employed. Options available to the clinician include insertion of colonic stents (Table 1), simple dilatation, endoscopic laser ablation and cryosurgery. However, despite these recent innovations, the role of surgery to assist palliation should not be discounted and may be the only suitable option (Table 2). Chemotherapeutic and radiotherapeutic treatments in isolation have been excluded from this discussion.

Where are we now?

Stents

An ideal colonic stent should be able to be easily inserted transrectally, negotiate the colonic folds, be deployed comfortably, remain in position and allow a sufficient channel for faecal material to pass. There are numerous stents commercially available; most have a mesh design and are constructed from steel or

Table 1. The role of colorectal stents.	
Stents	
Uses	Palliation (56%)
	Bridge to surgery (44%)
Clinical success	88%
Mortality	0.5%
Morbidity	Perforation 4%
	Migration 10%
	Re-obstruction 10%
	Bleeding 5%
	Pain 5%
Cost	Less than half of surgical decompression

Table 2. Morbidity and mortality from emergency surgery for colonic obstruction.	
Emergency surgery	
Mortality	6%-30%
	Left-sided obstruction 12.9%
Morbidity	10-36%
	Often 2-stage procedure
Colostomy	30% never reversed
	Associated morbidity and quality of life implications

nitinol. Nitinol stents are constructed from a nickel and titanium alloy. They have "shape memory", reverting to a predetermined configuration after deployment, usually after 2-5 days. The inherent flexibility of nitinol permits some colonic peristalsis. Self-expanding metal stents (SEMS) differ in their final expanded diameter and length after deployment. The Food and Drug Administration (FDA) in the United States have approved three stents for use in malignant colonic obstruction: the Enteral Wallstent (Boston Scientific, Microvasive Corporation, Natick, Massachusetts, USA), the BARD Memotherm stent (BARD, Billerica, Massachusetts, USA) and the colonic Z-stent (Wilson-Cook Medical, Winston-Salem, North Carolina, USA). Though the latter two have larger deployment diameters, the Enteral Wallstent has a longer and smaller diameter delivery system making it suitable for endoscopic placement and as such it may be preferred for more proximal colonic lesions.

Stent placement

A combined approach as advocated by Soonawalla et al (1998) with both a surgical endoscopist and an interventional radiologist is recommended for successful insertion of a SEMS [3]. The nature and position of the obstructing lesion may permit non-fluoroscopically-guided SEMS placement, where the endoscope first visualises the lesion. The SEMS may then be deployed, either using a stent delivered through the working channel of the endoscope over a guide wire placed across the lesion, or alternatively a guide wire may be placed across the lesion under fluoroscopic control. In fluoroscopic SEMS placement, the passage of a second safety wire proves useful in case the initial guide wire should become displaced during stent placement. The stent position can be checked fluoroscopically and endoscopically. Characteristic features of correct placement include "flaring" of the ends and the appearance of a central "waist" (Figures 1-4).

Early attempts at colonic decompression with Lecluk et al's (1986) [4] use of a nasogastric tube and Keen and Orsay's (1992) [5] use of a chest tube were unsuccessful as the tubes were of small calibre and were prone to obstruction. Dohmoto (1991) first described the use of a metal stent to relieve malignant rectal obstruction [6]. This was followed by sporadic similar reports, predominantly for the palliation of obstructing lesions.

An early report by Spinelli et al (1993) showed successful stent placement in 12 of 13 (92%) patients [7]. At a mean follow-up of 7 months, 10 (83%) had a patent stent lumen with no reports of discomfort. Rey et al (1995) used SEMS in 12 patients with rectal or rectosigmoid carcinomas as an alternative to laser ablation [8]. Initial treatments were performed with an Nd:YAG laser in order to allow free passage of a colonoscope. Stent placement was successful in 11 of the 12 (92%) patients. Failure occurred in the

7 Invasive palliative therapies for colorectal cancer

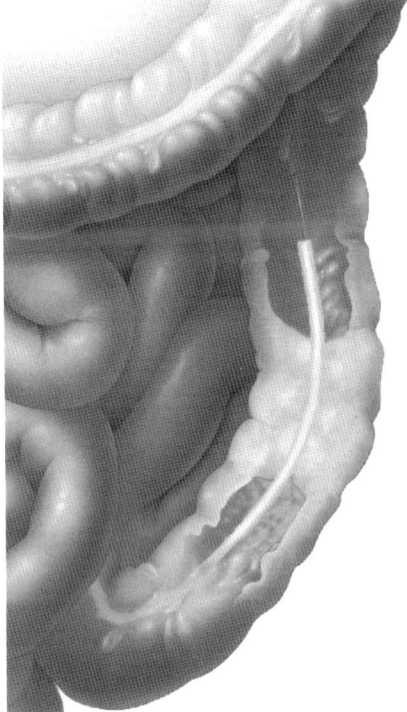 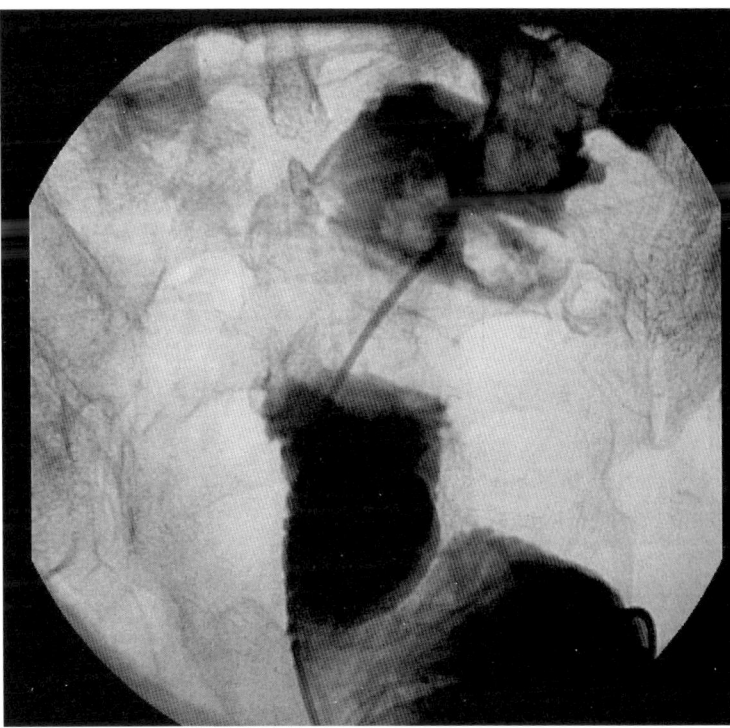

Figure 1. Insertion of guide wire through colonic stricture (diagram reproduced with permission from Boston Scientific Ltd.).

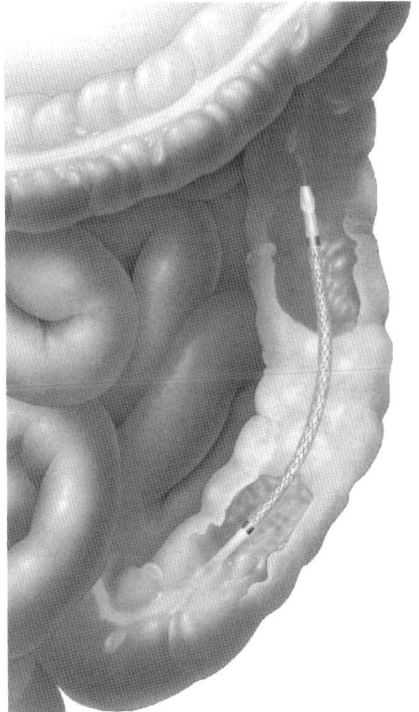 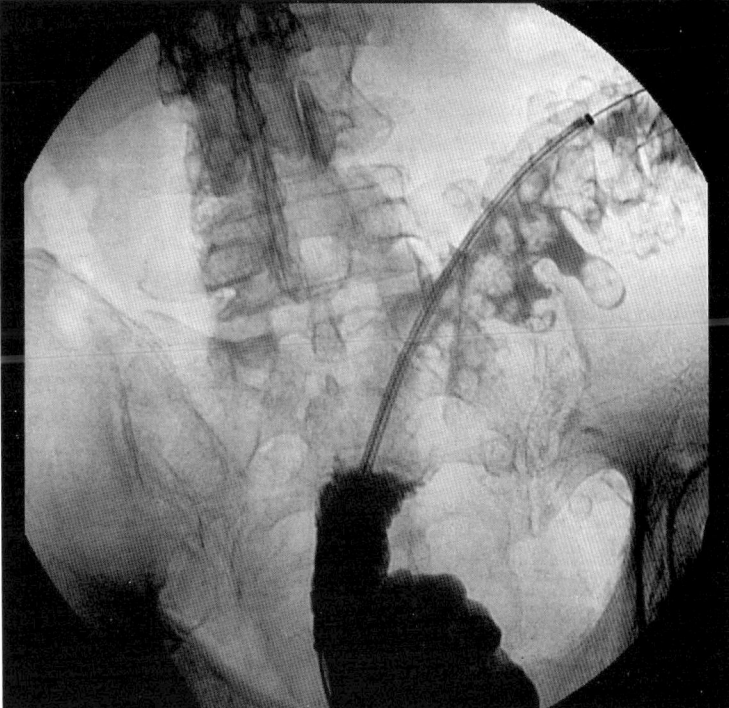

Figure 2. Insertion of stent over guide wire (diagram reproduced with permission from Boston Scientific Ltd.).

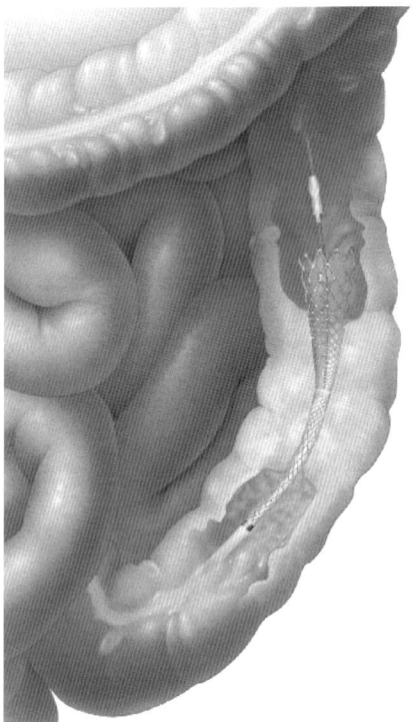
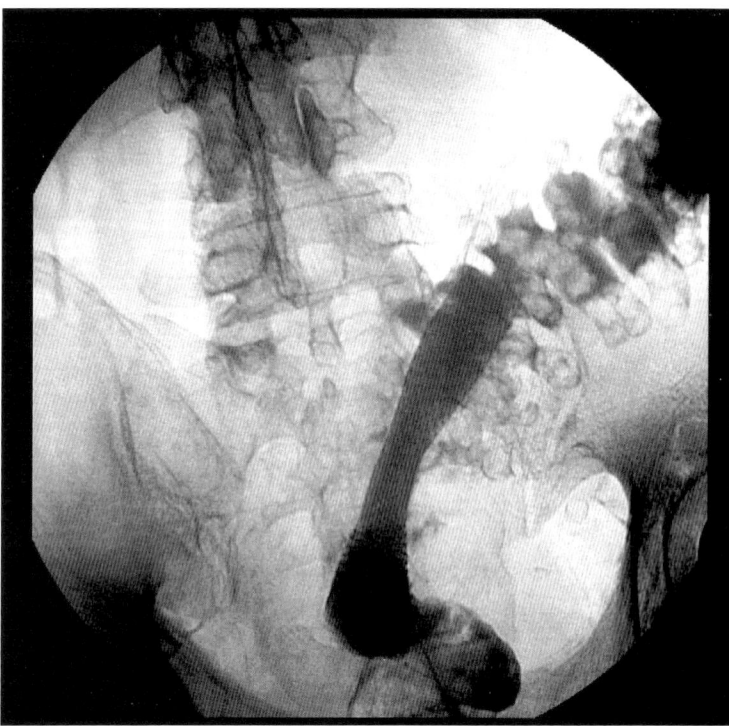

Figure 3. Deploying the stent (diagram reproduced with permission from Boston Scientific Ltd.).

remaining patient due to colonic distortion and diverticulosis. Though stent migration occurred in three patients, replacement stents were placed. The authors demonstrated that in their series stent placement reduced the number of laser sessions required to achieve adequate palliation. Dohmoto et al (1997) employed three varieties of stent prostheses in 19 patients with non-resectable or metastatic rectal cancer: plastic tubes (n=8), SEMS (n=6) or endocoil stents (n=5) [9]. Prior to insertion, laser canalisation or balloon dilatation was employed. At a median follow-up of 6 months eight patients had died whereas those remaining alive had no evidence of recurrent obstruction. Dislocation of the endoprosthesis occurred in two of eight plastic tubes and one of five mesh stents. Recurrent obstruction from tumour ingrowth did occur in those with self-expanding mesh stents, whereas those with endocoil stents showed no evidence of treatment failure. Turegano-Fuentes et al (1998) reported relief of obstruction in seven of 11 (64%) patients with left-sided colonic obstruction and either advanced pelvic disease, peritoneal carcinomatosis and/or multiple parenchymatous metastatic disease [10]. Surgical intervention was prevented in six (55%), five of whom died with an unobstructed colon from 26 days to 7 months after SEMS placement. Tack et al (1998) also described the use of an Nd:YAG laser to create a channel for SEMS placement [11]. In their series, nine of ten (90%) patients with advanced obstructing rectosigmoid carcinomas had successful stent placement and the patients remained free of obstruction for 103 ± 31 days. The remaining patient's stent deployment was complicated by sigmoid perforation requiring surgery. Of those that had successful SEMS placement, migration occurred at 38 ± 10 days and re-obstruction from tumour ingrowth occurred in another patient. De Gregorio et al's (1998) multicentre study of 24 patients treated palliatively showed successful stent placement in all patients and in 23 (96%) there was relief of obstruction within 24 hours [12]. Complications developed in ten (42%) patients; these included rectal bleeding (2), abdominal pain (3), stent malposition (2), faecal impaction of the stent (2) and tumour ingrowth (1). Malposition of the stent required surgical reinsertion of a further stent. In Paul et al's (1999) series, in which 16 consecutive patients had SEMS inserted successfully, similar complications were seen and reintervention was required in three (20%) of the 15 cases in whom colonic obstruction was initially

7 Invasive palliative therapies for colorectal cancer

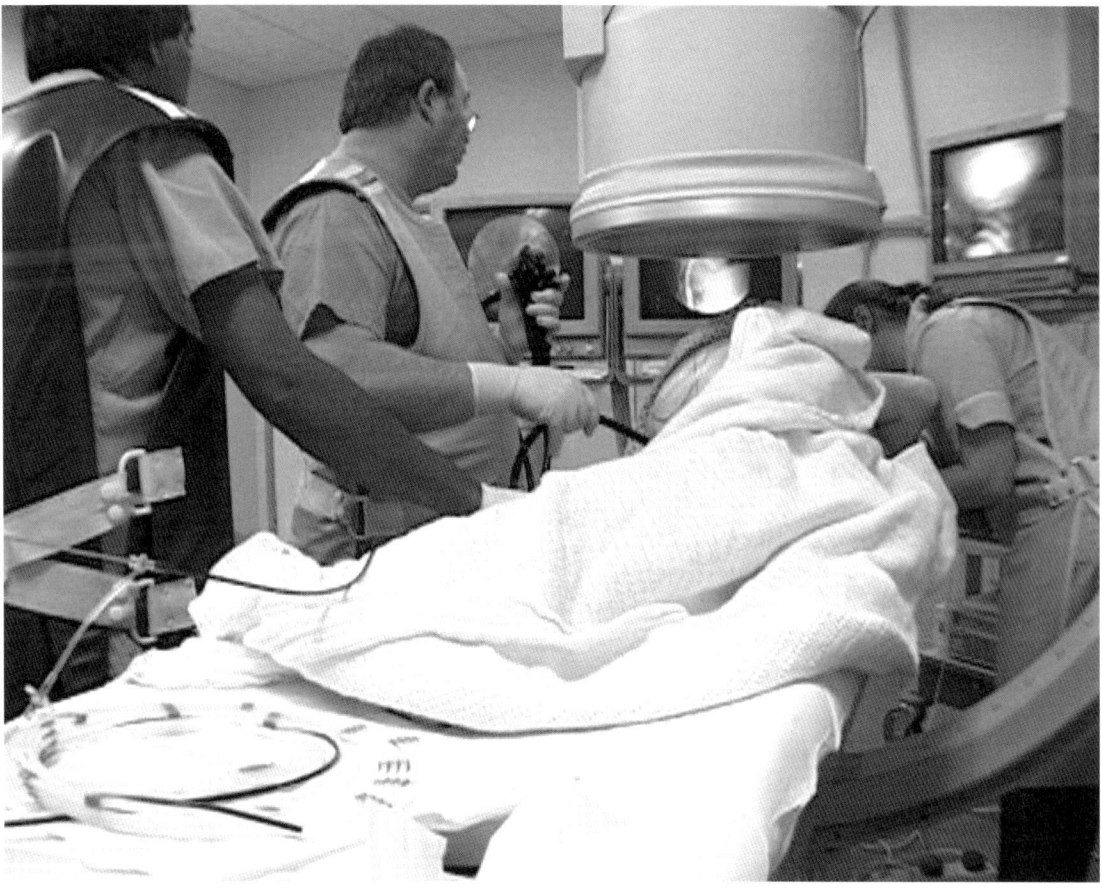

Figure 4. Endoscopist and radiologist working in tandem to obtain placement of guide wire across colorectal stricture.

relieved [13]. In a larger series by Fernandez et al (1999) involving 41 patients with advanced malignancy, the obstruction was relieved within 24-96 hours in 38 (93%) [14]. Whilst there was increasing evidence of the benefits of SEMS as an alternative palliative measure to treat colonic obstruction, the incidence of reported complications and the necessity for reintervention in a proportion of cases was noted.

This century's literature has described increasing uses of SEMS with refinements in techniques and indications for use (Tables 1 & 2). Whilst Coco et al (2000) showed successful stent placement in three patients with recurrent rectal cancer and pelvic recurrences, patients complained of rectal tenesmus during the first 48 hours [15]. Though this troublesome side effect was treated with non-steroidal anti-inflammatory drugs, it showed that SEMS, if selected for rectal cancers, can result in marked anorectal irritation. SEMS use does not exclude further surgery in the palliative setting. Law et al (2000) reported 18 patients in whom SEMS were used for palliation, three of whom required the subsequent formation of a stoma [16]. In Miyayama et al's (2000) series, where one covered and ten uncovered nitinol stents were deployed in eight patients with left-sided colonic cancers, re-obstruction occurred in two cases [17]. These required either a subsequent formation of a colostomy or ileostomy. Six complications occurred in four patients and included migration (1), bleeding (2), pain requiring analgesia (1) and fever (2). In Ben Soussan et al's (2001) series, in which 16 (94%) of 17 patients had successful stent placement, relief occurred in 13 (74%) within 48 hours [18]. However, subsequent colostomies were necessary in five patients due to complications which included perforation, stent migration and dislocation of the stent. SEMS remained effective in relieving obstruction over long periods in the majority of cases where expertise was available. Covered stents may be more effective in preventing tumour ingrowth which can lead to re-obstruction. In Repici et al's (2000) series, in which 15 of 16 (93%) had successful SEMS placement with covered stents, there was no obstruction seen at a median follow-up of 21 (range 1-46) weeks [19]. Spinelli and Mancini (2001) showed that, of 36 patients in whom SEMS were placed successfully, 33 were followed for a median of 7 (3 weeks-33 months) with 28 (78%) experiencing restoration of luminal patency with disappearance of obstructive symptoms [20]. SEMS may also be used for treating colonic obstruction from other intra-abdominal malignancies. Araki et al (2002) reported five cases in which colonic obstruction from recurrent malignancy (three of colonic origin, one of ovarian origin and one from gastric cancer) were treated successfully with SEMS [21]. One stent obstructed and two patients experienced bleeding which was treated with argon plasma coagulation. Xinopoulos et al's (2002) study consisted of 11 patients who presented with advanced malignant colonic obstruction [22]. Eight had colorectal adenocarcinoma; in two the malignancy was ovarian in origin and in the remaining patient the obstruction was due to an infiltrating bladder carcinoma. SEMS placement with the additional use of a Diomed laser in five cases to deal with late tumour ingrowth proved successful in all cases. Palliation even of fistulating colorectal malignancies is possible with the use of covered stents. Grunshaw and Ball described the use of a covered oesophageal stent to occlude an enterorectal fistula with recurrent inoperable colonic carcinoma [23].

The use of SEMS in the UK has gained increasing popularity in recent years as evidence regarding efficacy has increased. Aviv et al (2002) reported successful placement of 16 stents in 13 of 15 (87%) patients, most of whom were almost obstructed [24]. Though stent migration and ingrowth was noted, the median survival in the group was two (range 0.5-12) months. Seymour et al (2002) identified 20 patients with obstruction: ten with metastatic disease, four with fixed rectal cancers and six with comorbidity not permitting safe surgery [25]. Stents were successful in 18 (90%) cases with a median duration of palliation of 80 (range 14-257) days. One late complication described was due to migration and fracturing of a low rectal stent causing tenesmus. Clark et al (2003) collected prospective data on 16 patients of whom 13 (81%) underwent successful stent placement [26]. In two cases insertion of overlapping stents was necessary. In the three unsuccessful cases a guide wire could not be placed across the lesion. Two were benign strictures and in the remaining case the colonic compression was due to an ovarian malignancy.

Recent work has focused on comparisons of SEMS against surgery. Law et al (2003) compared the outcome for obstructing colonic lesions distal to the splenic flexure in 31 patients treated with emergency surgery against 30 patients treated with SEMS over a 5-year period from 1997 [27]. The two groups were similar in terms of age, sex distribution and presence of comorbidity. The authors concluded that SEMS were associated with a shorter hospital stay, less likelihood of intensive care and a lower incidence of stoma creation when compared with emergency surgery. A similar study by Johnson et al (2004) evaluated 18 patients with obstructing left-sided colonic cancer treated successfully with SEMS compared with 18 historical controls treated with a palliative stoma [28]. Those in the stent group were older with greater comorbidities. Though both groups of patients gained relief of obstructive symptoms, there were no differences in survival or in-hospital mortality. The median length of palliation was 92 days for stenting and 121 days for stoma formation. Those with a stoma required a longer stay in ITU but total hospital stay in the two groups was similar. The authors concluded that stenting could relieve obstruction in very frail patients who would otherwise be managed conservatively.

A recent small randomised trial compared efficacy, safety and cost of endoscopic palliative treatment with SEMS in 15 patients with stoma creation in another 15 patients in the management of inoperable malignant left-sided colonic obstructions [29]. SEMS were placed successfully in 14 (93%), though in six tumour ingrowth was observed which was treated successfully with laser ablation. The cost-effectiveness analysis showed that, although the stoma creation procedure was less expensive, the authors suggested that the SEMS provided a better quality of life for the patient. A similar cost analysis in the UK affirmed the cost saving of SEMS vs. stoma formation (Osman et al 2000) [30]. There is now a need for a national randomised trial comparing SEMS and surgery.

Complications of colorectal stents

Khot *et al* (2002) conducted a systematic review of the efficacy and safety of colorectal stents by examining the literature from January 1990 to December 2000 [31]. Twenty-nine case series were included. Stent insertion was attempted in 598 cases; technical success was achieved in 551 (92%) and clinical success, defined by colonic decompression within 96 hours without endoscopic or surgical reintervention, was achieved in 525 (88%). Three hundred and two of 336 (90%) were adequately palliated and 223 of 262 (85%) went on to have a successful bridge to surgery. Technical failure was seen in 47 of 598 (8%) cases and was predominantly related to inability to place a guide wire across the lesion (36 cases). Other main causes of technical failure included stent malposition and perforation of the colonic wall. Clinical failure was mainly due to perforation, persistence of obstructive symptoms and adhesions of the colonic wall.

Stent migration occurs in approximately 10% of cases, usually after 3 days post-deployment. Most cause no symptoms and are often identified on routine radiological follow-up. In those patients in whom stents migrate, further stents can be inserted, particularly in those being treated palliatively. In some cases stents that dislodge into the lower rectum require manual or endoscopic removal. Factors that predispose to stent migration include laser pre-treatment, chemotherapy or the presence of benign tumours. Perforation of the colonic wall as a complication can be immediate, at the time of insertion, or post-deployment. It has the potential disadvantage of shedding malignant cells into the peritoneal cavity. It occurs in approximately 4% of cases and prior balloon dilatation is a contributing factor [31]. The risk of perforation is in part related to the physical characteristics of the tumour and in part to clinical experience. Scurtu *et al* (2003) described colonic perforation in five of six cases, two in the first 24 hours after the procedure and the remainder at 3, 5 and 10 months [32]. Clinical re-obstruction after placement of a SEMS may be due to tumour ingrowth or overgrowth of the stent, stent migration or faecal impaction. Pain occurs in 5% of patients with SEMS placed and simple analgesics can often help. If a SEMS is placed within 6cm of the anal verge the patient may experience significant discomfort and tenesmus. Though bleeding is uncommon it is thought to arise in the most part from the friable tumour; occasionally, the stent may cause some mucosal damage but transfusion is rarely required.

Lasers

Laser (light amplification by stimulated emission of radiation) photocoagulation of colorectal malignancies in the palliative setting has been advocated as a major alternative to surgery. Reports have been optimistic throughout the last two decades but regular use in the clinical setting is not widespread. The Neodynium: yttrium-aluminum-garnet (Nd:YAG) laser is most commonly employed and is used to treat bleeding and obstructing colorectal cancers (Figure 5). The procedure can be conducted under sedation, sometimes requiring simple bowel preparation and in selected cases day-case therapy is possible. Mathus-Vliegen and Tytgat (1986) investigated 63 patients [33]: 15 of 16 (94%) had obstruction and were decompressed, and in 28 of 32 (88%) with bleeding, haemostasis was achieved. Restenosis necessitating colostomy formation occurred in three patients. Two patients suffered post-treatment haemorrhage requiring blood transfusion and one patient developed a pararectal abscess. Several interventional sessions are often required to achieve resolution of symptoms. Naveau *et al* (1986) treated 45 patients with rectal carcinoma palliatively and showed cessation of bleeding in 89% and restoration of luminal patency in 80% with a minimum of three sessions; total destruction of intraluminal tumour was possible in 40% [34]. Bown *et al* (1986) advocated laser therapy as the only safe non-surgical therapy for lesions above the peritoneal reflection [35]. In their series of 17 patients presenting with obstruction, bleeding, diarrhoea or incontinence improvement was seen in 15 (88%). Walfisch *et al* (1989) treated seven patients with metastatic colonic obstruction along with benign strictures and large villous tumours [36]. No lesion was beyond 30cm from the anal verge and in the lowermost lesions prior manual debulking facilitated laser therapy. All patients achieved symptomatic improvement and, though perforation was identified in one patient, this responded to

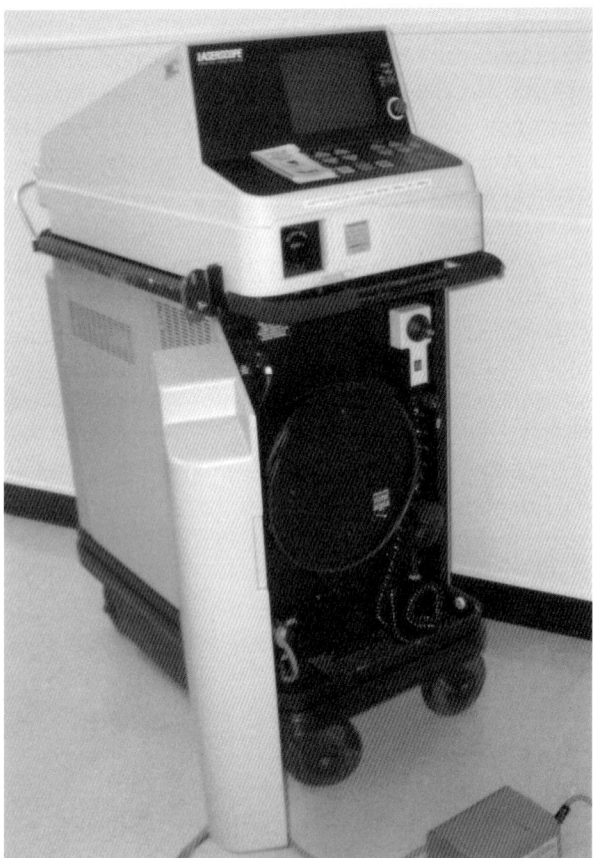

Figure 5. Illustration of a Neodynium: yttrium-aluminum-garnet (Nd:YAG) laser used to ablate obstructing rectosigmoid carcinoma. Reproduced with permission from LASERSCOPE, San Jose, CA, USA.

antibiotics. Laser therapy is not time-consuming: Mandava et al (1991) reported a mean duration of treatment of 40 (range 30-90) minutes in 27 patients with rectal or sigmoid cancers treated palliatively [37]. The cancers had a maximum distance from the anal verge of 25cm and a mean lesion length of 5cm. Mesko et al (1993) reported that in 53 patients treated palliatively the mean treatment session time was 35 (range 25 to 90) minutes [38].

Chia et al (1991) reported 20 cases with rectal carcinoma in whom adequate palliation was achieved [39]. However, whilst obstruction was relieved with one session, haemostasis took on average two sessions. Though most symptoms, such as obstruction and bleeding, can be treated successfully, larger lesions often require repeat sessions. Mlkvy et al (1994) showed that of 126 patients treated, 112 had larger tumours and of these, 84 had tumours that occupied three quarters of the lumen [40]. These 112 patients required an average of 3.7 sessions to achieve symptom improvement. Schulze and Lyng (1994) showed that in 55 patients with either disseminated or complex rectosigmoid lesions or with severe comorbidity, 74% experienced symptomatic relief [41]. However, Nd:YAG laser induced five perforations and one case of bleeding. Bleeding can be so severe that it may necessitate surgery. Rantala and Ovaska (1995) in their series noted that of 20 patients palliated, one patient required an abdominoperineal resection for bleeding after laser treatment [42]. Sometimes laser therapy may not completely resolve symptoms but does improve them. Tan et al (1995) reviewed 26 cases treated with Nd:YAG laser therapy, 12 (46%) presenting with obstruction, ten (39%) with bleeding and four (15%) with diarrhoea [43]. Of those followed-up, 12 (46%) had total relief and 12 (46%) had partial relief. The mean interval for treatment sessions was 7.3 (range 1-20) weeks and two deaths were reported, one from cardiac failure and the other from stercoral perforation. After a mean follow-up of 51 (range 9-84) weeks, four remained alive. The mean follow-up of the others was 5 (range 0-23) months. Farouk et al (1997) conducted a study to assess the degree of symptom relief, complication rate and survival time in patients being treated palliatively in 41 consecutive patients [44]. Thirty-three received treatment for the primary tumour and eight for local recurrence following surgery. The mean survival time was 19 (range 1-60) months and 7 (range 18-41) months respectively. For both groups the mean number of treatments was two and the interval between treatments was 6 weeks. Four patients decided to undergo palliative surgery and five others eventually had a loop colostomy. The authors stated that, whilst laser ablation was effective in palliating symptoms, surgery may still be indicated if patients survived for longer than 24 months. Gevers et al (2000) conducted a retrospective analysis in 219 patients with rectal cancer from 1986 to 1995 referred for palliative laser therapy [45]. After initial resolution of symptoms in 198 (92%), therapy for obstruction was repeated at intervals from 2-4 months and those with bleeding, tenesmus or diarrhoea were only treated if symptomatic. The total number of treatments was significantly higher if obstruction was present at presentation and if tumours were circumferential. The survival rate in the group was 44.4% at 1 year and 20.4% at 2 years. Complications included perforation (4.1%), fistulae (3.2%), abscess formation (1.7%) and bleeding (4.1%) and the authors identified five deaths from laser ablation. Jakobs et al (2002) reviewed their experience with laser ablation for palliation of rectal cancer over a 10-year period in 83 consecutive patients [46]. Although 80 of 84 (96%) experienced initial resolution of symptoms, during later follow-up eight required surgery for treatment failures, such as recurrent obstruction or complications.

There have been several reports advocating radiotherapy to enhance palliation with lasers. Sargeant et al (1993) gave external beam radiotherapy after initial laser therapy to 13 patients in order to reduce the frequency of laser treatments required [47]. In this series further treatments were only required every 19 (range 6-53) weeks and the laser energy required reduced from 15,000 joules/month to 2000 joules/month after radiotherapy. Further evidence from Chapuis et al (2002) showed that the crude relapse rate of symptoms was significantly higher in the laser only group than in the laser plus radiotherapy group with no additional morbidity [48].

Cryosurgery

Cryosurgery has not gained wide acceptance in surgical fields. Yamamoto et al (1989) used this modality in 27 patients to control bleeding or recurrent tumour bulk without complications [49]. Recently, Meijer et al (1999) reported on 106 patients undergoing palliative cryosurgery for primary rectal cancer [50]. Sixty-six (62%) described complete relief of local symptoms, particularly of rectal bleeding or mucous discharge. In 17 (16%), palliation was moderate, and in 23 (22%) no palliation was achieved. Despite the lack of enthusiastic proponents it appears to be a simple and safe procedure.

Surgery

Surgery in the palliative setting is indicated to provide relief of disabling symptoms in those in whom disease is advanced, locally extensive, or when the comorbid risks of putative curative surgery are great. Symptoms that may be surgically palliated include obstruction, uncontrollable rectal bleeding or diarrhoea. Those arising from local tumour perforation, fistulae and invasion of local structures result in pain [51].

A colostomy is effective in palliating impending or actual obstruction and a trephine stoma can be constructed with minimal risk to the patient (Figure 6) [52, 53]. Alternatively, laparoscopic techniques allow for accurate mobilisation of bowel and facilitate a rapid assessment of intrabdominal disease. For obstructing left colonic malignancies sigmoid colostomies are favoured over transverse colostomies as they prolapse less.

Endoscopic transanal excision of rectal cancer (ETAR) performed with a urological resectoscope is a relatively minimally invasive approach. Hamy et al (2003) reported on 46 patients who underwent this technique from 1992 to 2000 [54]. Twenty-four patients (52%) had locally advanced rectal cancer with a tumour length greater than 5cm. The mortality rate was 2% and morbidity occurred in 8%. The mean postoperative stay was 5.5 (range 3-16) days and the median survival time was 14 (range 0-62) months. However, eight patients went on to have a colostomy.

Resection is dependent on surgical experience and accuracy of pre-operative assessment of advanced disease. The associated morbidity of surgical resection must be balanced against the expected quality of life envisaged in the postoperative period and a multidisciplinary approach is essential. Surgical options include colectomy, Hartmann's procedure or abdominoperineal resection. Law et al (2000) analysed 24 patients who underwent total pelvic exenteration from 1983 to 1998 for locally advanced rectal cancer [55]. Bowel continuity was restored in 60%, though over half of the patients experienced complications. The overall 5-year survival was 44%. Advances in pre-operative imaging and chemoradiotherapy have resulted in even better patient selection.

Laparoscopic surgery is emerging as an established technique in the surgical palliative setting. Milsom et al (2000) conducted a prospective

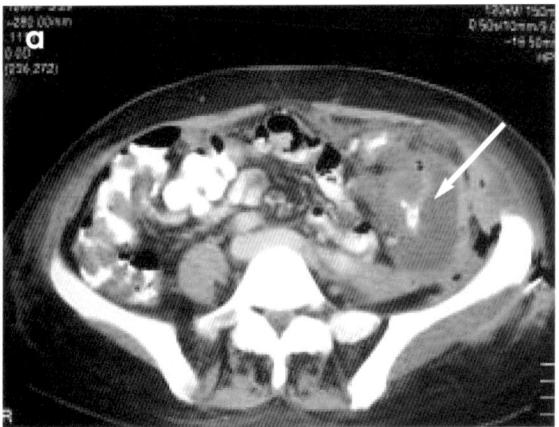

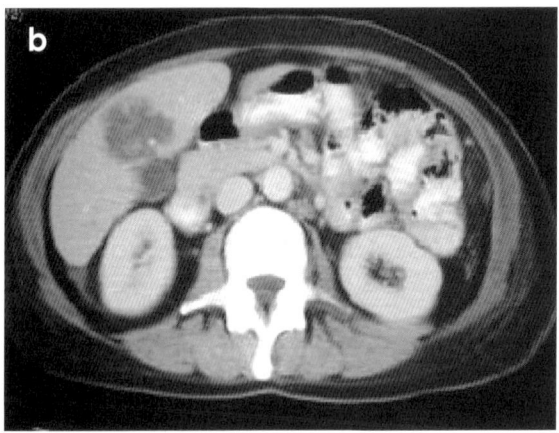

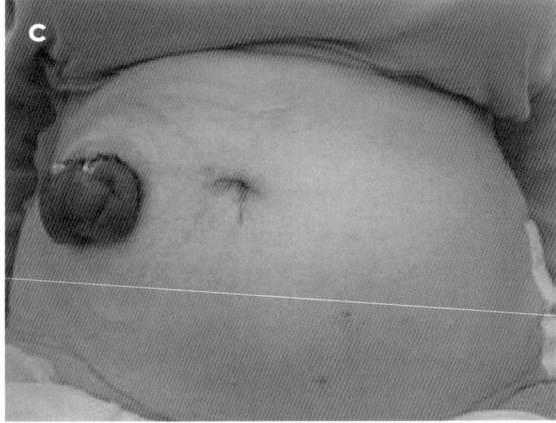

Figure 6. a) CT scan demonstrating disseminated sigmoid carcinoma with enterocutanous fistula; b) with liver metastases; and c) subsequent laparoscopically assisted formation of palliative colostomy. Reproduced with permission from Mr. H Wegstapel, Consultant Surgeon, Medway Maritime Hospital, Gilligham, UK.

analysis of 30 patients with incurable rectal cancer with 15 undergoing resection of a single segment of bowel, one had two segments excised due to synchronous lesions, and stomas were formed in 11 patients [56]. Three patients were converted to an open procedure. Morino *et al* (2002) presented four endolaparoscopic cases in whom the malignant obstruction was relieved by initial placement of a SEMS followed by laparoscopic resection after a delay of 4 or 5 days [57]. The patients were discharged 5-7 days after surgery. Hasegawa *et al* (2003) randomised 59 patients with T2 or T3 lesions to either laparoscopic (n=29) or open (n=30) colectomy [58]. Whilst the operation time was longer, blood loss and postoperative analgesic requirements were less in the laparoscopic group than in the open group. In the laparoscopic arm an earlier return of bowel motility and earlier discharge from the hospital was noted. Postoperative complications did not differ between the two groups. The authors concluded that laparoscopic surgery for advanced colorectal cancer is feasible with a favourable short-term outcome.

Where are we going?

There are numerous strategies available for the clinician invasively to palliate colorectal carcinoma. The choice of which modality to employ is entirely dependent on the experience of the clinician using those techniques and availability of local infrastructure to support such clinical services. Whilst laser therapy and cryosurgery seemed promising they have not been widely accepted. Stenting can be established in most centres but requires considerable training to avoid complications during the procedure. Surgery, though accessible in all centres, may not be suitable for all cases. It is imperative that established techniques are validated and lessons learnt. Recent developments in cancer service provision, such as multidisciplinary meetings, allow for a frank exchange of ideas and optimum palliation of colorectal symptoms. Some clinical issues of invasive palliative treatments may only be resolved by randomised trials.

References

1. Smith JJ, Tekkis PP, Thompson MR, et al. ACPGBI Colorectal Cancer Study 2004. Dendrite Clinical Systems, Oxfordshire 2004.
2. Tekkis PP, Poloniecki JD, Thompson MR, et al. ACPGBI Colorectal cancer study 2002. Part A: Unadjusted outcomes. Dendrite Clinical Systems, Oxfordshire, 2002.
3. Soonawalla Z, Thakur K, Boorman P, et al. Use of self-expanding metallic stents in the management of obstruction of the sigmoid colon. Am J Roentgenol 1998; 171(3): 633-6
4. Lecluk S, Ratan J, Klausner JM, et al. Endoscopic decompression of acute colonic obstruction. Avoiding staged surgery. Ann Surg 1986; 203: 292-4.
5. Keen RR, Orsay CP. Rectosigmoid stent for obstructing colonic neoplasms. Dis Colon Rectum 1992; 35: 912-3.
6. Dohmoto M. New Method - endoscopic implantation of rectal stent in palliative treatment of malignant stenosis. Endoscopica Digestiva 1991; 3: 1507-12.
7. Spinelli P, Dal Fante M, Mancini A. Rectal metal stents for palliation of colorectal malignant stenosis. Bildgebung 1993; 60 Suppl 1: 48-50.
8. Rey JF, Romanczyk T, Greff M. Metal stents for palliation of rectal carcinoma: a preliminary report on 12 patients. Endoscopy 1995; 27(7): 501-4.
9. Dohmoto M, Hunerbein M, Schlag PM. Application of rectal stents for palliation of obstructing rectosigmoid cancer. Surg Endosc 1997; 11(7): 758-61.
10. Turegano-Fuentes F, Echenagusia-Belda A, Simo-Muerza G, et al. Transanal self-expanding metal stents as an alternative to palliative colostomy in selected patients with malignant obstruction of the left colon. Br J Surg 1998; 85: 232-5.
11. Tack J, Gevers AM, Rutgeerts P. Self-expandable metallic stents in the palliation of rectosigmoidal carcinoma: a follow-up study. Gastrointest Endosc 1998; 48: 267-71.
12. De Gregorio MA, Mainar A, Tejero E, et al. Acute colorectal obstruction: stent placement for palliative treatment - results of a multicenter study. Radiology 1998; 209: 117-20.
13. Paul DL, Pinto P, I, Fernandez LR, et al. Palliative treatment of malignant colorectal strictures with metallic stents. Cardiovasc Intervent Radiol 1999; 22: 29-36.
14. Fernandez Lobato R, Pinto I, Paul L, et al. Self-expanding prostheses as a palliative method in treating advanced colorectal cancer. Int Surg 1999; 84: 159-62.
15. Coco C, Cogliandolo S, Riccioni ME, et al. Use of a self-expanding stent in the palliation of rectal cancer recurrences. A report of three cases. Surg Endosc 2000; 14(8): 708-11.
16. Law WL, Chu KW, Ho JW, et al. Self-expanding metallic stent in the treatment of colonic obstruction caused by advanced malignancies. Dis Colon Rectum 2000; 43(11):1522-7.
17. Miyayama S, Matsui O, Kifune K, et al. Malignant colonic obstruction due to extrinsic tumor: palliative treatment with a self-expanding nitinol stent. Am J Roentgenol 2000; 175(6):1631-7.
18. Ben Soussan E, Savoye G, Hochain P, et al. Expandable metal stents in palliative treatment of malignant colorectal stricture. A report of 17 consecutive patients. Gastroenterol Clin Biol 2001; 25(5): 463-7.
19. Repici A, Reggio D, De Angelis C, et al. Covered metal stents for management of inoperable malignant colorectal strictures. Gastrointest Endosc 2000; 5: 735-40.
20. Spinelli P, Mancini A. Use of self-expanding metal stents for palliation of rectosigmoid cancer. Gastrointest Endosc 2001; 53(2): 203-6.
21. Araki Y, Sato Y, Kido K, et al. Endoluminal ultraflex stent for palliative treatment of malignant rectosigmoidal obstruction. Kurume Med J 2002; 49(3): 81-5.
22. Xinopoulos D, Dimitroulopoulos D, Tsamakidis K, et al. Treatment of malignant colonic obstructions with metal stents and laser. Hepatogastroenterology 2002; 49: 359-62.
23. Grunshaw ND, Ball CS. Palliative treatment of an enterorectal fistula with a covered metallic stent. Cardiovasc Intervent Radiol 2001; 24(6): 438-40.
24. Aviv RI, Shyamalan G, Watkinson A, et al. Radiological palliation of malignant colonic obstruction. Clin Radiol 2002; 57: 347-51.
25. Seymour K, Johnson R, Marsh R, et al. Palliative stenting of malignant large bowel obstruction. Colorectal Dis 2002; 4(4): 240-5.
26. Clark JS, Buchanan GN, Khawaja AR, et al. Use of the Bard Memotherm self-expanding metal stent in the palliation of colonic obstruction. Abdom Imaging 2003; 28(4): 518-24.
27. Law WL, Choi HK, Chu KW. Comparison of stenting with emergency surgery as palliative treatment for obstructing primary left-sided colorectal cancer. Br J Surg 2003; 90(11): 1429-33.
28. Johnson R, Marsh R, Corson J, et al. A comparison of two methods of palliation of large bowel obstruction due to irremovable colon cancer. Ann R Coll Surg Engl 2004; 86(2): 99-103.
29. Xinopoulos D, Dimitroulopoulos D, Theodosopoulos T, et al. Stenting or stoma creation for patients with inoperable malignant colonic obstructions? Results of a study and cost-effectiveness analysis. Surg Endosc 2004; 18(3): 421-6.
30. Osman HS, Rashid HI, Sathananthan N, et al. The cost effectiveness of self expanding metal stents in the management of malignant left-sided large bowel obstruction. Colorectal Dis 2000; 2: 233-7.
31. Khot U, Wenk Lang A, Murali K, et al. Systematic review of the clinical evidence on colorectal self-expanding metal stents. Br J Surg 2002; 89: 1096-102.
32. Scurtu R, Barrier A, Andre T, et al. Self-expandable metallic stent for palliative treatment of colorectal malignant obstructions: risk of perforation. Ann Chir 2003; 128(6): 359-63.
33. Mathus-Vliegen EM, Tytgat GN. Laser photocoagulation in the palliation of colorectal malignancies. Cancer 1986; 57(11): 2212-6.
34. Naveau S, Roulot D, Zourabichvili O, et al. Palliative treatment of adenocarcinoma of the rectum by Nd-YAG laser. Immediate and long-term results. Study of factors related to the initial destruction of the tumor. Gastroenterol Clin Biol 1986; 10(10): 651-5.
35. Bown SG, Barr H, Matthewson K, et al. Endoscopic treatment of inoperable colorectal cancers with the Nd-YAG laser. Br J Surg 1986; 73(12): 949-52.

36. Walfisch S, Stern H, Ball S. Use of Nd-Yag laser ablation in colorectal obstruction and palliation in high-risk patients. *Dis Colon Rectum* 1989; 32(12): 1060-4.
37. Mandava N, Petrelli N, Herrera L, *et al.* Nava H. Laser palliation for colorectal carcinoma. *Am J Surg* 1991; 162(3): 212-4.
38. Mesko TW, Petrelli NJ, Rodriguez-Bigas M, *et al.* Nava H. Endoscopic laser treatment for palliation of colorectal adenocarcinoma. *Surg Oncol* 1993; 2(1): 25-30.
39. Chia YW, Ngoi SS, Goh PM. Endoscopic Nd:YAG laser in the palliative treatment of advanced low rectal carcinoma in Singapore. *Dis Colon Rectum* 1991; 34(12): 1093-6.
40. Mlkvy P, Vrablik V, Kralik G, *et al.* Endoscopic ND:YAG laser treatment of rectosigmoidal cancer. *Neoplasma* 1994; 41(5): 285-9.
41. Schulze S, Lyng KM. Palliation of rectosigmoid neoplasms with Nd:YAG laser treatment. *Dis Colon Rectum* 1994; 37(9): 882-4.
42. Rantala A, Ovaska J. Palliative laser treatment of rectal cancer. *Scand J Gastroenterol* 1995; 30(2): 177-9.
43. Tan CC, Iftikhar SY, Allan A, *et al.* Local effects of colorectal cancer are well palliated by endoscopic laser therapy. *Eur J Surg Oncol* 1995; 21(6): 648-52.
44. Farouk R, Ratnaval CD, Monson JR, *et al.* Staged delivery of Nd:YAG laser therapy for palliation of advanced rectal carcinoma. *Dis Colon Rectum* 1997; 40(2): 156-60.
45. Gevers AM, Macken E, Hiele M, *et al.* Endoscopic laser therapy for palliation of patients with distal colorectal carcinoma: analysis of factors influencing long-term outcome. *Gastrointest Endosc* 2000; 51(5): 580-5.
46. Jakobs R, Miola J, Eickhoff A, *et al.* Endoscopic laser palliation for rectal cancer - therapeutic outcome and complications in eighty-three consecutive patients. *Z Gastroenterol* 2002; 40(8): 551-6.
47. Sargeant IR, Tobias JS, Blackman G, *et al.* Radiation enhancement of laser palliation for advanced rectal and rectosigmoid cancer: a pilot study. *Gut* 1993; 34(7): 958-62.
48. Chapuis PH, Yuile P, Dent OF, *et al.* Combined endoscopic laser and radiotherapy palliation of advanced rectal cancer. *ANZ J Surg* 2002; 72(2): 95-9.
49. Yamamoto Y, Sano K, Kimoto M. Cryosurgical treatment for anorectal cancer. A method of palliative or adjunctive management. *Am Surg* 1989; 55(4): 252-6.
50. Meijer S, Rahusen FD, van der Plas LG. Palliative cryosurgery for rectal carcinoma. *Int J Colorectal Dis* 1999; 14(3): 177-80.
51. Fazio VW. Indications and surgical alternatives for palliation of rectal cancer. *J Gastrointest Surg* 2004; 8(3): 262-5.
52. Senapati A, Nicholls RJ. Formation of a loop stoma. *Br J Surg* 1991; 78(1): 23.
53. Senapati A, Phillips RKS. The trephine colostomy: a permanent left iliac fossa end colostomy without recourse to Laparotomy. *Ann R Coll Surg Engl* 1991; 73: 305-6
54. Hamy A, Tuech JJ, Pessaux P, *et al.* Palliation of carcinoma of the rectum using the urologic resectoscope. *Surg Endosc* 2003; 17(4): 627-31.
55. Law WL, Chu KW, Choi HK. Total pelvic exenteration for locally advanced rectal cancer. *J Am Coll Surg* 2000; 190(1): 78-83.
56. Milsom JW, Kim SH, Hammerhofer KA, *et al.* Laparoscopic colorectal cancer surgery for palliation. *Dis Colon Rectum* 2000; 43(11): 1512-6.
57. Morino M, Bertello A, Garbarini A, *et al.* Malignant colonic obstruction managed by endoscopic stent decompression followed by laparoscopic resections. *Surg Endosc* 2002; 16(10): 1483-7.
58. Hasegawa H, Kabeshima Y, Watanabe M, *et al.* Randomized controlled trial of laparoscopic versus open colectomy for advanced colorectal cancer. *Surg Endosc* 2003; 17(4): 636-40.

Chapter 8

Colorectal liver metastases

Robert Hutchins MS FRCS, Consultant Hepatopancreatobiliary Surgeon
Barts and the London NHS Trust
Honorary Senior Lecturer, Institute of Cancer, London, UK

Jina Krissat MD, Liver Surgeon, Centre Hepatobiliaire, Hopital Paul-Brousse, Paris, France

Satya Bhattacharya MS MPhil FRCS, Consultant Hepatopancreatobiliary Surgeon
Barts and the London NHS Trust, London, UK

What is the problem?

Fifteen to thirty percent of patients with colorectal cancer are found to have synchronous liver metastases. A similar proportion will go on to develop metastatic liver disease usually within the first 2-5 years of their disease. Unlike other solid tumours, the resection of colorectal liver metastases is now fully justified on the basis of long-term results from many series [1-12] (Table 1). Most centres can now perform this type of procedure with a mortality of less than 5% and, indeed, the commonest cause of death (historically bleeding) has now been overtaken by sepsis related to low volume residual liver, a reflection of the increasingly aggressive approach of most units.

However, only 20% of patients are suitable for liver resection and 60% of those resected fail due to disseminated disease (50%) or liver recurrence (50%). The goal of liver surgeons and oncologists worldwide is to increase the proportion of patients who can be offered resection and to reduce the failure rate after operation. To this end, new technologies have been introduced into the armamentarium of liver surgeons and both neoadjuvant and adjuvant strategies are being developed.

The historical viewpoint of liver surgery is of resecting a solitary metachronous lesion by either right or left hepatectomy (unfortunately still considered as the only possible therapeutic option by some oncologists). Better understanding of the anatomical segments of the liver alongside developments such as the ultrasonic dissector, harmonic scalpel, radiofrequency probes, argon coagulator, plasma coagulator and tissue glues now allow for multiple lesions and/or bilobar lesions to be resected. The limiting factor for resection now is if the lesions cannot be removed in their entirety, leaving behind sufficient functional volume with an intact vascular and biliary system (this may be reconstructed if necessary). The exact margin of clearance is debatable. A margin of at least 1cm has been suggested as necessary [2,3,13]. However, lesser margins even down to 0cm have been reported to equate to better long-term survival than can be achieved with chemotherapy [1,6,11,12,14,15]. The exact margin is also confused by the type of resection carried out. Radiofrequency-assisted resections may "sterilise" 2-5mm of remaining liver tissue and the ultrasonic dissector has a tendency to wash away some of the achieved margin.

Extrahepatic disease generally has been viewed as a contra-indication to curative resection. There are now series of long-term survivors with resection of limited pulmonary metastases. Hilar lymphadenopathy is generally thought of as representing spread of

Table 1. Recent large series of resection of colorectal liver metastases.

Authors	Country	Year	No. of patients	Peri-operative mortality (%)	5-year survival (%)	Recurrence rate (%)
Rosen et al [1]	USA	1992	280	4	25	-
Scheele et al [2]	Germany	1995	434	4.4	39	60
Nordlinger et al [3]	France	1996	1568 *	2.3	28	55
Rees et al [4]	UK	1997	107	1	30	69
Bismuth et al [5]	France	1997	243	0.8	39	-
Ohlsson et al [6]	Sweden	1998	111	3.6	25	76
Fong et al [7]	USA	1999	1001	2.8	37	-
Sugihara et al [8]	Japan	2000	330	0	44	71
DeMatteo et al [9]	USA	2000	267	0.4	43	51
Seifert et al [10]	Germany	2000	120	5.8	31	62
Minagawa et al [11]	Japan	2001	235	0	38	73
Choti et al [12]	USA	2002	226	0.9	40	62

* multicentre study

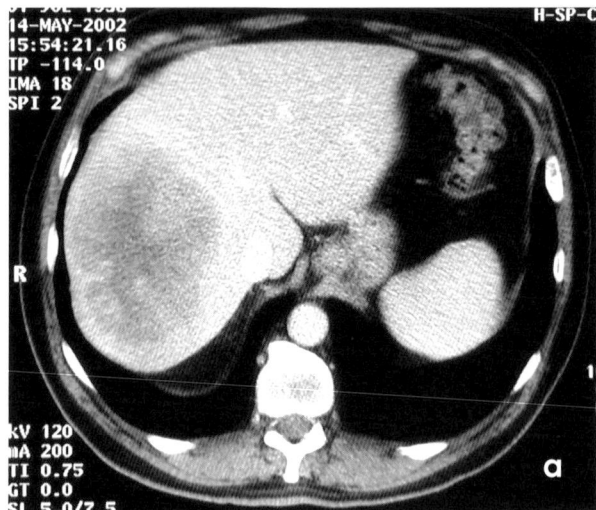 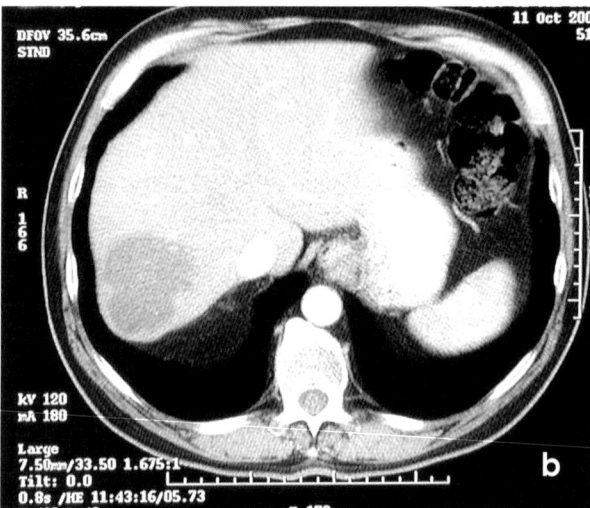

Figure 1. a) Large metastatic deposit in the right lobe of the liver from previously resected colon cancer. There were concerns about the proximity of the tumour to the inferior vena cava and the confluence of the right and left portal veins. b) Significant tumour response was seen after systemic chemotherapy with six cycles of 5-fluorouracil and oxaliplatin. The lesion was then successfully resected with adequate margins.

disease from the liver to its draining lymph node bed. Few long-term survivors have been reported once these nodes are involved. Many centres would consider this a contra-indication to liver resection. However, against this are now 5-year survivors (albeit less than 10%) even with combined resection of liver and limited peritoneal disease [16].

Where are we now?

Strategies to improve resection rates

Portal vein embolisation

Portal vein embolisation was developed from the observation that primary liver tumours involving a main portal venous branch induced atrophy of the affected liver and compensatory hypertrophy of the unaffected side. The portal vein can be approached by direct liver puncture and a variety of particles, glue, alcohol or microspheres used to occlude the venous supply of the segments to be resected. Within 4-6 weeks, sufficient hypertrophy of the unaffected side will have occurred to allow for a larger volume of residual functional liver to remain after resection. This approach is used if the volume of the remaining liver after resection is less than 40% in a cirrhotic or 25% in a normal liver. It is extremely safe and well tolerated with sufficient hypertrophy reported in up to 68-78% [17,18]. Five-year survival after portal vein embolisation can be achieved in 35% [19]. The place of chemotherapy in and around portal vein embolisation is unknown. Initial experience would suggest that it does not affect the potential hypertrophic effect of embolisation and may lead to a decrease in tumour size (unpublished data).

Neoadjuvant chemotherapy

The goal of neoadjuvant chemotherapy is to downstage initially unresectable tumours and render them suitable for resection (Figure 1). No randomised trial of this approach has been carried out but evidence certainly exists that tumour response rates with 5-folinic acid (5-FU) and oxaliplatin or 5-FU and irinotecan-based therapies are in the order of 50%. Survival after neoadjuvant therapy and resection has been reported to be as high as with liver resection alone [20]. One of the earliest studies of this approach (which included pulmonary metastectomy and re-hepatectomy) was reported by Bismuth et al [21]. In this series 16% of patients considered to have initially unresectable disease were downstaged to a resectable option. Of the 53 patients who had liver surgery the 5-year survival was 40% (Table 2).

Staged hepatectomy

Insufficient parenchyma to allow resection of all lesions may not preclude liver resection on a planned staged basis. This allows sufficient hypertrophy between resections to perform a second-stage procedure usually 3-6 months after the first operation. The success of this radical approach is unknown but early results would suggest its feasibility and safety [27].

Strategies to reduce recurrence

Neoadjuvant chemotherapy

Is there a role for neoadjuvant chemotherapy in the setting of initially resectable lesions? The rationale behind this therapy would be to limit the amount of liver removed at operation and perhaps to improve the outcome especially in poor prognosis groups. The outcome of liver resections for metastatic colorectal disease appears to depend on the number of lesions, size of lesions, margin of clearance, pre-operative CEA, blood requirements/losses, Dukes' stage of initial lesion and extent of resection.

Reducing the volume of liver resected may allow for further hepatectomy to be performed in the future. On the assumption that 60% of patients will fail treatment, this is not an unreasonable consideration. This approach is only acceptable if lesser resections lead to a similar long-term outcome. There is now evidence to support this more conservative approach [9,11,28].

A period of neoadjuvant therapy may also select out those patients who rapidly go on to develop widespread metastases despite treatment. It may also improve the outcome of those patients who, while having resectable lesions, fall into the poorer prognostic groups. A recent study from Tanaka et al has compared the efficacy of neoadjuvant chemotherapy before hepatectomy in those patients with multiple (>5) bilobar lesions with surgery alone.

Table 2. Neoadjuvant chemotherapy prior to resection of colorectal liver metastases.

Authors	Year	No. of patients	Regimen	Route	Outcome
Bismuth et al [21]	1996	53	5-FU/leucovorin/ oxaliplatin	IV	40% 5-year survival
Fowler et al [22]	1992	11	5-FU/leucovorin	IV	3 disease-free at 15, 18, 31 months
Elias et al [23]	1995	9	5-FU/mitomycin C or epirubicin	IA	6 disease-free at a mean of 20 months
Shankar et al [24]	1999	12	5-FU/leucovorin	IV	53% 3-year survival
Link et al [25]	1999	50	5-FU/folic acid/ mitoxantrone/ mitomycin C	IA	Median survival 27.4 months
Tanaka et al [26] *	2003	48	5-FU/folic acid/ oxaliplatin or irinotecan	IV	38.9% 5-year survival vs 20.7% 16.4% 2-year disease-free survival vs 0% δ

δ=from the time of diagnosis of liver metastases; 5-FU=5-fluorouracil; IV=intravenous; IA=intra-arterial; * retrospective study comparing patients with multiple bilobar liver metastases receiving neoadjuvant chemotherapy + surgery, versus surgery alone

The 5-year survival from diagnosis of liver lesions was better in the combined treatment group (38.9 v 20.7% respectively) and the 2-year disease-free survival after hepatectomy was 16.4% in the chemotherapy group compared with 0% in the surgery alone group [26].

Adjuvant chemotherapy (Table 3)

Hepatic metastases derive their blood supply from the hepatic artery unlike hepatocytes which are mainly supplied by portal venous radicals. Hepatic arterial infusion of chemotherapy therefore appears an attractive option to treat micrometastases or liver only recurrence. Initial studies suggested a response rate of 42-62% compared with 10-21% for systemic chemotherapy [38,39]. However, this treatment has not been shown to increase survival over systemic chemotherapy. A large number of both randomised and historical studies have examined the role of regionally-based treatment as adjuvant therapy following liver resection with conflicting results. Some small studies have suggested improved survival. A larger study by Lorenz et al failed to find any advantage with regional therapy [32]. In this study, however, only 74% of those assigned to regional treatment actually received this therapy. On analysing patients actually given treatment, the median disease-free survival was improved from 23.3 to 44.8 months.

The limiting factor with regional therapy is systemic recurrence. A more logical approach therefore might be to incorporate both regional and systemic therapies together. Kemeny et al randomised 72 patients after hepatectomy to receive combined treatment and 82 to receive systemic chemotherapy alone [36]. Six cycles were given during the first year after resection. Median survival was significantly increased from 59.3 to 72.2 months in favour of the combined treatment modality group, as was the 2-year disease-free survival (90% v 60%).

At present, however, the role of adjuvant therapy and its mode of delivery remains an unanswered question. Also unknown is the type of chemotherapeutic agent to be given. Most early studies were based on fluoropyrimidines and not

8 Colorectal liver metastases

Table 3. Adjuvant chemotherapy after surgical resection of colorectal liver metastases.

Authors	Year	No. of patients	Drugs	Route	Control	Outcome (%)
Lygidakis et al [29]	1995	20	5-FU, MMC, δ-IFN, IL-2, LV, epirubicin, carboplatin	HAI	Randomised	MS: 20 vs 11 months
Tsuji et al [30]	1995	12	5-FU	HAI	Randomised	3-yr S: 69% vs 25%
Asahara et al [31]	1998	10	5-FU	HAI	Historic	3-yr DFS: 100% vs 42%
Lorenz et al [32]	1998	108	5-FU, FA	HAI	Randomised	MDFS: 21.6 vs 24 months
Rudroff et al [33]	1999	14	5-FU, MMC	HAI	Randomised	5-yr DFS: 23 vs 15 months
Tono et al [34]	1999	9	5-FU	HAI	Randomised	3-yr DFS: 67 vs 20 months
Ambiru et al [35]	1999	78	5-FU, MMC, aclarubicin	HAI	Historic	5-yr DFS: 35 vs 9 months
Kemeny et al [36]	1999	74	FUDR, IV 5-FU+ LV	HAI+ IV	Randomised *	2-yr DFS: 57 vs 42 months
Figueras et al [37]	2001	99	5-FU, FA	IV	Historic	5-yr S: 53% vs 25%

HAI=hepatic arterial infusion; IV=systemic chemotherapy; 5-FU=5-fluorouracil; MMC=mitomycin C; FUDR= floxuridine; LV=leucovorin; IFN=interferon; IL=interleukin; FA=folinic acid; S=survival; MS=median survival; DFS=disease-free survival; MDFS=median disease-free survival; * vs systemic chemotherapy

newer agents with better response rates such as oxaliplatin or irinotecan.

Treatment of recurrence

There is evidence to support an aggressive surgical policy of offering repeat resection for recurrent liver metastases. Repeat hepatectomy can provide long-term outcome similar to primary liver resections and can be carried out with acceptable mortality [40]. Repeat resection is only possible in about one third of patients because of either diffuse liver disease or extrahepatic recurrence. Systemic chemotherapy remains the mainstay of treatment of those who cannot be offered further surgical intervention.

Ablative therapies

Initial experience with cryotherapy for liver tumours suggested a high morbidity for this procedure. However, as ablative therapies have developed and interstitial laser therapy as well as radiofrequency ablation introduced, it has become apparent that the initial problems with cryotherapy were secondary to its learning curve and the technical difficulties encountered with destructive therapy within the liver. The role of this treatment however, has still not been established. Suggestions that it is equivalent to surgical resection are probably unfounded [41]. Although the initial survival curves matched well, long-term outcome in this study was far superior with surgical resection. Ablation remains, however, an extremely useful local treatment providing good control of disease. It obviously fails to control systemic disease and therefore may be more useful combined with other treatment modalities. It has also been used in the setting of combination resection/ablation for multiple lesions and to avoid second or third hepatectomy with good outcome.

Where are we going?

It is likely that in the future the role of adjuvant and neoadjuvant therapies will become clearer with the results of EORTC multicentre trials currently underway. In one of these studies, surgery alone for resectable disease is being compared to surgery plus "sandwich" neoadjuvant 3-monthly and adjuvant 3-monthly chemotherapy. The role of ablative therapy may also become clearer with the chemotherapy versus chemotherapy plus radioablation CLOCC study. The goal of the liver surgeon to produce bloodless liver surgery will continue to provide innovative technologies which will benefit not only liver surgeons but other specialities. Examples of this include the application of radiofrequency-assisted surgery to urology and orthopaedics.

Further developments in targeted treatment may arise from the use of monoclonal antibody therapy. It has already been demonstrated that in those patients who fail with second-line chemotherapy, the combination of cetuximab (an epithelial growth factor receptor [EGFR] anatagonist) with irinotecan can improve response rates and survival [42]. This opens the door for adjuvant therapy based on the resected tumour's proteome pattern in order to reduce recurrence rates. Further monoclonal antibody treatments based again on EGFR and its tyrosine kinase downstream signalling pathway include gefitinib and erlotonib.

The other major goal of both liver and colorectal surgeons will be the ability to predict those patients who will go on to develop recurrence within their liver on a certain basis. The development of both genomic and proteomic technologies will almost certainly help provide this important information to improve the outcome further of patients with this disease.

References

1. Rosen CB, Nagorney DM, Taswell HF, *et al*. Perioperative blood transfusion and determinants of survival after liver resection for metastatic colorectal carcinoma. *Ann Surg* 1992; 216: 493-505.
2. Scheele J, Stang R, Altendorf-Hofmann A, Paul M. Resection of colorectal liver metastases. *World J Surg* 1995; 19: 59-71.
3. Nordlinger B, Jaeck D, Guiguet M. Surgical resection of hepatic metastases: multicentric retrospective study by the French Surgical Association. In: *Treatment of hepatic metastases*. Nordlinger B, Jaeck D, Eds. Springer, Paris, 1992: 129-46.
4. Rees M, Plant G, Bygrave S. Late results justify resection for multiple hepatic metastases from colorectal cancer. *Br J Surg* 1997; 84: 1136-40.
5. Bismuth H, Krissat J, Adam R. Evidence for metastasectomy for colorectal liver metastases. In: *The effective management of metastatic colorectal cancer*. Cunningham D, Allen-Mersh TG, Miles A, Eds. Radcliffe Medical Press, Oxford, 1999: 12-24.
6. Ohlsson B, Stenram U, Tranberg KG. Resection of colorectal liver metastases: 25-year experience. *World J Surg* 1998; 22: 268-77.
7. Fong Y, Fortner J, Sun RL, Brennan MF, Blumgart LH. Clinical score for predicting recurrence after hepatic resecion for metastatic colorectal cancer. Analysis of 1001 consecutive cases. *Ann Surg* 1999; 230: 309-21.
8. Sugihara K, Yamamoto J. Surgical treatment of colorectal liver metastases. *Annales Chirurgiae et Gynaecologiae* 2000; 89: 221-4.
9. DeMatteo RP, Palese C, Jarnagin WR, Sun RL, Blumgart LH, Fong Y. Anatomic segmental hepatic resection is superior to wedge resection as an oncologic operation for colorectal liver metastases. *J Gastrointest Surg* 2000; 4(2): 178-84.
10. Seifert JK, Bottger TC, Weigel TF, Gonner U, Junginger T. Prognostic factors following liver resection for hepatic metastases from colorectal cancer. *Hepatogastroenterology* 2000; 47: 239-46.
11. Minagawa M, Makuuchi M, Torzilli G, *et al*. Extensions of the frontiers of surgical indications in the treatment of liver metastases from colorectal cancer. *Ann Surg* 2000; 231: 487-99.
12. Choti MA, Sitzmann JV, Tiburi MF, Sumetchotimetha W, Rangsin R, *et al*. Trends in long-term survival following liver resection for hepatic colorectal metastases. *Ann Surg* 2002; 235: 759-66.
13. Cady B, Jenkins RL, Steele GD, *et al*. Surgical margins in hepatic resection for colorectal metastases. A critical and improvable determinant of outcome. *Ann Surg* 1998; 227(4): 566-71.
14. Stephenson KR, Steinberg SM, Hughes KS, Vetto JT, Sugarbaker PH, Chang AE. Peri-operative blood transfusions are associated with decreased time to recurrence and decreased survival after resection of colorectal liver metastases. *Ann Surg* 1988; 208: 679-87.
15. Shirabe K, Takenaka K, Gion T, *et al*. Analysis of prognostic risk factors in hepatic resection for metastatic colorectal carcinoma with special reference to surgical margins. *Br J Surg* 1997; 84: 1077-80.

16. Elias D, Ouellet JF, Bellon N, Pignon JP, Pocard M, Lasser P. Extrahepatic disease does not contraindicate hepatectomy for colorectal liver metastases. *Br J Surg* 2003; 90: 567-74.
17. Hemming AW, Reed AI, Howard RJ, et al. Preoperative portal vein embolization for extended hepatectomy. *Ann Surg* 2003; 237: 686-91.
18. Fujii Y, Shimada H, Endo I, et al. Effects of portal vein embolization before major hepatectomy. *Hepatogastroenterology* 2003; 50: 438-42.
19. Elias D, Ouellet JF, De Baere T, Lasser P, Roche A. Preoperative selective portal vein embolization before hepatectomy for liver metastases: long-term results and impact on survival. *Surgery* 2002; 131: 294-9.
20. Ong SY. Neoadjuvant chemotherapy in the management of colorectal metastases: a review of the literature. *Ann Acad Med Singapore* 2003; 32: 205-11.
21. Bismuth H, R RA, Levi F, et al. Resection of non-resectable liver metastases from colorectal cancer after neoadjuvant chemotherapy. *Ann Surg* 1996; 224: 509-22.
22. Fowler WC, Eisenberg BL, Hoffman JP. Hepatic resection following systemic chemotherapy for metastatic colorectal carcinoma. *J Surg Oncol* 1992; 51: 122-5.
23. Elias D, Debaere T, Mutillo I, Cavalcanti A, Coyle C, Roche A. Intraoperative use of radiofrequency treatments allows an increase in the rate of curative liver resection. *J Surg Oncol* 1998; 67: 190-1.
24. Shankar A, Renaut AJ, Lederman J, Lees W, Gillams A, Taylor I. Neoadjuvant therapy improves resectability rates for colorectal cancer. *Br J Cancer* 1999; 80: 110.
25. Link KH, Pillasch J, Formentini A, Sunelaitis E. Downstaging by regional chemotherapy of non-resectable isolated colorectal liver metastases. *Eur J Surg Oncol* 1999; 25: 381-8.
26. Tanaka K, Adam R, Shimada H, Azoulay D, Levi F, Bismuth H. Role of neoadjuvant chemotherapy in the treatment of multiple colorectal metastases to the liver. *Br J Surg* 2003; 90: 963-9.
27. Cavallari A, Vivarelli M, Bellusci R, et al. Liver metastases from colorectal cancer: present surgical approach. *Hepatogastroenterology* 2003; 50: 2067-71.
28. Yamamoto J, Sugihara K, Kosuge T, et al. Pathologic support for limited hepatectomy in the treatment of liver metastases from colorectal cancer. *Ann Surg* 1995; 221(1): 74-8.
29. Lygidakis NJ, Ziras N, Parissis J. Resection versus resection combined with pre- and postoperative chemotherapy-immunotherapy for metastatic colorectal liver cancer. A new look at an old problem. *Hepatogastroenterology* 1995; 42: 155-61.
30. Tsuji Y, Nishimura A, Katsuki Y, Yasuda T. Preventive chemotherapy for residual liver after resection of hepatic metastases from colorectal cancer. *Gan To Kagaku Ryoho* 1995; 22: 1493-6.
31. Asahara T, Kikkawa M, Okajima M, et al. Studies of postoperative transarterial infusion chemotherapy for liver metastases of colorectal carcinoma after hepatectomy. *Hepatogastroenterology* 1998; 45: 805-11.
32. Lorenz ML, Muller HH, Schramm H, et al. Randomized trial of surgery versus surgery followed by adjuvant hepatic arterial infusion with 5-fluorouracil and folinic acid for liver metastases of colorectal cancer. *Ann Surg* 1998; 228(6): 756-62.
33. Rudroff C, Altendorf-Hofmann A, Stangl R, Scheele J. Prospective randomised trial of adjuvant hepatic-artery infusion chemotherapy after R0 resection of colorectal metastases. *Langenbecks Arch Surg* 1999; 384: 243-9.
34. Tono T, Hasuike Y, Ohzato N, Takatsuka Y, Kikkawa N. Adjuvant regional chemotherapy for colorectal liver metastases. *Cancer* 2000; 88(7): 1549-56.
35. Ambiru S, Miyasaki M, H.Ito, Nakagawa K, Shimizu H, Nakajima N. Adjuvant regional chemotherapy after hepatic resection for colorectal metastases. *Br J Surg* 1999; 86: 1025-31.
36. Kemeny N, Huang Y, Cohen AM, et al. Hepatic arterial infusion of chemotherapy after resection of hepatic metastases from colorectal cancer. *N Engl J Med* 1999; 341(27): 2039-48.
37. Figueras J, Valls C, Rafecas A, Fabregat J, Ramos E, Jaurrieta E. Resection rate and effect of postoperative chemotherapy on survival after surgery for colorectal metastases. *Br J Surg* 2001; 88: 980-5.
38. Rougier P, Laplanche A, Huguier M, Hay JM, Ollivier JM, Escat J. Hepatic arterial infusion of floxuridine in patients with liver metastases from colorectal carcinoma: long-term results of a prospective randomised trial. *J Clin Oncol* 1992; 10: 1112-8.
39. Kemeny N, Daly J, Reichman B, Geller N, Botet J, Oderman P. Randomized study of intrahepatic versus systemic infusion of fluorodeoxyuridine in patients with liver metastases from colorectal carcinoma. *Ann Intern Med* 1987; 107: 459-65.
40. Adam R, Pascal G, Azoulay D, Tanaka K, Castaing D, Bismuth H. Liver resection for colorectal metastases: the third hepatectomy. *Ann Surg* 2003; 238: 871-83.
41. Oshowo A, Gillams A, Harrison E, Lees WR, Taylor I. Comparison of resection and radiofrequency ablation for treatment of solitary colorectal liver metastases. *Br J Surg* 2003; 90: 1240-3.
42. Cunningham D, Humblet Y, Siena S, et al. Cetuximab monotherapy and cetuximab plus irinotecan in irinotecan-refractory metastatic colorectal cancer. *N Engl J Med* 2004; 351: 337-45.

Chapter 9

Evaluation and management of local recurrence

Sue Clark MD FRCS (Gen Surg), Consultant Colorectal Surgeon
Barts and the London NHS Trust, London, UK

Sina Dorudi PhD FRCS, Professor of Surgical Oncology
Barts and the London, Queen Mary's School of Medicine and Dentistry
Honorary Consultant Colorectal Surgeon
Barts and the London NHS Trust, London, UK

What is the issue?

Rectal cancer is one of the commonest malignancies in Europe and North America, occurring in approximately 8,000 people each year in the UK. Historically, up to 40% of patients developed pelvic recurrence following surgery for this tumour [1]. In recent years there have been considerable advances in the prevention of local recurrence by improved pre-operative staging, meticulous surgical technique and the use of adjuvant therapy, so that local recurrence rates of 2-4% can be achieved [2].

Despite all of this, a proportion of patients still develop locally recurrent disease within the pelvis, which can result in distressing and disabling symptoms that are not easily palliated. Many of these are otherwise healthy, without distant metastases, and are amenable to surgical resection, which provides the only chance of cure. There have been a number of reports of such surgery resulting in acceptable morbidity and mortality and 5-year survival of around 35%.

The important issues that arise are:

- Minimising the risks of local recurrence occurring in the first place.
- Determining whether intensive follow-up following rectal cancer surgery not only allows early detection of local recurrence but also improves prognosis.
- Identifying optimal investigations for a patient with suspected local recurrence.
- Selection for and planning of treatment aimed at cure.
- Providing palliation if cure is not possible.

Where are we now?

Cause of local recurrence

Recurrence confined to the pelvis is a local failure of primary treatment. The published rates of local recurrence after "curative" surgery for rectal cancer range from 2-32%. Most occur within 2 years of surgery and without treatment the median survival is around 7 months [3], with 5-year survival less than 4%.

Recurrence after anterior resection (AR) occurs outside the bowel in 80-96% [4,5], and is usually due to incomplete removal of the mesorectum containing tumour deposits [6]. Most cases of suture line recurrence are actually due to extramural disease growing in towards the bowel lumen, though disease at this site may also be caused by inadequate longitudinal resection margins or by implantation of exfoliated cells.

Risk factors for recurrence

The tumour

Rectal cancers that exhibit aneuploidy are twice as likely to recur locally as those whose cells are diploid [7], and the presence of p53 mutations has also been shown to be associated with a poorer prognosis [8].

Poorly differentiated cancers [9], those with lymphatic, venous or perineural invasion on histology [10], or with reduced stromal reaction are more likely to recur than those without these features.

Advanced Dukes' stage was strongly related to an enhanced risk of local recurrence in one large series of patients who had undergone abdominoperineal excision [11], which occurred in 9% with Dukes' A disease, 17% with Dukes' B and 41% with Dukes' C.

Cancers that are obstructing or have perforated are more likely to recur [9], as are low rectal cancers compared with those in the mid or upper rectum.

Surgical technique

Incomplete removal of the primary tumour or mesorectal lymph nodes containing tumour deposits leads to local recurrence. Involvement of the circumferential resection margin on histopathological examination of the resected specimen is associated with a high frequency of local recurrence (78% [95% CI 62-94]) compared with clear margins (10% [4-16])[12]. The technique of total mesorectal excision has reduced recurrence rates where it has been introduced. In one personal series [6] of 115 patients, the local recurrence rate was less than 4%.

Dissection of the lateral pelvic lymph nodes has attracted some interest, but is associated with high levels of morbidity without reduction in local recurrence or improvement in survival. It seems that involvement of these nodes signifies advanced disease which has usually already metastasised, so that there is little to be gained from their removal [13].

Local resection of rectal cancers can be performed under some circumstances, but is only recommended if the tumour is smaller than 3cm, well or moderately differentiated, and T1 or T2 on pre-operative staging. Even then local recurrence rates are high, with one study finding local recurrence in 28% after local excision of T1 and T2 tumours compared with 4% after radical surgery for T1N0 and T2N0 tumours [14]. This is presumably a result of the fact that spread to lymph nodes has occurred in 0-12% of T1 tumours and 12-28% of T2 tumours [15], but goes undetected and untreated after local excision.

Diagnosis

The aim of assessment of a patient with possible local recurrence of a rectal cancer is to confirm the presence of pelvic disease, assess its resectability, and to identify disease elsewhere.

Surveillance

There is controversy surrounding the value of intensive follow-up after resection of rectal cancer. It is unclear whether detection of local recurrence before it causes symptoms results in improved survival by allowing early aggressive surgery. A full discussion of this topic is presented elsewhere.

A rise in carcinoembryonic antigen (CEA) on follow-up testing triggered "second-look" surgery in a number of studies, but improved imaging methods mean that further investigation is now more usually employed.

Clinical presentation

The clinical presentation of localised pelvic recurrence depends to an extent on the nature of the previous surgery, together with the site of recurrence.

After AR there may be alteration of bowel habit or even obstructive symptoms, rectal bleeding, passage of mucus and tenesmus. The fact that these symptoms may develop and that access to the pelvis for digital and endoscopic examination is more straightforward after anterior resection than after abdominoperineal excision (APE) means that recurrence is often detected earlier.

After APE a discharging perineal sinus, perineal pain, induration or even a fungating tumour may occur.

Weight loss suggests more widespread disease; urinary symptoms may occur if there is bladder involvement; sciatic nerve pain can be caused by either nerve compression or invasion; lymphatic infiltration causes oedema of lower limbs.

A full history and physical examination, paying particular attention to comorbidities, is an essential part of assessment, not only of the possible recurrent cancer, but also of fitness for major surgery.

Endoscopy

Flexible and rigid endoscopy may allow visualisation and biopsy of the anastomosis and neorectum, but full colonoscopy should be undertaken if at all possible to exclude metachronous colorectal cancer.

Imaging

Imaging both aids in the diagnosis of recurrent rectal cancer and also identifies the site and extent of the tumour and any distant metastases.

Computed tomography (CT)

CT identifies anatomical abnormalities and allows imaging-guided needle biopsy of areas of suspected recurrence. Small lesions may be missed, and in the absence of histological confirmation it can be very difficult to make a definitive diagnosis.

Serial scans may be helpful, as normal postoperative changes can be very difficult to differentiate from recurrent disease [16]. A soft tissue mass may be due to recurrent tumour, organised haematoma, granulation tissue or fibrosis [17], and radiotherapy may result in streaking or a presacral mass [18]. A further limitation is that metastatic disease cannot be identified in normal sized lymph nodes [16].

Locally recurrent cancer can be detected with a sensitivity of 69-88% and a specificity of 50% [19,20,21]. The sensitivity of CT for the detection of local recurrence is significantly greater after APE than AR [22].

This imaging modality was reliable for determining need for sacrectomy or hysterectomy, but overestimated bladder involvement and had an accuracy of only 25% in predicting unresectability of a fixed lesion after radiotherapy in one study from the Mayo Clinic [23].

It should be remembered, however, that much of the published literature was based on studies done before the introduction of current multislice spiral CT, which may well produce superior results.

Magnetic resonance imaging (MRI)

MRI allows better definition of anatomical structures than CT, can also guide percutaneous biopsy, and its multiplanar capability can be very useful when assessing resectability of a pelvic tumour. An advantage of MRI is that most tumours have intermediate or high signal intensity on T2-weighted sequences, while the signal intensity from fibrous tissue is low [24]. However, active inflammation and fluid collections may also exhibit high signal intensity, making these difficult to differentiate from recurrent tumour. Overall, the sensitivity of MRI in the detection of local recurrence in the pelvis is 80-90%, with a specificity approaching 100% [25].

Ultrasound

Transrectal or transvaginal ultrasound can detect small extraluminal recurrences. Difficulty in distinguishing normal and abnormal lymph nodes and limitations of resolution are drawbacks. Ultrasound can be used to guide biopsy of pelvic masses via the rectum, vagina or even perineum [26].

Positron emission tomography (PET)

PET is a functional, non-invasive imaging modality based on the principle that there is an increase in glycolysis in malignant compared with normal tissue. Fluorine-18 labelled 2-fluoro-2-deoxy-D-glucose (18F-FDG) is an analogue of glucose which is taken up by cells but is not metabolised. It accumulates at a rate proportional to the metabolic activity of the cell and the fluorine-18 decays by positron emission, the source of which is detected by a PET scanner over a period of 30-40 minutes [27].

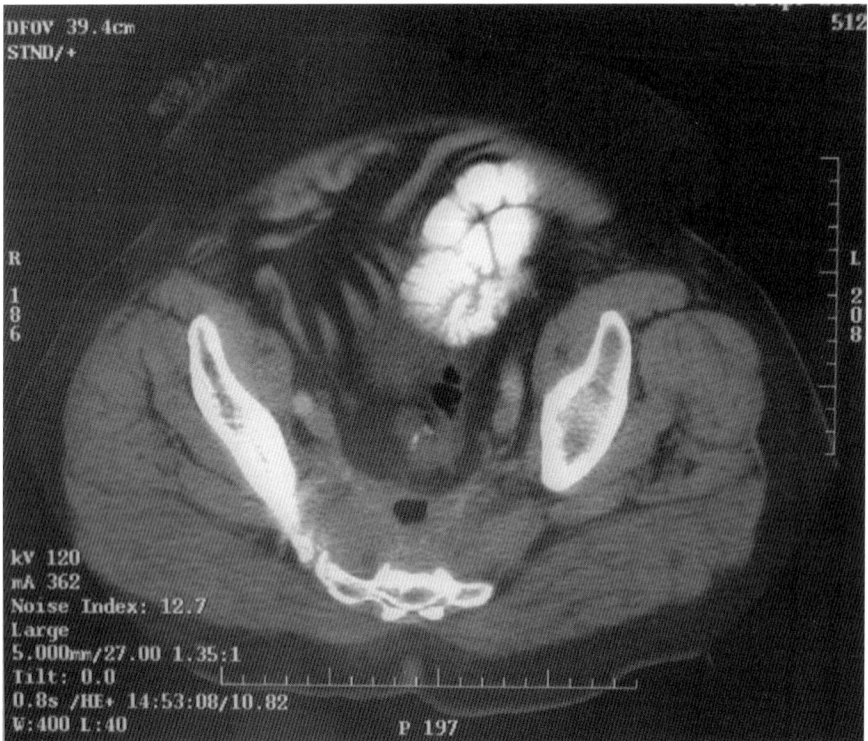

Figure 1. CT scan showing recurrent tumour in the pelvis.

PET scanning cannot distinguish malignant tissue from active inflammation in which glucose metabolism is also enhanced. Other limitations of PET include a lack of sensitivity when tumour deposits are small (0.5-1cm), especially in areas of movement such as the lung bases. Inflamed tissue and organs with a normally high rate of glucose metabolism (e.g. brain and heart) show up as "hot spots", as do areas of FDG excretion (the kidneys and bladder). There is also some degree of FDG uptake in normal small bowel and colon, as well as increased uptake after radiotherapy and a possible decrease due to chemotherapy (so-called "stunning").

Studies of PET in recurrent rectal cancer have shown sensitivities in the range 90-100% [28,29], with specificity around 75%. Detection of liver metastases approaches 100% and 90% for metastases at other sites [29]. In one study [30] of 22 patients with a rising CEA and normal CT, PET identified the site of tumour recurrence in 17 of them.

While the presence of malignant tissue can be detected with great sensitivity, its relationship with surrounding structures cannot be identified. Because of this PET is used in combination with CT or MRI, either as separate investigations (Figures 1 and 2) or, increasingly, in combination scanners.

PET scanning now has an established role in:

- restaging of patients with apparently isolated local recurrence of rectal cancer;
- characterisation of equivocal lesions detected by conventional imaging; and
- identification of recurrence detected by rising serum CEA in the face of normal conventional imaging.

Immunoscintigraphy

Radiolabelled monoclonal antibodies can be detected either with a conventional gamma camera or intra-operatively with a hand-held probe, and aroused great interest before the advent of PET scanning. The

9 Evaluation and management of local recurrence

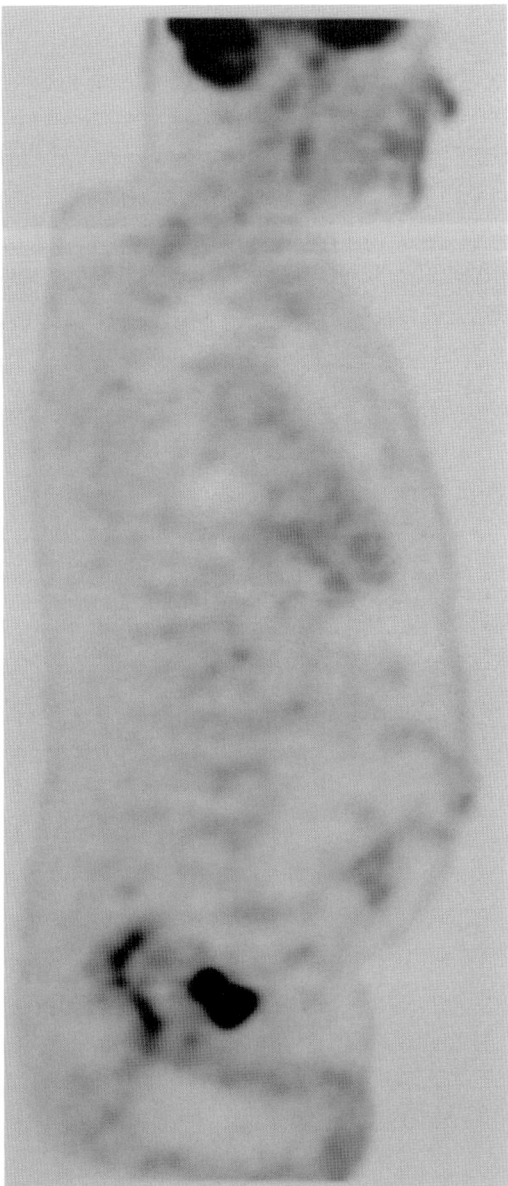

Figure 2. PET scan from the same patient in Figure 1 showing recurrent tumour in the pelvis, with no distant metastases.

first approach allows conventional nucleotide imaging, while the latter can guide biopsies and surgery. This can aid in identifying the extent of disease, and in one series patients with resectable local recurrence were found to require more extensive resection when a handheld probe and radiolabelled antibody was used than suggested by conventional imaging [31]. The sensitivity of this technique in the detection of local recurrence is around 74% [32], and it has the advantage that tumour deposits in normal sized lymph nodes are often positive [33]. A number of different antibody and isotope combinations have been investigated, but no clear role has been established.

Biopsy

It is essential to obtain histological evidence of recurrence prior to treatment, although this can be difficult. If there is mucosal involvement, endoscopic biopsies are usually sufficient. Masses which are palpable per rectum or per virginam or perineal masses can be core biopsied via these routes. CT-guided biopsy may be needed for less accessible recurrences.

Examination under anaesthetic

Examination under anaesthetic with rectal and vaginal examination allows assessment of the size and position of the tumour, together with its fixity to the sacrum, pelvic side walls or anterior pelvic organs. Biopsies can be taken.

Multidisciplinary management

The management of recurrent rectal cancer is challenging for both the medical team and the patient and their family. The aim of treatment is to achieve resection with microscopically tumour-free margins. This often requires multimodality treatment including pre-operative chemoradiotherapy and extended resection involving a range of surgical specialities, and is often followed by further chemotherapy.

Patterns of recurrence

Localised perineal recurrence

Recurrence in the perineal wound after APE may be amenable to local excision via a posterior approach, provided it does not encroach on the peritoneum. The coccyx and lower sacrum may also need to be excised.

Anterior recurrence

Local recurrence with anterior invasion into the bladder, prostate, seminal vesicles, vagina, Fallopian tubes, ovaries or uterus requires *en bloc* resection of the involved organs and tumour.

Central recurrence

If there is recurrence at the site of the anastomosis without involvement of the pelvic side walls, sacrum or anterior pelvic organs, this may be amenable to APE or AR. This pattern of recurrence was common in the past, but is unusual where total mesorectal excision is practised.

Lateral and posterior recurrence

While pelvic side wall or sacral involvement is associated with a poor prognosis, pelvic exenteration with sacrectomy can be done with reasonably low peri-operative morbidity and mortality [34,35].

Pre-operative assessment

Identification of extra-pelvic disease

CT of the chest and abdomen are the investigations most often used, though PET scanning may have a role in equivocal cases. At least 50% of those with local recurrence have detectable disease outside the pelvis[36], which has been considered a contra-indication to re-resection. Advances in the management of liver metastases, and now even lung metastases, mean that resection in these circumstances is now less controversial.

Colonoscopy to assess for metachronous colorectal cancer should be performed if possible.

Assessment of resectability of pelvic disease

CT, MRI and examination under anaesthetic are the mainstays of local staging. Plain films of the lumbosacral spine can show sacral erosion by tumour, though this is usually seen just as well on CT. An intravenous urogram to identify the course of the ureters can be helpful.

Recurrent disease is not resectable if there is extensive involvement of the pelvic side walls, of the sacrum at the level of S1 or S2, or if the tumour extends through the greater sciatic notch. It may be difficult to be certain about resectabilty without embarking on a trial dissection, but adverse features include bilateral ureteric obstruction and sciatic pain.

Fitness for surgery

Comorbid conditions should be investigated and optimised, and must be fully considered in weighing up the risks and benefits of such major surgery. Long-term morbidity is considerable, but needs to be taken in the context of the pain, infection and fistula formation resulting from uncontrolled pelvic tumour growth.

Patients and their families should have access to extensive counselling and support. It is essential that patients and their families are fully informed of the magnitude of surgery and its effect on quality of life. Most patients will require a permanent colostomy. They should have the opportunity to discuss this with a stoma therapist.

Pre-operative treatment

The aim of preoperative therapy is locally to downstage disease, with combined chemoradio-therapy being more effective than radiotherapy alone. In one series, the R0 resection rate for recurrent rectal cancer rose from 52% after radiotherapy alone to 72% (with complete response in 8%) after the introduction of chemoradiotherapy [37]. A variety of regimens is used, the most common being 45-50 Gy given in 20-25 fractions (5 consecutive days per week for 4 weeks).

External beam radiotherapy is delivered by a linear accelerator using a three- or four-field technique. The target volume is defined from CT and MRI images and includes all identifiable disease and extends up to L5. 5-fluorouracil is given by an infusion during the first and fifth weeks of radiotherapy.

Another study of this type of treatment [38] in 35 patients with locally recurrent rectal cancer found that 28 (80%) subsequently underwent potentially curative surgery, and clear margins were achieved in 17 (61%). Postoperative complications occurred in 14 (44%).

Increasingly, patients have already been given radiotherapy prior to their first resection. The management of these previously irradiated individuals is more difficult [39], and is lacking an evidence base. Such patients will usually have been given 25 Gy over 5 days ("short course") or 40-50 Gy over 5-6 weeks ("long course"). This amounts to about 70% of the maximum tolerable dose of many tissues, but the small bowel is more sensitive. If the interval since previous radiotherapy is at least a few months, it may be possible to give a further 30 Gy over 3-4 weeks provided the small bowel can be excluded. Such a dose is too low to result in radical tumour eradication, even if combined with sensitizing chemotherapy, but may eradicate some subclinical tumour deposits.

Once pre-operative chemoradiotherapy is complete, an interval of 4-8 weeks allows it to reach its maximal effect. The tumour should then be restaged before surgery.

Surgery

Surgery is tailored to individual requirements, adhering to the principle of *en bloc* resection, and aiming to excise the tumour with clear margins. This may require excision of vagina, uterus, prostate, bladder, seminal vesicles, distal ureters and part of the sacrum and can involve colorectal surgeons, urologists, plastic surgeons, spinal surgeons, gynaecologists and even vascular surgeons.

Dissection may be difficult because of loss of anatomical tissue planes, scarring, indistinct tumour margins and the risks of damaging ureters and iliac vessels, and can take 4-14 hours, with considerable blood loss.

Preparation and set-up

Surgery is performed in the Lloyd-Davies position, although the patient is later turned prone if sacrectomy is to be performed. Great care is needed to avoid lower limb pressure sores and compartment syndrome, and in very prolonged procedures the legs should be lowered periodically.

An examination under anaesthetic is performed, followed by cystoscopy and insertion of ureteric catheters or stents to aid identification of the ureters.

Dissection

Access to the abdomen is via a midline incision taken down to the pubic symphysis. Care is taken to preserve the inferior epigastric vessels in case a rectus abdominis flap is needed. After adhesiolysis, a careful laparotomy is performed to look for peritoneal seedlings and other unidentified metastases.

Pelvic dissection commences at the level of the aortic bifurcation, with identification of both ureters and iliac vessels, which are isolated with slings. If access to the pelvis is very difficult, the pubis can be divided and opened with a rib retractor [40]. The ureters are dissected up to the bladder and the iliac arteries are cleared to the origin of the internal iliac to allow proximal vascular control. The internal iliac arteries can be ligated prior to sacrectomy.

Dissection continues in the presacral plane. If the sacrum is involved this is continued to a level below S2, aiming to divide the sacrum 2cm above the tumour. Anterior and lateral mobilisation is then done, leaving the tumour attached to the sacrum (Figure 3). If necessary the bladder is mobilised and the obturator nodes swept medially with the specimen and an ileal conduit formed. If ureteric involvement is unilateral partial excision with proximal uretero-ureterostomy allows conservation of the urinary tract.

The prostate and seminal vesicles may need to be taken *en bloc* in men, and the uterus, Fallopian tubes, ovaries and posterior vagina in women.

Frozen sections can be helpful in determining completeness of resection and the site of any residual tumour. If the disease is not resectable, debulking may relieve compressive symptoms and proximal faecal or urinary diversion may be helpful.

If sacrectomy is to be performed the abdomen is closed and the patient is turned into the prone jack-knife position. A vertical incision is made over the sacrum to include the anus or perineal scar and the gluteal muscles are retracted laterally to expose the sacrum, which is cleared at the chosen level of section. The sacrum is then divided and the distal part, with the tumour attached, is removed.

Closure of the perineum

The perineum can be closed primarily, provided it can be done without tension. If this is not possible, omentum can be brought down to fill the pelvic and perineal defect, reducing bleeding and fluid accumulation. Subsequent skin grafting can allow healing in the irradiated area. The omentum is often not suitable, in which case a myocutaneous flap can be used.

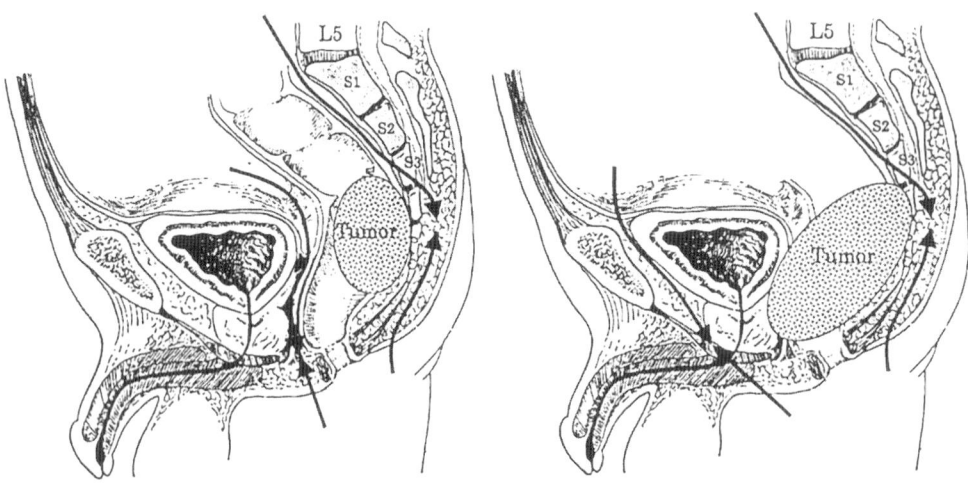

Figure 3. Diagram showing planes of dissection for a recurrent tumour invading the lower sacrum. Reproduced with permission from Springer, © 2002. Yamada K, Ishizawa T, Niwa K, Chuman Y, Aikou T. Pelvic exenteration and sacral resection for locally advanced primary and recurrent rectal cancer. *Dis Colon Rectum* 2002; 45: 1078-84.

The most common is a rectus abdominis flap [41]. In a study comparing myocutaneous flap closure with primary skin and omental closure [42], the use of a flap was associated with lower overall morbidity, fewer wound complications and more rapid wound healing.

A rectus abdominis flap cannot be used if two stomas are created. An alternative technique has been described in which a mesh is used, covered on the peritoneal side with omentum and on the perineal side with a gracilis flap [43].

Intra-operative radiotherapy (IORT)

IORT offers localised treatment to the site of tumour resection while sparing normal structures such as small bowel, and may be particularly useful when resection margins are involved [44]. IORT can be given instead of further external beam radiotherapy in previously irradiated patients, or as a further 10 Gy in addition. The results in a retrospective study of 51 such patients from the Mayo Clinic were poor, with a 5-year survival of 12%, although local control within the radiation field was 72% at 2 years, and better in those who were given external beam radiotherapy in addition to IORT [45].

There have been no randomised controlled trials, but some centres have published their results using this IORT, with 33% disease-free survival after sacrectomy with clear surgical margins in one [46]. In another series of 42 patients who had undergone palliative resection and IORT 3- and 5-year survival rates were 43% and 19% respectively [47].

IORT requires expensive specialist facilities and is only available in a few centres [48]. Brachytherapy, either in the form of a permanent implant [49] or remote afterloading [50] has also been used. A group in the Netherlands has reported a 3-year survival rate of 60% and local control rate of 73% using such a technique [51], and another group in Los Angeles used brachytherapy in patients where surgical excision margins were positive, with some success [52].

While bowel can be excluded from the IORT field, nerves and ureters are not so easily avoided, and complications include ureteric stenosis and peripheral neuropathy.

Postoperative complications

As well as the usual complications of major abdominopelvic surgery, particular problems encountered are:

- Perineal wound infection and non-healing.
- Enterocutaneous fistulation.
- Sacral plexus neuropathy.

Palliative therapy

In most studies palliative surgery offers no benefit over non-operative management in terms of survival [53,54] and in view of its magnitude and risks is not recommended.

Radiotherapy results in temporary palliation [55] only, with a duration of between 6-9 months. Advances, notably the use of chemoradiotherapy, mean that the outcome of palliative medical therapy is improving. In one recent series [53], 20% of patients with locally recurrent rectal cancer managed non-surgically were alive at 5 years, and it may be that a proportion of these had a complete response. However, these modalities are used without surgery with palliative intent.

Outcome

Results from different series vary widely, probably due to differences in philosophy, selection criteria and adjuvant therapies (Table 1). With careful patient selection a median survival of 21-30 months [60,61] and 5-year survival of up to 50% can be achieved [62]. An operative mortality of 8% has been reported after en bloc resection of one or more organs, with 32% 5-year survival [63], as well as a 16% rate of local recurrence and a cancer-specific 5-year survival of 62% [64].

These results compare favourably to liver and pulmonary resections for metastatic disease, and should be taken in the context of the pain and disabling symptoms which can develop if pelvic recurrence is left untreated. Direct comparison with palliative therapy is difficult, but surgery offers the only real chance of long-term survival, and can also provide effective palliation in some with debilitating symptoms [35], although it is not recommended that surgery is undertaken with palliative intent as it offers no survival benefit.

Policy-making is increasingly driven by analyses of quality of life and cost-effectiveness. One retrospective study [65] divided 68 patients into three groups. Those in one group underwent resection with curative intent, resulting in a median survival of 42 months at a mean cost of USD 71,000 per patient. A second group were treated with palliative surgery at a cost of USD 45,000. Their median survival (17 months) differed little from those treated conservatively (median survival 18 months, mean cost

Table 1. Outcome of surgery for locally recurrent rectal cancer.

Centre	n	Postoperative morbidity (%)	5-year survival after R0 resection (%)	Local re-recurrence (%)
Mayo Clinic [47]	224	21	34	47 at 5 years
Cleveland Clinic [56]	43	19	42	28
Netherlands [57]	33	-	60 (at 3 years)	27
Minnesota [53]	87	25	35	25
Memorial Sloan Kettering [58]	131	-	35	-
Japan [59]	42	60	23	-

USD 20,000). The incremental cost utility ratio of surgery compared with non-operative management was USD 110,000 per quality-adjusted life year saved.

Prognostic factors

The prognosis is best if recurrence is confined to the neorectum, worsens if other pelvic organs are involved, and is even poorer if there is pelvic side wall or sacral involvement [59]. Previous sphincter-saving surgery, young age [53], clear resection margins and absence of vascular invasion in the resected specimen [66] are associated with better results.

In one study, patients with pre-operative CEA less than 10mg ml^{-1} had a significantly better survival that those with CEA above this level (45% and 15% respectively), and bone marrow involvement, positive resection margins and lymph node metastases were also associated with a poorer prognosis [65].

The pattern of recurrence may also be important, with one series having a 38% 5-year survival after resection of central recurrence, 10% after sacrectomy and zero in those with lateral pelvic wall involvement [59].

Where are we going?

Minimising the problem

Population screening, so that rectal cancers are identified early, together with better staging, universal application of the technique of total mesorectal excision and improvements in adjuvant therapies for the management of primary tumours will still further reduce the rates of local recurrence.

Better investigation

A better understanding of tumour biology and improved accuracy of prognosis after initial surgery for rectal cancer should allow intensive follow-up to be targeted towards those who might develop local recurrence and would be suitable for surgery should they do so. The resolution of CT scanners is likely to improve further, and various contrast media for MRI are being studied, which may improve the sensitivity of this type of scan. A new generation of CT/PET and MRI/PET scanners will be able to provide coregistered images, combining the high sensitivity and specificity of PET with the anatomical resolution of CT and MRI.

Better treatment

There is increasing evidence that specialisation and volume of surgery improves outcomes in complex cases. The management of locally recurrent rectal cancer involves large multidisciplinary teams, as well as facilities such as PET scanners, brachytherapy or IORT. Centralisation of this work to a handful of regional centres would allow teams to develop expertise with an adequate caseload.

Adjuvant treatments with addition of new drugs such as oxaliplatin may achieve further improvement in the complete resection rate. Novel therapies such as anti-angiogenesis factors and antibodies to growth factors may also have a role.

PET scanning may have a place in predicting response to treatment, allowing changes in treatment where it is suboptimal [27], though investigation of this is at a very preliminary stage.

Better evidence

The current literature on the management of recurrent rectal cancer is difficult to interpret and apply. Most of it is retrospective, and series vary in their selection criteria, adjuvant therapies used and follow-up.

Great advances have been made in the treatment of liver metastases over recent years, and that of pelvic recurrence lags behind. Better studies are needed, especially randomised trials of modalities such as IORT. Rationalisation of services will facilitate such work.

References

1. Abulafi AM, Williams NS. Local recurrence of colorectal cancer: the problem, mechanisms, management and adjuvant therapy. *Br J Surg* 1994; 81: 7-19.
2. Dahlberg M, Glimelius B, Pahlman L. Changing strategy for rectal cancer is associated with improved outcome. *Br J Surg* 1999; 86: 379-84.
3. Gunderson LL, Sosin H. Areas of failure found at reoperation (second or symptomatic look) following "curative surgery" for adenocarcinoma of the rectum. *Cancer* 1974; 34: 1278-92.
4. McDermott FT, Hughes ESR, Pih IE, et al. Local recurrence after potentially curative resection for rectal cancer in a series of 1008 patients. *Br J Surg* 1985; 72: 34-7.
5. Pilipshen SJ, Heilweil M, Quan SHO, et al. Patterns of pelvic recurrence following definitive resections for rectal cancer. *Cancer* 1984; 53: 1354-62.
6. Heald RJ, Ryall RDH. Recurrence and survival after total mesorectal excision for rectal cancer. *Lancet* 1986; I: 1479-82.
7. Scott NAS, Rainwater LM, Wieand HS, et al. The relative prognostic value of flow cytometric DNA analysis and conventional clinicopathological criteria in patients with operable rectal carcinoma. *Dis Colon Rectum* 1987; 30: 513-20.
8. Hamelin R, Laurent-Puig P, Olschwang S, et al. Association of p53 mutations with short survival in rectal cancer. *Gastroenterology* 1994; 106: 42-8.
9. Phillips RKS, Hittinger R, Blesovsky L, et al. Local recurrence following "curative" surgery for large bowel cancer. II: the rectum and rectosigmoid. *Br J Surg* 1984; 71: 17-20.
10. Michelassi F, Block GE, Vannucci L, et al. A 5- to 21-year follow-up and analysis of 250 patients with rectal adenocarcinoma. *Ann Surg* 1988; 208: 379-89.
11. Gilbertsen VA. The results of surgical treatment of cancer of the rectum. *Surg Gynecol Obstet* 1962; 114: 13-19.
12. Adam II, Mohamdee MO, Martin IG, et al. Role of circumferential margin involvement in the local recurrence of rectal cancer. *Lancet* 1994; 344: 707-11.
13. Billingham RP. Extended lymphadenectomy for rectal cancer: cure vs quality of life. *Int J Surg* 1994; 79: 11-22.
14. Mellgren A, Sirivongs P, Rothenberger DA, et al. Is local excision adequate therapy for early rectal cancer? *Dis Colon Rectum* 2000; 43: 1064-74.
15. Sitzler PJ, Seow-Choen F, Ho YH, et al. Lymph node involvement and tumour depth in rectal cancers: an analysis of 805 patients. *Dis Colon Rectum* 1997; 440: 1472-6.
16. Thoeni RF. Colorectal cancer: cross-sectional imaging for staging of primary tumour and detection of local recurrence. *Am J Roentgenol* 1991; 156: 909-15.
17. Adalsteinsson B, Pahlman A, Hemmingsson A, et al. Computed tomography in early diagnosis of local recurrence of rectal carcinoma. *Acta Radiol* 1987; 28: 41-6.
18. Rifkin MD, Ehrlich SM, Marks G. Staging of rectal carcinoma: prospective comparison of endorectal US and CT. *Radiology* 1989; 170: 319-22.
19. Thompson WM, Halvorsen RA, Foster WL Jr, et al. Preoperative and postoperative CT staging of rectosigmoid carcinoma. *Am J Roentgenol* 1986; 146: 703-10.
20. Freeney PC, Marks WM, Ryan IA, et al. Colorectal carcinoma evaluation with CT: preoperative staging and detection of postoperative recurrence. *Radiology* 1987; 158: 347-53.
21. Chen YM, Ott DI, Wolfman N, et al. Recurrent colorectal carcinoma: evaluation with barium enema examination and CT. *Radiology* 1987; 163: 307-10.
22. Mendez RJ, Rodriguez R, Kovacevich T. CT in local recurrence of rectal carcinoma. *J Comput Assist Tomogr* 1993; 17: 741-4.
23. Farouk R, Nelson H, Radice E, et al. Accuracy of computed tomography in determining respectability for locally advanced primary or recurrent colorectal cancers. *Am J Surg* 1998; 175: 283-7.
24. Krestin GP, Steinbrich W, Friedmann G. Recurrent rectal cancer: diagnosis with MR imaging versus CT. *Radiology* 1988; 168: 307-11.
25. Charnnsangavej C. New imaging modalities for follow-up of colorectal carcinoma. *Cancer* 1993; 71: 4236-4240.
26. Beynon I, Mortensen MIM, Foy DMA, et al. The detection and evaluation of locally recurrent cancer with rectal endosonography. *Dis Colon Rectum* 1989; 32: 509-17.
27. Tutt ANJ, Plunkett TA, Barrington SF, et al. The role of positron emission tomography in the management of colorectal cancer. *Colorectal Dis* 2004; 6: 2-9.
28. Takeuchi O, Saito N, Koda K, et al. Clinical assessment of positron emission tomography for the diagnosis of local recurrence in colorectal cancer. *Br J Surg* 1999; 85: 932-7.
29. Arulampalam TH, Costa DC, Loizidou M, et al. Positron emission tomography and colorectal cancer. *Br J Surg* 2001; 88: 176-89.
30. Flanagan FL, Dehdashti F, Ogunbiyi OA, et al. Utility of FDG-PET for investigating unexplained plasma CEA elevation in patients with colorectal cancer. *Ann Surg* 1998; 227: 319-23.
31. Cohen AM, Martin EW Jr, Lavery I, et al. Radioimmunoguided surgery using iodine 125 B723 in patients with colorectal cancer. *Arch Surg* 1991; 126: 349-52.
32. Collier BD, Abdel-Nabi H, Doerr RI. Immunoscintigraphy performed with In-111-labeled CYT-103 in the management of colorectal cancer: comparison with CT. *Radiology* 1992; 185: 179-86.
33. Neal CE, Abdel-Nabi H. Clinical immunoscintigraphy of recurrent colorectal carcinoma. *Appl Radiol* 1994; 23: 32-9.
34. Wanebo HI, Koness I, Turk PS, et al. Composite resection of posterior pelvic malignancy. *Ann Surg* 1992; 215: 685-95.
35. Temple WI, Ketcham AS. Sacral resection for control of pelvic tumours. *Am J Surg* 1992; 163: 370-4.
36. Wiggers T, de Vries MR, Veeze-Kuypers B. Surgery for local recurrence of rectal carcinoma. *Dis Colon Rectum* 1996; 39: 323-8.
37. Glimelius B. Chemoradiotherapy for rectal cancer - is there an optimal combination? *Ann Oncol* 2001; 12: 1039-45.
38. Rodel C, Grabenbauer G, Matzel KE, et al. Extensive surgery after high dose preoperative chemoradiotherapy for locally advanced recurrent rectal cancer. *Dis Colon Rectum* 2000; 43: 312-19.

39. Glimelius B. Recurrent rectal cancer. The pre-irradiated primary tumour: can more radiotherapy be given? *Colorectal Dis* 2003; 5: 501-3.
40. Patil UB, Ackerman NB, Waterhouse K. The transpubic approach in the management of problems of the lower genitourinary and intestinal tracts. *Surg Gynecol Obstet* 1982; 155: 97-101.
41. Kroll SS, Pollock R, Jessup JM, *et al*. Transpelvic rectus abdominis flap reconstruction of defects following abdominoperineal resection. *Ann Surg* 1989; 55: 632-7.
42. Radice E, Nelson H, Mercill S, *et al*. Primary myocutaneous flap closure following resection of locally advanced pelvic malignancies. *Br J Surg* 1999; 86: 349-54.
43. Borel Rinkes IH, Wiggers T. Gracilis muscle flap in the treatment of persistent, infected pelvis necrosis. *Eur J Surg* 1999; 165: 390-1.
44. Magrini S, Nelson H, Gunderson LL, *et al*. Sacropelvic resection and IORT in the management of recurrent rectal and anal cancer. *Dis Colon Rectum* 1995; 38: 7.
45. Haddock MG, Gunderson L, Nelson H, *et al*. Intraoperative irradiation for locally recurrent colorectal cancer in previously irradiated patients. *Int J Radiat Oncol Biol Phys* 2001; 49: 1267-74.
46. Willett CG, Shellito PC, Tepper JE, *et al*. Intraoperative electron beam radiation therapy for recurrent locally advanced rectal and rectosigmoid carcinoma. *Cancer* 1991; 67: 1504-8.
47. Suzuki K, Dozois RR, Devine RM, *et al*. Curative reoperations for locally recurrent rectal cancer. *Dis Colon Rectum* 1996; 39: 730-36
48. Rutten HJ, Mannaerts GH, Martijn H, *et al*. Intraoperative radiotherapy for locally recurrent rectal cancer in The Netherlands. *Eur J Surg Oncol* 2000; 18: 199-206.
49. Meigooni AS, Nath R. Dosimetry of Pd-103 model 200 sources for intestinal brachytherapy. *Endocurie Hyperthermic Oncology* 1989; 5: 64.
50. Kaufman N, Non D, Shank B, *et al*. Remote afterloading intraluminal brachytherapy in the treatment of rectal, rectosigmoid and anal cancer: a feasibility study. *Int J Radiat Oncol Biol Phys* 1989; 17: 663-8.
51. Mannaerts GH, Rutten HJ, Martijn H, *et al*. Comparison of intraoperative radiation therapy-containing multimodality treatment with historical treatment modalities for locally recurrent rectal cancer. *Dis Colon Rectum* 2001; 44: 1749-58.
52. Kuehne J, Kleisli T, Biernacki P, *et al*. Use of high-dose-rate brachytherapy in the management of locally recurrent rectal cancer. *Dis Colon Rectum* 2003; 46: 895-9.
53. Garcia-Aguilar J, Cromwell JW, Marra C, *et al*. Treatment of locally recurrent rectal cancer. *Dis Colon Rectum* 2001; 44: 1743-8.
54. Ogunbiyi OA, McKenna K, Birnbaum EH, *et al*. Aggressive surgical management of recurrent rectal cancer - is it worth it? *Dis Colon Rectum* 1997; 40: 150-5.
55. Pacini P, Cionini L Pirtoli L, *et al*. Symptomatic recurrences of carcinoma of the rectum and sigmoid. The influence of radiotherapy on the quality of life. *Dis Colon Rectum* 1986; 29: 865-8.
56. Lopez-Kostner F, Fazio VW, Vignali A, *et al*. Locally recurrent rectal cancer. Predictors of success of salvage surgery. *Dis Colon Rectum* 2001; 44: 173-8.
57. Wiggers T, Mannaerts GH, Marinelli AW, *et al*. Surgery for locally recurrent rectal cancer. *Colorectal Disease* 2003; 5: 504-7.
58. Salo JC, Paty PB, Guillem J, *et al*. Surgical salvage of recurrent rectal carcinoma after curative resection: a 10-year experience. *Ann Surg Oncol* 1999; 6: 171-7.
59. Yamada K, Isahizawa T, Niwa Y, *et al*. Patterns of pelvic invasion are prognostic in the treatment of locally advanced rectal cancer. *Br J Surg* 2001; 88: 988-93.
60. Estes NC, Thomas IH, Jewell WR, *et al*. Pelvic exenteration: a treatment for failed rectal cancer surgery. *Ann Surg* 1993; 59: 420-2.
61. Brophy PF, Hoffman IP, Eisenberg BL. The role of palliative pelvic exenteration. *Am J Surg* 1994; 167: 386-90.
62. Boey I, Wong I, Ong GB. Pelvic exenteration for locally advanced colorectal carcinoma. *Ann Surg* 1982; 195: 513-8.
63. Bonfanti G, Bozzetti F, Dolci R, *et al*. Results of extended surgery for cancer of the rectum and sigmoid. *Br J Surg* 1982; 69: 305-7.
64. Devine RM, Dozois RR. Surgical management of locally advanced adenocarcinoma of the rectum. *World J Surg* 1992; 16: 486-9.
65. Miller AR, Cantor SB, Peoples GE, *et al*. Quality of life and cost effectiveness of therapy for locally recurrent rectal cancer. *Dis Colon Rectum* 2000; 43: 1695-1703.
66. Shoup M, Guillem JG, Alektiar KM, *et al*. Predictors of survival in recurrent rectal cancer after resection and intraoperative radiotherapy. *Dis Colon Rectum* 2002; 45: 585-92.

Chapter 10

The TME debate in light of the Dutch radiotherapy trial

Gisella Salerno BSc MRCS, Surgical Research Fellow
Brendan Moran MCh FRCSI, Consultant Colorectal Surgeon
North Hampshire Hospital, Basingstoke, UK

What is the problem?

Cancer of the rectum, defined as tumours within 15cm from the anal verge, accounts for 30% of all colorectal malignancies. Thus, there are approximately 13,000 new cases of rectal cancer annually in the UK.

The main aims in treating rectal cancer are cure and prolongation of good quality cancer-specific survival, with preservation and restoration of normal function if possible. Surgery is the mainstay of treatment and total mesorectal excision (TME) is now considered the "gold standard" with fewer local recurrences and better overall survival. Local recurrence is a particular problem after rectal cancer surgery and is defined as disease in the pelvis, including recurrence at the site of the anastomosis and in the perineum [1]. Local recurrence results in severe morbidity with debilitating symptoms of pelvic pain, ureteric obstruction, bowel fistulation and poor bowel and urinary function. Palliative treatment has limited success. Local recurrence markedly impairs quality of life and eventually leads to death in most cases. The 5-year survival of patients with local recurrence is less than 5%, with a median survival of 7 months. It is often due to failure of complete removal of tumour, or its initial field of spread in the mesorectum, both of which can be influenced by surgical technique. Thus, in reality, local recurrence may in many cases represent persistent disease rather than recurrence. Predictors of risk of local recurrence are outlined in Table 1.

Table 1. Predictors of local recurrence.

- Size of the primary and involvement of the circumferential resection margin (CRM) by tumour [2,3]
- Distal location of tumour: the nearer the anal verge, the higher the risk [2,3]
- Extramural vascular invasion [4-6]
- Tumour differentiation [4,5]
- Nodal status [4,5]
- Extent of extramural spread [3-5]
- Peritoneal involvement by tumour [4,5,7]

Reported local recurrence rates vary from 2.6% to 32% and are probably most influenced by surgical technique [8]. The lowest recurrence rates and best survival have been consistently reported with TME [9,10]. Local recurrence is influenced by the pathology of the tumour and can be reduced by optimal surgical technique and by pre-operative radiotherapy.

Table 2. Involved circumferential resection margin (CRM) and outcome.

Study group	Distance from tumour to CRM (mm)	Local recurrence (%)	Distant metastases (%)	Survival for curative operations (%)
Birbeck, Leeds (5-year follow-up) [2]	<1	38.2	-	40
	>1	10	-	79
Quirke 1986 (median follow-up 23 months) [3]	<1	64	-	-
	>1	9	-	-
Norwegian (median follow-up 29 months) [11]	<1	22	40	63
	>1	5	12	81
Dutch TME (median follow-up 2 years) [12]	<1	16.4	37.6	69.7
	1-2	15	21	84.8
	>2	10.3	17.2	87

The evidence for TME

The concept of circumferential clearance

Rectal cancer spreads proximally along the lymphatic drainage associated with the vascular pedicle and circumferentially in the pelvis. Work by Quirke has shown that a positive circumferential resection margin (CRM), defined as tumour within 1mm of the edge of the resected specimen, and depth of extramural invasion are independent predictors of local recurrence and poor prognosis [3]. There are a number of reports outlining the detrimental effect of tumour within 1mm of the CRM as described in Table 2. In the Norwegian report, only 5% of patients with an uninvolved CRM developed local recurrence, so it is assumed that radiotherapy would have overtreated 97% of the patients with clear margins.

Nagtegaal reports in the Dutch trials that a CRM of ≤2mm should be referred to as an involved margin as local recurrence was higher in this group (16% versus 6% in the group with a clear CRM of >2mm) [12]. She also reports that margins of ≤1mm are predictive of an increased risk of distant metastases (37% versus 15% if the involved CRM is >1mm). The significant increase in local recurrence with a CRM of 1-2mm was not seen in the Norwegian or Leeds studies.

Simunovic et al report data from 150 consecutive patients who underwent TME with selective use of pre-operative radiotherapy [13]. The local recurrence rate was significantly lower in the non-irradiated group (2.6%) compared to the irradiated group (17.1%). Only patients with tumours deemed at risk of local recurrence from threatened or involved circumferential margins, using clinical assessment of tumour size, tethering or fixity, were considered for pre-operative irradiation. It was concluded that the majority of patients with operable rectal cancer could probably be spared the risk of irradiation, if pre-operative assessment and surgery are optimal.

Jatzko et al report that patients with positive lymph nodes had a higher risk of local recurrence [14,15]. However, others found that lymph node involvement was not associated with higher local recurrence, perhaps attributable to the beneficial effects of TME [11,13].

Of the independent risk factors, the only one that can be manipulated by treatment is the CRM.

The surgical technique

TME involves a number of technically challenging steps, which aims to maximise circumferential clearance. The skill of the surgeon is important which means that it is difficult to subject this to a randomised controlled trial (RCT). Surgeons trained in TME are no longer prepared to randomise to the "standard" technique of rapid manual extraction of the tumour. The evidence base depends on historical case series.

TME surgery has decreased the rate of local recurrence from 30-40% to 5-15% [10, 16]. The variability suggests that surgery is important. A recent paper from Stockholm has been the first report of a direct benefit in a whole population following a video-based surgical training programme [35]. Workshops were started in 1994 and the study population included all patients who underwent abdominal operations for rectal cancer during 1995-1996. For patients with curative abdominal resections, there were no differences between Stockholm I and II studies and the TME project in terms of 30-day mortality, anastomotic leakage, or all complications, despite the decrease in abdominoperineal excisions from 55-60% to 27%.

Local recurrence was significantly lower in the TME group compared with the Stockholm I and II groups (6% vs 15% vs 14% respectively) as was cancer-related death (9% vs 15% and 16% respectively) [17]. The CRM positivity rate was 4% - the lowest reported incidence so far in any published series. Therefore, improvement in treatment results related to surgical technique and reported by individual surgeons has been reproduced in a population-based study [9, 16].

Where are we now?

TME training

Ideally, surgeons with training and experience should operate on rectal cancer. Colorectal-trained surgeons and surgeons performing >21 resections annually are more likely to perform a sphincter-preserving resection [18].

Martling et al [19] compared outcome from abdominal resection for rectal cancer between two teams of surgeons from a cohort of 652 patients from the aforementioned Swedish TME project and recruited between 1995-1996. One group included high volume surgeons (more than 12 rectal cancer operations per year) and the other low volume surgeons (12 operations or fewer per year). The outcome was significantly better in patients treated by high volume surgeons, with local recurrence rates of 4% versus 10% and rates of rectal cancer deaths of 11% compared with 18% in the low volume group. Also, workshop participants more commonly performed TME, sphincter-preserving surgery, and used radiotherapy. This is probably explained by the fact that knowledge of the "TME concept" includes proper pre-operative staging, pre-operative radiotherapy where the CRM is at risk of tumour infiltration, meticulous surgical dissection, and pathological evaluation of the circumferential resection margin. After adjustment for use of radiotherapy in the multivariate analysis, the differences in local recurrence and rectal cancer death were still significantly better in patients operated on by high volume surgeons.

Further evidence for the beneficial effect of training and the practice of TME has recently been published by the Dutch [20] and Norwegian Rectal Cancer Study Groups [21]. The Dutch Group attempted to measure the impact of TME training by comparing the patients who did not have radiotherapy in the recently published study to patients in a previously published randomised study (Cancer Recurrence and Blood Transfusion [CRAB] trial) who had not had radiotherapy. The local recurrence rates significantly dropped from 16% to 9% [20].

Similarly, in the Norwegian Rectal Cancer Project, initiated in 1993, over the period 1994-97 the proportion of patients undergoing TME increased from 78% to 92%. The local recurrence rate for patients undergoing a curative resection was 6% in the TME group and 12% in the conventional surgery group. Four-year survival rate was 73% after TME and 60% after conventional surgery [21]. Standardisation of surgical technique and TME in another Norwegian centre reported a reduction in local recurrence (LR) from 9% at 5 years after an R0 TME resection compared with 24% LR in the conventional surgery period [22].

A more recent paper from Denmark has shown improved survival after the introduction of TME in 1996 [23]. The only other factors influencing survival following curative surgery on a multivariate Cox proportional hazard regression model were: gender, age, surgical procedure (low anterior resection [LAR] and abdominoperineal excision [APE] had a higher survival than Hartmann's procedure) and anastomotic leakage.

Evidence for pre-operative radiotherapy

There is ongoing debate as to the value of pre-operative radiotherapy. The rationale for using combinations of radiotherapy and chemotherapy is based on the risks of relapse after surgery alone. Much of the evidence for this comes from the Swedish and Stockholm Rectal Cancer Trials [24-26]. In 1988, a meta-analysis of the available randomised trials failed to show an overall significant survival benefit with pre-operative radiotherapy [27]. A further meta-analysis in 2000 concluded that in patients with resectable rectal cancer, pre-operative radiotherapy significantly improved overall and cancer-specific survival compared with surgery alone [28]. However, the irradiation schedules used varied greatly between trials, histological staging of patients undergoing radiotherapy was not accurate, and overall complications in the immediate postoperative period were significantly increased. By excluding the Swedish data from this meta-analysis there was loss of significance. A summary of the current randomised trials showing significant differences between local recurrence in pre-operative radiotherapy and surgery, versus surgery alone, is shown in Table 3.

The Swedish Rectal Cancer Trial showed a relative survival benefit of 21%, with an increase in the 5-year survival from 48% to 58% and a reduction in local recurrence from 27% to 11% [24, 72]. With local recurrence rates of less than 10%, there are no data demonstrating a beneficial effect with the routine addition of radiotherapy [29]. This would mean that in order further to reduce local recurrence many patients would need to be treated to achieve significant further reduction [30].

Therefore, after extensive analysis of the treatment of rectal cancer, the Dutch Colorectal Cancer Group concluded that one major aspect of treatment that could be randomised was pre-operative radiotherapy and that patients should be operated on by trained TME surgeons. With addition of radiotherapy, local recurrence was reduced from 8.2% to 2.4% after a median follow-up of 2 years in the Dutch TME Trial in 1784 patients who underwent a macroscopically complete resection [31]. However, the surgery alone arm had high local recurrence rates suggesting inadequate surgery in a significant proportion. The Dutch trial had attempted to standardise the surgery and provide quality control measures through workshops and live video demonstrations. Despite this "standardisation" of surgery, the involved margin rate in what were considered mobile tumours was 18.3%.

Quality control of the TME specimen can now be estimated by naked eye assessment of the

Table 3. Rectal cancer: randomised trials showing significant reduction in local recurrence (LR) and survival results with pre-operative short course radiotherapy (RT) and surgery versus surgery alone.

Trial	No. patients (n)	LR with RT	LR with surgery alone	LR (p value)	Survival (p value)
St. Marks RCG [32]	475	17%	24%	<0.05	Not significant
NWRCG [33]	284	12.8%	36.5%	<0.001	Not significant
EORTC 76-81 [34]	466	15%	30%	0.003	Not significant
MRC II [35]	279	40%	50%	0.04	Not significant
Stockholm I [26]	849	10.8%	22.8%	<0.01	Not significant
Stockholm II [24]	479	5.4%	12.9%	<0.01	Not significant
Swedish RCT [25]	1165	11%	27%	<0.001	0.004
Dutch TME Trial (2-year follow-up) [31]	1861	2.4%	8.2%	<0.001	Not significant

completeness of the mesorectal envelope. From the 180 patients in the Dutch TME trial for whom information was available, 24% were classified as incomplete and 19% as nearly complete. Patients in the incomplete group had an increased risk of local and distant recurrence, with a 36.1% versus 20.3% 2-year recurrence in the group with a complete mesorectum. This could be attributable mainly to the local recurrence (15% versus 8.7%), although this difference was not significant. No difference was found in survival rates at 2 years. However, in patients with a negative resection margin, the overall recurrence rate was increased in the group with an incomplete mesorectum (28.6% versus 14.9%); both local and distant recurrence contributed to this effect. Therefore, the quality of the mesorectum does have additional value in patients without CRM involvement. Survival rates were also different between the groups: 90.5% versus 76.9% in the patients with a complete compared with an incomplete mesorectum (p<0.05) [31].

Problems with neoadjuvant radiotherapy

Pre-operative radiotherapy is associated with toxicity, early complications and long-term side effects. Early complications include perineal wound breakdown, diarrhoea, proctitis, urinary tract infection, small bowel obstruction, leucopenia and venous thrombosis. In one retrospective study, 63% of patients undergoing pre-operative long course radiotherapy and APE or LAR had grade 1-2 toxicity and 33% of patients experienced grade 3 toxicity [36]. The toxicity of pre-operative radiotherapy was also emphasised by two recently published meta-analyses. The Italian meta-analysis showed an increase in septic complications from 15.2% to 21% (p<0.001), and other complications from 17.8% to 21% (p=0.03), leading to an overall postoperative rate of adverse events of 42.3 vs. 57.4% (p<0.001). Mortality at 30 days did not differ [28]. The second meta-analysis from the UK yielded similar results [37]. The risk of death from non-rectal cancer was 15% higher in the irradiated group, mainly from infective and vascular complications. In patients 75 years and older, the outcome with radiotherapy was worse and side effects more than counterbalanced the benefits.

An audit in the North Trent Region (UK) showed a higher than expected anastomotic leak rate (15%) and perineal wound infection rates (18%) following the introduction of pre-operative radiotherapy [38]. There are also concerns when the radiotherapy field includes the anus, if attempting a restorative procedure after the resection of low rectal cancer. We know that radiotherapy damages the myenteric plexus of the internal sphincter, consequently reducing the anal resting pressure, diminishing the recto-anal inhibitory reflex and causing damage to the pudendal nerve [39]. Hence, there may be a contributory negative effect of radiotherapy on the function and integrity of the colo-anal anastomosis with or without formation of a colonic pouch.

Other problems with radiotherapy apart from the side effects include cost and variability in access.

The problem of local recurrence

At least 50% of the patients with local recurrence have detectable distant metastases at the time of diagnosis, making them unsuitable for curative local treatment. A multimodality approach in planning surgery for locally recurrent rectal cancer is suggested [40].

The role of radiotherapy in recurrent disease is limited as it has often been given prior to the primary surgery, in tumours with adverse features. Therefore, problems arise with dose accumulation toxicity and scarring of tissues seen on MRI, which make the extent of tumour growth difficult to assess. Positron emission tomography (PET) may prove useful in distinguishing fibrosis from recurrence and in finding unsuspected metastatic disease, especially in retroperitoneal lymph nodes and the liver [41]. Due to the cumulative effects of radiotoxicity, some centres have tried additional focused, intra-operative radiotherapy (IORT) of 10Gy. However, toxicity was considerable, including radionecrosis, perineal wound infection, voiding problems, fistula formation and sacral plexus neuropathy [42]. Nevertheless, the authors quote a 60% overall 3-year survival rate with a local control rate of 73%, when pre-operative radiotherapy and salvage surgery was used. The combination of chemotherapy with long course radiotherapy increased the R0 resection rate from 52% to 72% in an uncontrolled series of patients. This is thought to be due to the radiosensitizing properties of oxaliplatin.

Surgery for pelvic recurrence after resection of rectal cancer has high morbidity and mortality (up to 72% and 10% respectively). However, radiotherapy is not curative for recurrence and although it may achieve palliation of symptoms in 60-80%, its effects usually last only 3 to 6 months [43].

There seems to be less chance of re-resection after AP excision compared with LAR [44]. Nevertheless, although surgical resection is not always curative, it can provide some palliation of intractable pain and prevent or treat complications such as obstruction, perforation, bleeding and sepsis.

Where are we going?

Downstaging and downsizing with long course radiotherapy (LRT), chemoradiotherapy (CRT) but not short course radiotherapy (SRT)

Attempts have been made to reduce the rate of positive CRM, and so reduce local recurrence and improve survival of low rectal tumours by giving the patient neoadjuvant combined chemoradiation or radiotherapy alone. Pre-operative radiotherapy is commonly utilised in low anterior resection, which may compensate for the limitations of surgical technique resulting from a narrow pelvis and short distal surgical margins [45]. Radiotherapy probably destroys micro-foci of tumour outside the main tumour mass. Administered with chemotherapy, radiotherapy produces a 30-40% histological response in the primary tumour, allowing short distal margins and anal sphincter preservation [46].

The superiority of pre-operative over postoperative radiotherapy was reported in 1985 and it was suggested that pre-operative therapy would approximately halve the local recurrence rate in any given group at risk [47]. Today, the routine use and efficacy of radiotherapy and chemotherapy remain controversial, though a consensus is that irradiation reduces local recurrence but the survival benefit remains unproven.

Pre-operative neoadjuvant radiotherapy for potentially resectable, but fixed or tethered, rectal cancer is generally accepted in clinical practice.

However, controversy continues as to the role of radiotherapy in resectable, mobile rectal cancer, and the UK CRO7 study is addressing this issue. For locally advanced rectal cancer, two UK trials have evaluated the effect of long course, pre-operative radiotherapy and have shown effective downstaging with reduction in local recurrence but no difference in overall survival [48]. Nonetheless, it is debatable as to whether it is oncologically safe to perform a low anastomosis on tissue which had previously had tumour, prior to its downstaging with neoadjuvant therapy. Minsky et al reported on a small series where 83% of patients with low rectal cancer, who would have required an APE, had sphincter-preservation surgery after pre-operative radiotherapy. Despite a 10% complete pathologic response, 4-year overall local recurrence was high at 23% and 4-year disease-free survival was 66% [49]. So it may be that radiotherapy can enable more sphincter-saving operations by sterilising the area of anastomosis and delaying the time to local and distant metastases.

Evidence for the use of pre-operative chemotherapy in addition to radiotherapy was reported in 2001 when Frykholm et al published a small randomised controlled trial of patients with fixed rectal carcinomas who were randomised to pre-operative radiotherapy or chemoradiotherapy (CRT). This trial showed a significant improvement in resectability and reduction in local failure with the use of CRT [50]. The feasibility of a pre-operative strategy involving capecitabine, oxaliplatin and radiotherapy has been demonstrated and is being evaluated as part of the phase II "EXPERT" trial at the Royal Marsden Hospital.

With pre-operative irradiation of clinically mobile lesions, pathological complete response rates of 10-20% have been reported, and with pre-operative chemoradiation, these have been higher at 30-35% [51]. However, when the curative potential of irradiation alone was evaluated in patients with clinically mobile lesions who were medically unfit or refused to have an abdominoperineal excision, complete clinical regression was noted in 50% but 40% relapsed locally [52]. There is some evidence from the randomised Lyons R90-01 trial that long course radiotherapy with a delay of 6 to 8 weeks for surgery results in a significantly better tumour response and pathological downstaging of rectal cancer. In the same trial, there was a non-significant increase in the number of sphincter-preserving operations in the long interval group compared with the short interval group (76% versus 68% respectively) [53]. The Stockholm III trials are underway assessing whether a delay to surgery after pre-operative short course radiotherapy has any effect on downstaging and downsizing rectal cancer.

Difficulties with rectal cancer below 6cm from the anal verge. APE versus ultralow AR

Cancers of the distal rectum pose a problem of local tumour control and sphincter preservation. APE was long considered the standard treatment of tumours within 6cm from the anal verge, providing local control in most patients, but the loss of sphincter function can cause psychological problems. Consequently, there is an increasing practice of sphincter-preserving surgery with LAR. LAR is possible without compromising oncological safety as pathological assessment of rectal cancer has shown that spread is mainly circumferentially and not distally. Therefore, the rate of anterior resection for low rectal tumours is now 76% to 83% in some centres with a rate of APE as low as 5.5% in some institutions [49, 54, 55].

Most surgeons consider a distal margin of 1-2cm safe, as distal intramural spread rarely exceeds 1cm [56-58]. In fact, preliminary data suggest that distal intramural spread may carry little importance in determining local recurrence of rectal cancer [59]. Histopathological studies have shown that distal spread for more than 2cm, as measured on a fixed operative specimen, occurs in only 2% of patients, all of whom have Dukes' stage C tumours, the majority of which are poorly differentiated and are associated with poor survival [60].

The optimal surgical treatment of rectal cancer in the lower one third remains controversial with an absence of randomised trials. Recent literature has shown that the local recurrence of low rectal cancers is higher, compared with middle and upper rectal cancers. In one series, the 5-year local recurrence for low rectal, mid rectal and upper rectal tumours after low AR was 7%, 2% and 0% respectively [6]. In a retrospective analysis of 1008 cases, local recurrence was less common after resection of upper rectal tumours (14%) than middle (21%) or lower third tumours (26%) [61]. This translates to a poorer survival with a 5-year survival of 69% for the curative resections and 19% in the subgroup developing local recurrence. This may be due to the mesorectum tapering out completely below the levator sling, accounting for a higher chance of the tumour spreading to perirectal tissues. Therefore, there is a higher risk for the resection margin to have tumour involvement with a higher risk of local recurrence. In addition, cancers of the low rectum present with more of the adverse risk factors prognostically significant for local recurrence, including lymphatic and vascular invasion, perineural invasion and positive nodal disease [62].

In the Basingstoke series of 683 consecutive cases of rectal cancer, 45% of patients had cancers in the lower rectum. Of the patients who had a curative LAR for tumours below 6cm, the 5-year local recurrence rate was 7% and the systemic recurrence rate was 27%, compared with 17% and 27% in patients who had curative APE [6]. Local recurrence after APE tends to be higher than for LAR in most series comparing rectal cancers of all stages, with a range of 10% to 33% from a review by Dehni et al [63]. This is in contrast with a local recurrence rate of 4% to 8% for anterior resection in all stages of rectal cancer, using the TME technique, which has been reproduced by Enker in the USA [64].

Inferior cancer cure rates with APE may be due to less precision in the excision of the surrounding tissues, and thus a definable dissection plane, than TME for higher tumours. It may be that adjuvant radiotherapy should be considered for all low rectal tumours. To avoid "waisting" of the APE specimen and therefore reduce the risks of a positive resection margin, visceroparietal plane dissection should stop at the pelvic floor and perineal dissection should encompass the tumour with a wide resection margin, including the ischiorectal fat and taking a wide cuff of levators above the level of puborectalis. This would enable a cylinder of tissue to be excised, in keeping with the more traditional description of an APE by Ernest Miles [69]. Additionally, the higher rates of positive margins and local recurrence with AP excisions may be due to the alternative lymphatic drainage of low rectal cancers through the internal iliac lymphatic vessels.

MRI is equivalent to histopathology T staging

There are recent data which suggest that a CRM at risk of tumour involvement can be reliably seen on the pre-operative MRI scan and that this correlates with the post-surgery histological specimen of the rectal tumour [65]. Recent unpublished data from the prospective, multicentred MRI and Rectal Cancer European Equivalence Study (MERCURY) confirm accurate prediction both of the T staging and CRM within 1mm of the resection margin. Previous studies reported a varying accuracy for T staging between 67% and 83%, with a considerable interobserver variability [66]. However, it has been shown that the distance of tumour to the circumferential margin (CRM) is the most powerful predictor of local recurrence and not the T stage. In a large series of MR evaluation of CRM, there was higher accuracy for predicting tumour-free resection margins (95%) than for the prediction of T stage [67]. Therefore, an accurate pre-operative staging system can be used with MRI to detect which rectal cancers are close to the surgical resection margin and may benefit from downstaging with pre-operative neoadjuvant therapy.

Conclusions

Though radiotherapy may reduce local recurrence rates, its associated toxicity, early complications, long-term side effects and costs suggest that it is best reserved for patients at high risk of recurrence. Nicholls and Hall have identified two groups of tumours, locally not extensive and locally extensive [8]. The former group includes those tumours which are confined to the bowel wall or with less than 5mm penetration into the extra-rectal tissues, where the survival is high and recurrence is low. This includes T1, T2 and less extensive T3 and Dukes' A and less extensive B tumours. Tumours that have extended more than this (T3 and T4) would be locally extensive with a high risk of local recurrence and poor survival. The same subdivision of T3 tumours into T3a (up to 5mm tumour invasion beyond the muscularis propria) and T3b (more than 5mm) was made by Merkel *et al* who noted a locoregional recurrence rate at 5 years of 10.4% for pT3a and 26.3% for pT3b tumours and a 5-year survival of 85.4% for pT3a and 54.1% for pT3b [68]. The use of MRI is the most promising modality to select out cases where the surgical resection margin is threatened, with consideration of pre-operative radiotherapy in this group.

In summary, the optimal treatment for rectal cancer is surgery with selective use of pre-operative neoadjuvant therapy. The outcomes can be evaluated from local recurrence rates and overall survival. Although the recent Dutch Rectal Cancer Trial showed a significant reduction in local recurrence with radiotherapy, there was a high proportion of involved margins after TME on mobile tumours, which implies that either surgery, staging or both were sub-optimal. Finally, whilst demonstrating a benefit of SRT in some patients for local recurrence, no effect was seen on survival at 5 years [70]. Thus, there is evidence accumulating to suggest that TME surgery is the major factor in reduction of local recurrence after rectal cancer surgery. TME is based on sound pathological principles, encompassing circumferential and distal mesorectal clearance, carefully dissecting in a plane that encompasses the embryological hindgut. It seems unlikely that this technique will ever be subjected to a randomised controlled trial, but population-based evidence is accumulating to support this technique and the benefits of training.

References

1. Marsh PJ, James RD, Schofield PF. Definition of local recurrence after surgery for rectal carcinoma. *Br J Surg* 1995; 82(4): 465-8.
2. Birbeck KF, Macklin CP, Tiffin NJ, Parsons W, Dixon MF, Mapstone NP, et al. Rates of circumferential resection margin involvement vary between surgeons and predict outcomes in rectal cancer surgery. *Ann Surg* 2002; 235(4): 449-57.
3. Quirke P, Durdey P, Dixon MF, Williams NS. Local recurrence of rectal adenocarcinoma due to inadequate surgical resection. Histopathological study of lateral tumour spread and surgical excision. *Lancet* 1986; 2(8514): 996-9.
4. Hermanek P. [Current aspects of a new staging classification of colorectal cancer and its clinical consequences]. *Chirurg* 1989; 60(1): 1-7.
5. Hermanek P. [International documentation system for colorectal cancer – reporting pathological findings]. *Verh Dtsch Ges Pathol* 1991; 75: 386-8.
6. Croxford MA, Salerno G, Watson M, et al. Colorectal 23-28. *Br J Surg* 2004; 91(S1): 63-5.
7. Shepherd NA, Baxter KJ, Love SB. Influence of local peritoneal involvement on pelvic recurrence and prognosis in rectal cancer. *J Clin Pathol* 1995; 48(9): 849-55.
8. Nicholls RJ, Hall C. Treatment of non-disseminated cancer of the lower rectum. *Br J Surg* 1996; 83(1): 15-8.
9. Enker WE. Total mesorectal excision - the new golden standard of surgery for rectal cancer. *Ann Med* 1997; 29(2): 127-33.
10. Heriot AG, Grundy A, Kumar D. Preoperative staging of rectal carcinoma. *Br J Surg* 1999; 86(1): 17-28.
11. Wibe A, Rendedal PR, Svensson E, Norstein J, Eide TJ, Myrvold HE, et al. Prognostic significance of the circumferential resection margin following total mesorectal excision for rectal cancer. *Br J Surg* 2002; 89(3): 327-34.
12. Nagtegaal ID, Marijnen CA, Kranenbarg EK, van de Velde CJ, van Krieken JH. Circumferential margin involvement is still an important predictor of local recurrence in rectal carcinoma: not one millimeter but two millimeters is the limit. *Am J Surg Pathol* 2002; 26(3): 350-7.
13. Simunovic M, Sexton R, Moran BJ, Heald RJ. Optimal preoperative assessment and surgery for rectal cancer may greatly limit the need for radiotherapy. *Br J Surg* 2003; 90(8): 999-1003.
14. Enker WE. Total mesorectal excision - the new golden standard of surgery for rectal cancer. *Ann Med* 1997; 29(2): 127-33.
15. Jatzko GR, Jagoditsch M, Lisborg PH, Denk H, Klimpfinger M, Stettner HM. Long-term results of radical surgery for rectal cancer: multivariate analysis of prognostic factors influencing survival and local recurrence. *Eur J Surg Oncol* 1999; 25(3): 284-91.
16. Heald RJ, Moran BJ, Ryall RD, Sexton R, MacFarlane JK. Rectal cancer: the Basingstoke experience of total mesorectal excision, 1978-1997. *Arch Surg* 1998; 133(8): 894-9.
17. Martling AL, Holm T, Rutqvist LE, Moran BJ, Heald RJ, Cedermark B. Effect of a surgical training programme on outcome of rectal cancer in the County of Stockholm. Stockholm Colorectal Cancer Study Group; Basingstoke Bowel Cancer Research Project. *Lancet* 2000; 356(9224): 93-6.
18. Porter G. Surgeon-related factors and outcome in rectal cancer treatment. *International Journal of Surgical Investigation* 1999; 1(3): 257-8.
19. Martling AL, Cedermark B, Johansson H, Rutqvist L, Holm T. The surgeon as a prognostic factor after the introduction of total mesorectal excision in the treatment of rectal cancer. *Br J Surg* 2002; 2002(89): 8.
20. Kapiteijn E, Putter H, van de Velde CJ. Impact of the introduction and training of total mesorectal excision on recurrence and survival in rectal cancer in The Netherlands. *Br J Surg* 2002; 89(9): 1142-9.
21. Wibe A, Moller B, Norstein J, Carlsen E, Wiig JN, Heald RJ, et al. A national strategic change in treatment policy for rectal cancer - implementation of total mesorectal excision as routine treatment in Norway. A national audit. *Dis Colon Rectum* 2002; 45(7): 857-66.
22. Nesbakken A, Nygaard K, Westerheim O, Mala T, Lunde OC. Local recurrence after mesorectal excision for rectal cancer. *Eur J Surg* Oncol 2002; 28(2): 126-34.
23. Harling H, Bulow S, Kronborg O, Moller LN, Jorgensen T. Survival of rectal cancer patients in Denmark during 1994-99. *Colorectal Dis* 2004; 6(3): 153-7.
24. Randomized study on preoperative radiotherapy in rectal carcinoma. Stockholm Colorectal Cancer Study Group. *Ann Surg Oncol* 1996; 3(5): 423-30.
25. Improved survival with preoperative radiotherapy in resectable rectal cancer. Swedish Rectal Cancer Trial. *N Engl J Med* 1997; 336(14): 980-7.
26. Cedermark B, Johansson H, Rutqvist LE, Wilking N. The Stockholm I trial of preoperative short term radiotherapy in operable rectal carcinoma. A prospective randomized trial. Stockholm Colorectal Cancer Study Group. *Cancer* 1995; 75(9): 2269-75.
27. Buyse M, Zeleniuch-Jacquotte A, Chalmers TC. Adjuvant therapy for colorectal cancer: why we still don't know. *JAMA* 1988; 259: 3571-78.
28. Camma C, Giunta M, Fiorica F, Pagliaro L, Craxi A, Cottone M. Preoperative radiotherapy for resectable rectal cancer: a meta-analysis. *JAMA* 2000; 284(8): 1008-15.
29. Ross A, Rusnak C, Weinerman B, Kuechler P, Hayashi A, MacLachlan G, et al. Recurrence and survival after surgical management of rectal cancer. *Am J Surg* 1999; 177(5): 392-5.
30. Zaheer S, Pemberton JH, Farouk R, et al. Surgical treatment of adenocarcinoma of the rectum. *Ann Surg* 1998; 227: 800-11.
31. Kapiteijn E, Marijnen CAM, Nagtegaal ID, Putter H, Steup WH, Wiggers T, et al. Pre-operative radiotherapy combined with total mesorectal excision for resectable rectal cancer. *N Engl J Med* 2001; 345: 638-46.
32. Goldberg PA, Nicholls RJ, Porter NH, Love S, Grimsey JE. Long-term results of a randomised trial of short-course low-

dose adjuvant pre-operative radiotherapy for rectal cancer: reduction in local treatment failure. *Eur J Cancer* 1994; 30A(11): 1602-6.
33. Marsh PJ, James RD, Schofield PF. Adjuvant preoperative radiotherapy for locally advanced rectal carcinoma. Results of a prospective, randomized trial. *Dis Colon Rectum* 1994; 37(12): 1205-14.
34. Gerard A, Buyse M, Nordlinger B, Loygue J, Pene F, Kempf P, et al. Preoperative radiotherapy as adjuvant treatment in rectal cancer. Final results of a randomized study of the European Organization for Research and Treatment of Cancer (EORTC). *Ann Surg* 1988; 208(5): 606-14.
35. Randomised trial of surgery alone versus surgery followed by radiotherapy for mobile cancer of the rectum. Medical Research Council Rectal Cancer Working Party. *Lancet* 1996; 348(9042): 1610-4.
36. Allal AS, Bieri S, Pelloni A, Spataro V, Anchisi S, Ambrosetti P, et al. Sphincter-sparing surgery after preoperative radiotherapy for low rectal cancers: feasibility, oncologic results and quality of life outcomes. *Br J Cancer* 2000; 82(6): 1131-7.
37. Colorectal Cancer Collaborative Group. Adjuvant radiotherapy for rectal cancer: a systematic overview of 8,507 patients from 22 randomised trials. *Lancet* 2001; 358(9290): 1291-304.
38. Lele S, Radstone D, Eremin J, Kendal R, Hosie KB. Prospective audit following the introduction of short-course preoperative radiotherapy for rectal cancer. *Br J Surg* 2000; 87(1): 97-9.
39. Da Silva GM, Berho M, Wexner SD, Efron J, Weiss EG, Nogueras JJ, et al. Histologic analysis of the irradiated anal sphincter. *Dis Colon Rectum* 2003; 46(11): 1492-7.
40. Wiggers T, Mannaerts GH, Marinelli AW, Martijn H, Rutten HJ. Surgery for locally recurrent rectal cancer. *Colorectal Dis* 2003; 5(5): 504-7.
41. Franke J, Rosenzweig S, Reinartz P, Hoer J, Kasperk R, Schumpelick V. [Value of positron emission tomography (18F-FDG-PET) in the diagnosis of recurrent rectal cancer]. *Chirurg* 2000; 71(1): 80-5.
42. Rutten HJ, Mannaerts GH, Martijn H, Wiggers T. Intraoperative radiotherapy for locally recurrent rectal cancer in The Netherlands. *Eur J Surg Oncol* 2000; 26 Suppl A: S16-20.
43. Gagliardi G, Hawley PR, Hershman MJ, Arnott SJ. Prognostic factors in surgery for local recurrence of rectal cancer. *Br J Surg* 1995; 82(10): 1401-5.
44. Saito N, Koda K, Takiguchi N, Oda K, Soda H, Nunomura M, et al. Surgery for local pelvic recurrence after resection of rectal cancer. *Int J Colorectal Dis* 1998; 13(1): 32-8.
45. Papillon J. [Sphincter preservation in cancer of lower rectum. The role of radiotherapy]. *Gastroenterol Clin Biol* 1988; 12(5): 416-9.
46. Luna-Perez P, Rodriguez-Ramirez S, Rodriguez-Coria DF, Fernandez A, Labastida S, Silva A, et al. Preoperative chemoradiation therapy and anal sphincter preservation with locally advanced rectal adenocarcinoma. *World J Surg* 2001; 25(8): 1006-11.
47. Holm T, Johansson H, Cedermark B, Ekelund G, Rutqvist LE. Influence of hospital- and surgeon-related factors on outcome after treatment of rectal cancer with or without preoperative radiotherapy. *Br J Surg* 1997; 84(5): 657-63.
48. Marsh RD, Chu NM, Vauthey JN, Mendenhall WM, Lauwers GY, Bewsher C, et al. Preoperative treatment of patients with locally advanced unresectable rectal adenocarcinoma utilizing continuous chronobiologically shaped 5-fluorouracil infusion and radiation therapy. *Cancer* 1996; 78(2): 217-25.
49. Minsky BD, Cohen AM, Enker WE, Paty P. Sphincter preservation with preoperative radiation therapy and coloanal anastomosis. *Int J Radiat Oncol Biol Phys* 1995; 31(3): 553-9.
50. Frykholm GJ, Pahlman L, Glimelius B. Combined chemo- and radiotherapy vs. radiotherapy alone in the treatment of primary, nonresectable adenocarcinoma of the rectum. *Int J Radiat Oncol Biol Phys* 2001; 50(2): 427-34.
51. Sebag-Montefiore D. Treatment of T4 tumours: the role of radiotherapy. *Colorectal Dis* 2003; 5(5): 432-5.
52. Gunderson LL, Haddock MG, Schild SE. Rectal cancer: preoperative versus postoperative irradiation as a component of adjuvant treatment. *Semin Radiat Oncol* 2003; 13(4): 419-32.
53. Francois Y, Nemoz CJ, Baulieux J, Vignal J, Grandjean JP, Partensky C, et al. Influence of the interval between preoperative radiation therapy and surgery on downstaging and on the rate of sphincter-sparing surgery for rectal cancer: the Lyon R90-01 randomized trial. *J Clin Oncol* 1999; 17(8): 2396.
54. MacFarlane JK, Ryall RD, Heald RJ. Mesorectal excision for rectal cancer. *Lancet* 1993; 341(8843): 457-60.
55. Heald RJ, Smedh RK, Kald A, Sexton R, Moran BJ. Abdominoperineal excision of the rectum - an endangered operation. Norman Nigro Lectureship. *Dis Colon Rectum* 1997; 40(7): 747-51.
56. Williams NS, Dixon MF, Johnston D. Reappraisal of the 5 centimetre rule of distal excision for carcinoma of the rectum: a study of distal intramural spread and of patients' survival. *Br J Surg* 1983; 70(3): 150-4.
57. Madsen PM, Christiansen J. Distal intramural spread of rectal carcinomas. *Dis Colon Rectum* 1986; 29(4): 279-82.
58. Moore HG, Riedel E, Minsky BD, Saltz L, Paty P, Wong D, et al. Adequacy of 1-cm distal margin after restorative rectal cancer resection with sharp mesorectal excision and preoperative combined-modality therapy. *Ann Surg Oncol* 2003; 10(1): 80-5.
59. Andreola S, Leo E, Belli F, Lavarino C, Bufalino R, Tomasic G, et al. Distal intramural spread in adenocarcinoma of the lower third of the rectum treated with total rectal resection and coloanal anastomosis. *Dis Colon Rectum* 1997; 40(1): 25-9.
60. Penfold JC. A comparison of restorative resection of carcinoma of the middle third of the rectum with abdominoperineal excision. *ANZ J Surg* 1974; 44(4): 354-6.
61. McDermott FT, Hughes ES, Pihl E, Johnson WR, Price AB. Local recurrence after potentially curative resection for rectal cancer in a series of 1008 patients. *Br J Surg* 1985; 72(1): 34-7.
62. Enker WE, Thaler HT, Cranor ML, Polyak T. Total mesorectal excision in the operative treatment of carcinoma of the rectum. *J Am Coll Surg* 1995; 181(4): 335-46.

63. Dehni N, McFadden N, McNamara DA, Guiguet M, Tiret E, Parc R. Oncologic results following abdominoperineal resection for adenocarcinoma of the low rectum. *Dis Colon Rectum* 2003; 46(7): 867-74; discussion 874.
64. Enker WE, Merchant N, Cohen AM, Lanouette NM, Swallow C, Guillem J, et al. Safety and efficacy of low anterior resection for rectal cancer: 681 consecutive cases from a specialty service. *Ann Surg* 1999; 230(4): 544-52; discussion 552-4.
65. Brown G, Radcliffe AG, Newcombe RG, Dallimore NS, Bourne MW, Williams GT. Preoperative assessment of prognostic factors in rectal cancer using high-resolution magnetic resonance imaging. *Br J Surg* 2003; 90(3): 355-64.
66. Blomqvist L, Holm T, Rubio C, Hindmarsh T. Rectal tumours - MR imaging with endorectal and/or phased-array coils, and histopathological staging on giant sections. A comparative study. *Acta Radiol* 1997; 38(3): 437-44.
67. Beets-Tan RG. MRI in rectal cancer: the T stage and circumferential resection margin. *Colorectal Dis* 2003; 5(5): 392-5.
68. Merkel S, Mansmann U, Siassi M, Papadopoulos T, Hohenberger W, Hermanek P. The prognostic inhomogeneity in pT3 rectal carcinomas. *Int J Colorectal Dis* 2001; 16(5): 298-304.
69. Miles WE. *Rectal Surgery: A practical guide to the modern surgical treatment of rectal diseases.* Cassell & Co. Ltd, 1939.
70. van de Velde CJ. Personal communication, 2004.

Chapter 11

Chemotherapy trials in colorectal cancer

Gary Middleton MD MRCP, Consultant Medical Oncologist
Royal Surrey County Hospital, Guildford, Surrey, UK

What is the issue?

The crucial roles of chemotherapy in both the adjuvant treatment of resected colorectal cancer and the therapy of advanced disease have been established beyond doubt. The past decade has seen the development of new chemotherapeutic agents and an explosion in the knowledge of the biology of the disease. Whilst the former have been comprehensively integrated into standard therapy, the translational integration of the latter into clinical care looks set to make the coming decade one of enormous progress in the management of the disease.

Where are we now?

In the setting of advanced colorectal cancer (ACRC), attempts to improve the therapeutic index of bolus 5FU, either by modulation or scheduling, were met with limited success [1,2]. Whilst it was acknowledged that monthly bolus 5FU/folinic acid regimens, which had become standard by the late 1990s, were not without substantial toxicity, especially stomatitis and diarrhoea, this had to be weighed against the inconvenience of infusional 5FU regimens.

The lack of an optimal fluoropyrimidine (FP) regimen was demonstrated by the fact that in the four pivotal phase III studies published in 2000 investigating the impact of the addition of irinotecan or oxaliplatin to FP therapy in the front-line treatment of ACRC, four different FP regimens were used as the control arms (Table 1).

This series of studies demonstrated that the additional drug undoubtedly improved activity and, in the case of irinotecan, this translated to a survival advantage. The lack of survival advantage with the addition of oxaliplatin was probably due to these two studies being underpowered (powered to detect a 20% improvement in response rate and a 3-month prolongation of progression-free survival [PFS] respectively) and significant cross-over from the FP-alone arm to a second-line oxaliplatin-containing regimen (57% and 28% respectively). In early 2000, the FDA approved irinotecan and 5FU (as the IFL regimen) as a standard of care in the first-line treatment of advanced disease but turned down a first-line application for oxaliplatin. However, subsequent data very significantly weakened the prominence of IFL as a standard regimen. Accrual to the study N9741 was terminated prematurely in April 2001. This study compared IFL with FOLFOX (5FU/leucovorin [LV] and oxaliplatin) and irinotecan/oxaliplatin. An excess of

Table 1. Phase III randomised controlled trials investigating the impact of the addition of oxaliplatin or irinotecan to FP therapy in ACRC.

Author	n	Regimens	RR	PFS	MOS	12/12 OS
Saltz [3]	683	IFL	50%*	7.0/12*	14.8/12*	-
		5FU + LV (LD)	28%	4.3/12	12.6/12	-
		Ir	29%	4.2/12	12.0/12	-
Douillard [4]	387	Ir + De G/Aio	49%*	6.7/12*	17.4/12*	69%
		De G/Aio	31%	4.4/12	14.1/12	59%
Giachetti [5]	200	Ox + Chrono 5FU/LV	50%*	8.7/12*	19.1/12	-
		Chrono 5FU/LV	16%	6.1/12	19.4/12	-
De Gramont [6]	420	FOLFOX 4	51%	9.0/12*	16.2/12	69%
		LV 5FU	22%	6.2/12	14.1/12	61%

* statistically significant

toxic deaths within 60 days was noticed on the IFL arm and an independent panel issued a report of its findings on the toxicity of this programme later that year [7]. There was a 3.5% early treatment-induced death rate due to gastrointestinal or vascular toxicity on the IFL arm, compared to 1.1% for FOLFOX and IROX. This, in a palliative setting, was unacceptable and indeed subsequently published survival figures demonstrated a survival advantage for the oxaliplatin-containing regimen over what had been, up until then, the US standard [8].

This excessive toxicity for a bolus 5FU-based regimen came as little surprise to many European commentators, where the preference had been for infusional-based regimens in combination with irinotecan. Indeed, the decision by the National Institute for Clinical Excellence not to recommend the use of irinotecan in combination with infusional 5FU-based treatment in the first-line setting when it published its Health and Technology Assessment report on irinotecan, oxaliplatin and raltitrexed in March 2002 [9], was met with much dismay in the oncological community. NICE did, however, recommend irinotecan as a monotherapy in patients who had failed a prior 5FU-containing regimen. The strength of the data with regard to its use in this setting was very strong [10]. When compared to supportive care alone, the drug provided a 2.6 times survival advantage at 1 year. This extra quantity of life was of good quality. There were statistically significant differences in the worst score during study for all components on the EORTC QL30 functional subscales, besides the emotional subscale, in favour of irinotecan and also an improvement in global quality of life. Pain-free survival, survival without weight loss and time to definitive quality of life deterioration were all improved on the irinotecan arm.

The question as to whether it is better to use the drug in combination with FP up front or to use it as salvage monotherapy can only be answered by comparing these two strategies directly with time to tumour control, quality of life and health economics as endpoints. The FOCUS programme closed in December 2003, with 2,135 patients randomised (Figure 1). The pairwise comparisons of arms A and C are crucial to resolving this issue. The best supportive care comparison results notwithstanding, irinotecan monotherapy is not a trivial treatment, with diarrhoea and neutropenia being prominent potential toxicities. The A versus B comparison looks to improve the therapeutic index of irinotecan when the drug is used in the second-line setting.

What of oxaliplatin? NICE will be issuing their review of the guidance on irinotecan and oxaliplatin in ACRC in August 2005. The N9741 data certainly go some way to making a robust case for a first-line recommendation in combination with FP. A critical

11 Chemotherapy trials in colorectal cancer

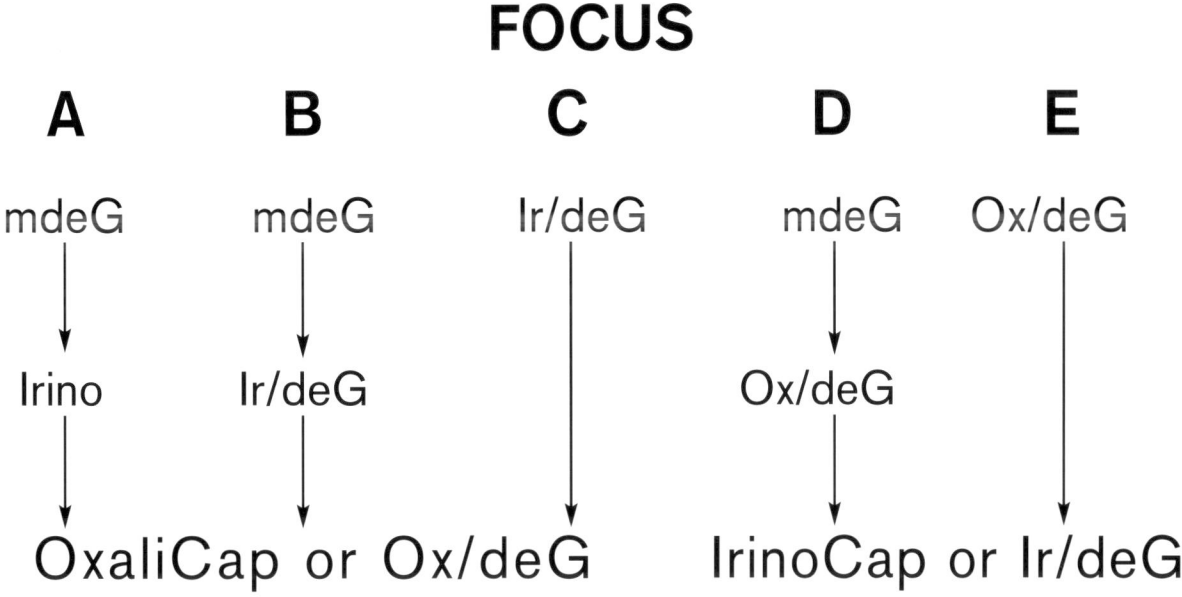

Figure 1. FOCUS trial schema following incorporation of planned cross-over (1/2003).

study, however, is LIFE, which grafted first-line oxaliplatin usage onto the NICE approved backbone of first-line FP and second-line irinotecan monotherapy. It randomised 725 patients to either 5FU/oxaliplatin or 5FU alone, with guaranteed second-line irinotecan, with overall survival as the primary endpoint. Overall survival data will be presented at ASCO 2005. The N9741 data alone were enough for the FDA to approve oxaliplatin for first-line usage in combination with FP. Indeed, in the USA, FOLFOX has become very much the first-line standard of care.

For many, the issue of first-line versus second-line usage of any individual drug is largely irrelevant. All three drugs are essential for the optimisation of outcomes in patients with ACRC. The 19.5-month median survival of FOLFOX treated patients in N9741 was the longest ever seen in a North American phase III ACRC chemotherapy trial: 60% of these patients received second-line irinotecan, making this effectively a result that could be obtained when patients are given all three active drugs. Axel Grothey has demonstrated a significant correlation of median overall survival with the percentage of patients who receive all three drugs during the course of their disease [11], and V308 published earlier this year a study comparing FOLFOX followed by FOLFIRI with the reverse sequence that showed median survivals of over 20 months for both arms [12]. It does not seem to matter when any individual drug is used, just as long as all three of them are used.

Advances in the advanced disease setting frequently form the platform for the development of more effective strategies treating early disease. Publication of the QUASAR study in 2000 marked the culmination of a decade of randomised trials, establishing 6 months of low-dose folinic acid-modulated bolus 5FU without levamasole as the standard of care, at least for curatively resected Dukes' C colorectal cancer patients [13-16].

The publication of the MOSAIC data was the first from a global series of studies which has been examining the impact of the addition of either irinotecan or oxaliplatin to FP in the adjuvant context [17]. Two thousand two hundred and forty-six patients who had undergone curative resection of Dukes' B or C colon cancer were randomised to bi-weekly 5FU/FA or FOLFOX. There was a statistically significant improvement in 3-year disease-free survival;

oxaliplatin-treated patients benefited from a 5.3% absolute improvement, which represents a 23% reduction in the risk of recurrence, compared to 5FU/LV alone. Three-year disease-free survival was used as the primary endpoint in this study. This has been validated as a surrogate for 5-year overall survival and unanimously approved by the Oncologic Data Advisory Committee for such a purpose [18]. The XELOXA programme, now closed, similarly has investigated the addition of oxaliplatin, but this time utilising oral FP by randomising Dukes' C patients to either bolus 5FU/FA or Xelox. The results of the analogous study to MOSAIC but utilising irinotecan, PETACC-3, are awaited.

Where are we going?

Impressive as the above results undoubtedly are, studies are already moving way beyond them. The publication in June 2004 of the results of a study randomising 813 patients to IFL ± bevacizumab, the anti-VEGF monocolonal antibody, was proof of principle that targeting the tumour vasculature was a valuable anti-cancer strategy [19]. Thirty years ago, Judah Folkman demonstrated that the induction of neovascularisation was essential to ensure continued growth of tumour nodules beyond 1-2mm [3], the limit of diffusion of oxygen and nutrients from any pre-existing blood supply. VEGF alone is sufficient to initiate the angiogenic switch, the rate limiting step in tumour progression, through its potent stimulation of dilatation and increased permeability of capillaries and venules. The addition of bevacizumab increased median overall survival from 15.6 to 20.3 months and PFS from 6.2 to 10.6 months. Similarly impressive results had been achieved earlier by the addition of bevacizumab to FP alone [20] and a major breakthrough was achieved when the 2-year median survival barrier for patients with ACRC was broken; the retrospective analysis of outcomes according to the post-progression therapy in this phase III trial documented a 25.1 month median survival for patients initially treated with IFL plus Avastin, who subsequently received oxaliplatin [21].

The question of whether these results are applicable to oxaliplatin/FP combinations in the first-line setting is being tested in the context of ongoing comparison trials of oral FP versus infusional FP in combination with oxaliplatin (Xelox versus FOLFOX ± bevacizumab - SWOG S0303/XELOX 1).

Larger tumour deposits have an established blood supply and anti-VEGF strategies which target neovascularisation may have limited efficacy here. Animal models suggest that small molecule inhibitors effective in the regression of such larger tumour deposits exert their effect through PDGF as opposed to VEGF [22]. They cause the dissociation of pericytes from endothelial cells and decrease pericyte numbers, cells which are strongly and, in this environment almost uniquely, PDGF positive. Dual VEGF and PDGF receptor antagonists are available and include the orally available PTK787. Such tyrosine kinase inhibitors would be expected to inhibit both neovascularisation and the integrity of pericyte: endothelial interactions, a potentially potent double impact on the vascularity of both micro- and macro-metastases. Confirm 1 is testing the impact of addition of PTK787 to up front FOLFOX 4 and Confirm 2 is the analogous second-line study following first-line irinotecan/FP failure.

Another major area of research in colorectal cancer therapeutics has been the epidermal growth factor receptor (EGFR). Upon binding its ligands, classically TGF-alpha and EGF, EGFR homodimerises or heterodimerises with other members of the erb-B family of type 1 receptor tyrosine kinases. This activates the tyrosine kinase, resulting in autophosphorylation and the subsequent activation of a number of phosphorylation-dependent cascades, including the ras-raf MAP kinase and PI3K-Akt pathways. The net effect of receptor activation is cellular proliferation through increased cyclin D1 activity (activated MAP kinase increases C-Jun levels, which activates AP-1 and increased Akt levels lead to decreased levels of P27 via inhibition of the Forkhead gene product pathway) and decreased apoptosis (via the inhibitory influence of Akt on Bad). The EGFR can either be inhibited by monocolonal antibodies directed against the extra-cellular ligand binding domain (cetuximab, Pentumomab) or small molecule inhibitors of the intracellular tyrosine kinase domain (gefitinib and erlotonib). Receptor inhibition also leads to a reduction of angiogenesis via decreased levels of beta-FGF and VEGF and increased endothelial cell apoptosis, as well as a reduction in tumour invasiveness via a decrease in matrix metalloproteinases activity, especially MMP-9.

EGFR is over-expressed in up to 80% of CRC. What is clear is that inhibition of the EGFR by cetuximab circumvents irinotecan resistance in a proportion of patients and has modest single-agent activity in resistant CRC. The Bond study, randomising over 300 patients with irinotecan-resistant CRC, showed a 22.9% response rate to the combination of irinotecan plus antibody, with a 10.8% response rate to cetuximab monotherapy [23]. Progression-free survival was significantly greater in the combination therapy arm. There was no correlation between the response rate and the intensity of EGFR expression (indeed, cetuximab activity has been demonstrated in patients who are negative for EGFR over-expression by standard immunohistochemical criteria [24]) but was highly correlated with the development of the characteristic acneiform rash (13% response rate in the monotherapy group with rash, compared with 0% for those not developing rash). These data raise a number of important questions:

- Does the small number of patients responding to cetuximab monotherapy represent a prospectively definable subset?

Response to EGFR inhibition using the small molecule tyrosine kinase inhibitors is highly correlated with the presence of mutations in the tyrosine kinase domain, which significantly enhances EGF-dependent activation of the receptor due to a greater affinity and prolonged binding of ATP to the activation site [25,26]. Such mutations do not, however, appear to be a feature of colorectal cancer [27,28]. Indeed, early results from Massachusetts General presented at ASCO 2004, have shown that the presence of tyrosine kinase domain mutations does not predict a response to cetuximab.

- What is the relevance of the rash?

The tight association of rash with response, and indeed survival, has also been seen with the small molecule tyrosine kinase inhibitors in non-small cell lung cancer. This is the principle side effect of these drugs and leads directly to the concept of dose escalation until the development of rash. This needs to be tested prospectively.

The first two are interrelated. EGFR activation can be inhibited by tyrosine kinase inhibitors in cells not harbouring mutations but at much higher doses than those with mutations. Pushing the dose may accrue a further population of patients responding to the drug who lack mutations. This might be true of colorectal cancer patients being treated with cetuximab where EGFR is a dominant oncogenic factor. Such patients might be distinguishable prospectively, for example, by detection of elevated tumoral pAkt levels or by the absence of any downstream activating event, for example, PI3 kinase amplification or ras mutation, which would abrogate EGFR inhibition either by antibody or a small molecule TK inhibitor. Whether this is a true molecular signature predictive of a response to cetuximab, as is seen in the situation of non-small cell lung cancer, remains to be established.

- The increased response rate and progression-free survival (PFS) advantage of irinotecan/cetuximab over cetuximab alone in irinotecan-resistant patients implies that cetuximab is, somehow, subverting irinotecan resistance. What is the potential mechanism?

There are two likely candidates which are not mutually exclusive and clearly there may be more than these. NFkB is important in inducible chemotherapy resistance. It negatively regulates apoptosis, both by upregulating molecules which promote cell survival, such as Bcl-Xl and Bfl-1, and by enhancing inhibitory factors such as IAP which binds to and inhibits caspase-8. Irinotecan activates NFkB in the majority of CRC cell lines and protection from apoptosis induced by irinotecan treatment can be inhibited by the inhibition of NFkB both in cell lines and in a xenograft model [29]. EGFR activation upregulates NFkB both through the cell death receptor pathway and the PI3K-Akt pathway and there are already published data showing that C225 (cetuximab is the humanised version of this antibody) overcomes gemcitabine resistance, at least in preclinical models, by downregulating NFkB and subsequently Bcl-Xl [30].

The second mechanism involves modulation of the damage caused by exposure to irinotecan. SN38 inhbits topoisomerase 1, resulting in subsequent DNA damage. DNA-dependent protein kinase is involved in the repair of double-stranded DNA breaks and anti-EGFR monoclonal antibody treatment causes a reduction of DNA-PK levels and activity by causing a physical interaction between EGFR and DNA-PK, preventing its nuclear translocation [31]. Thus, cetuximab may be accentuating the DNA damage caused by irinotecan.

- Does the addition of cetuximab to second-line irinotecan provide benefits over irinotecan alone?

The Bond study was essentially a salvage programme for patients with irinotecan-resistant disease. The EPIC study is randomising patients failing on or within 6 months of an oxaliplatin/FP front-line regimen to irinotecan or irinotecan/cetuximab.

- What is the role of cetuximab in combination with oxaliplatin and in the first-line management of patients with ACRC?

The NCRN sponsored COIN study will randomise previously untreated patients to oxaliplatin/FP ± cetuximab. A third arm of intermittent therapy with oxaliplatin/FP will extend observations from CR06B [32] to the combination setting and will particularly focus on trying to reduce, through drug holidays, oxaliplatin neuropathy. In the second-line, CA225014 is randomising patients who have progressed on an irinotecan-containing regimen to FOLFOX 4 ± cetuximab.

With regard to irinotecan first-line, Crystal is randomising chemo-naïve patients to FOLFIRI ± cetuximab and the global portfolio is completed by CALGB-80203, which plans to randomise 2,200 previously untreated patients to FOLFIRI, FOLFIRI and cetuximab, FOLFOX or FOLFOX and cetuximab.

With phase II studies already combining bevacizumab and cetuximab ongoing (MSKCC-03135) and pharmaceutical pipelines producing a burgeoning number of targeted agents, the most crucial development for oncology, particularly in a cash-strapped health economy, is to move rapidly into the era of individually tailored therapy, dependent upon the molecular signature of individual tumours. These therapies are likely to be niche products, active in just a small subset of patients and their rational selection is absolutely essential.

In spite of the relative immaturity of the advanced disease data using the antibody therapies, there has been a very swift move to bring these therapies into the context of early disease. AVANT, the successor to XELOXA, maintains the same chemotherapy randomisation as before but places it in a two by two factorial design of chemotherapy ± bevacizumab. QUASAR-2, the new NCRN adjuvant programme for high risk Dukes' B and Dukes' C patients, examines two questions in a three-way randomisation of patients to capecitabine (an oral FP choice alone significantly supported by the positive result from the X-ACT programme of capecitabine versus 5FU folinic acid bolus in Dukes' C patients demonstrating improved tolerability of the oral therapy, with a statistically significant hazard ratio of 0.78, in multivariate analysis in favour of capecitabine [33]), CapIri (the issue of the impact of the addition of irinotecan to oral FP) and CapIri plus bevacizumab.

With regard to cetuximab, an Intergroup study (NCCTG-N0147/ECOG-N0147) will randomise 4,800 Dukes' C patients to one of six arms: FOLFOX, FOLFIRI, FOLFOX for six cycles followed by FOLFIRI, FOLFOX plus cetuximab, FOLFIRI plus cetuximab or the sequential regimen plus cetuximab.

It hardly needs to be emphasised that should these strategies provide patient benefits in the adjuvant setting, the previous comments made concerning the urgent need to move towards patient-tailored therapies are even more cogent.

References

1. de Gramont A, Bosset J, Milan C, et al. Randomized trial comparing monthly low-dose leucovorin and fluorouracil bolus with bimonthly high-dose leucovorin and fluorouracil bolus plus continuous infusion for advanced colorectal cancer: a French Intergroup study. *J Clinic Oncol* 1997; 15: 808-15.
2. Meta-analysis Group In Cancer: efficacy of intravenous continuous infusion of fluorouracil compared with bolus administration in advanced colorectal cancer. *J Clin Oncol* 1998; 16: 301-8.
3. Saltz LB, Cox JV, Blanke C, et al. Irinotecan plus fluorouracil and leucovorin for metastatic colorectal cancer. *N Engl J Med* 2000; 343: 905-14.
4. Douillard JY, Cunningham D, Roth AD, et al. Irinotecan combined with fluorouracil compared with fluorouracil alone as first-line treatment for metastatic colorectal cancer: a multicentre randomised trial. *Lancet* 2000; 355: 1041-47.
5. Giachetti B, Perpoint B, Zidani R, et al. Phase III multicenter randomised trial of oxaliplatin added to chronomodulated fluorouracil-leucovorin as first-line treatment of metastatic colorectal cancer. *J Clin Oncol* 2000; 18: 136-47.
6. de Gramont A, Figer A, Seymour M, et al. Leucovorin and fluorouracil with or without oxaliplatin as first-line treatment in advanced colorectal cancer. *J Clin Oncol* 2000; 18: 2938-3947.
7. Rothenburg ML, Meropol NJ, Poplin EA, et al. Mortality associated with irinotecan plus bolus fluorouracil/leucovorin: summary findings of an independent panel. *J Clin Oncol* 2001; 20(4): 1145-6.
8. Goldberg RM, Sargent DJ, Morton RF, et al. A randomized controlled trial of fluorouracil plus leucovorin, irinotecan, and oxaliplatin combinations in patients with previously untreated metastatic colorectal cancer. *J Clin Oncol* 2004; 22: 23-30.
9. Full guidance on irinotecan, oxaliplatin and raltitrexed for advanced colorectal cancer. NICE Technology Appraisal March 2002; No 33.
10. Cunningham D, James RD, Punt CJA, et al. Randomised trial of irinotecan plus supportive care versus supportive care alone after fluorouracil failure for patients with metastatic colorectal cancer. *Lancet* 1998; 352: 1413-8.
11. Grothey A, Sargent D, Goldberg RM, Schmoll H: Survival of patients with advanced colorectal cancer improves with the availability of fluorouracil-leucovorin, irinotecan, and oxaliplatin in the course of treatment. *J Clin Oncol* 2004; 22: 1209-14.
12. Tournigand C, André T, Achille E, et al. FOLFIRI followed by FOLFOX6 or the reverse sequence in advanced colorectal cancer: a randomized GERCOR study. *J Clin Oncol* 2004; 22: 229-37.
13. QUASAR Collaborative Group: comparison of fluorouracil with additional levamisole, higher-dose folinic acid, or both, as adjuvant chemotherapy for colorectal cancer: a randomised trial. *Lancet* 2000; 355: 1588-96.
14. Moertel CG, Fleming TR, Macdonald JS, et al. Fluorouracil plus levamisole as effective adjuvant therapy after resection of Stage III colon carcinoma: a final report. *Ann Int Med* 1995; 122: 321-5.
15. O'Connell MJ, Mailliard JA, Kahn MJ, et al. Controlled trial of fluorouracil and low-dose leucovorin given for 6 months as postoperative adjuvant therapy for colon cancer. *J Clin Oncol* 1997; 15: 246-50.
16. O'Connell MJ, Laurie JA, Kahn MJ, et al. Prospectively randomized trial of postoperative adjuvant chemotherapy in patients with high-risk colon cancer. *J Clin Oncol* 1998; 16: 295-300.
17. Andre T, Boni C, Mounedji-Boudiaf L, et al. Oxaliplatin, fluorouracil and leucovorin as adjuvant treatment for colon cancer. *N Engl J Med* 2004; 350(23): 2406-8.
18. Sargent DJ, Wieand S, Benedetti J, et al. Disease-free survival (DFS) vs. overall survival (OS) as a primary endpoint for adjuvant colon cancer studies: individual patient data from 12,915 patients on 15 randomized trials. ASCO annual meeting, 2004.
19. Hurwitz H, Fehrenbacher L, Novotny W, et al. Bevacizumab plus irinotecan, fluorouracil, and leucovorin for metastatic colorectal cancer. *J Clin Oncol* 2004; 350 (23): 2406-8.
20. Kabbinavar F, Hurwitz HI, Fehrenbacher L, et al. Phase II, randomized trial comparing bevacizumab plus fluorouracil (FU)/leucovorin (LV) with FU/LV alone in patients with metastatic colorectal cancer. *J Clin Oncol* 2003; 21: 60-5.
21. Hedrick E, Hurwitz H, Sarkar S, et al. Impact of post-progression therapy on survival in AVF2107, a phase III trial of bevacizumab (Avastin^{TM}) in the first-line treatment of metastatic colorectal cancer. Proc ASCO 2004, #3517.
22. Bergers G, Song S, Meyer-Morse N, et al. Benefits of targeting both pericytes and endothelial cells in the tumour vasculature with kinase inhibitors. *J Clin Inv* 2003; 111: 1287-95.
23. Cunningham D, Humblet Y, Siena S, et al. Cetuximab monotherapy and cetuximab plus irinotecan in irinotecan-refractory metastatic colorectal cancer. *N Engl J Med* 2004; 351(4): 337-45.
24. Lenz H, Mayer RJ, Mirtsching B, et al. Activity of cetuximab in patients with colorectal cancer refractory to both irinotecan and oxaliplatin. Proc ASCO 2004, #3510.
25. Lynch TJ, Bell DW, Sordella R, et al. Activating mutations in the epidermal growth factor receptor underlying responsiveness of non-small-cell lung cancer to gefitinib. *N Engl J Med* 2004; 350(21): 2129-39.
26. Paez JG, Janne PA, Lee JC, et al. EGFR mutations in lung cancer: correlation with clinical response to gefitinib therapy. *Science* 2004; 304(5676): 1458-61.
27. Lee JW, Soung YH, Kim SY, et al. Absence of EGFR mutation in the kinase domain in common cancers besides non-small cell lung cancer. *Int J Cancer* 2005; 113(3): 510-1.
28. Bardelli A, Williams Parsons D, Silliman N, et al. Mutational analysis of the tyrosine kinome in colorectal cancers. *Science* 2003; 300: 949.
29. Cusack J, Liu R, Baldwin. A. Inducible chemoresistance to 7-Ethyl-10-[4-(1-piperidino)-1-piperidin} Carbonyloxycamptothecin (CPT-11) in colorectal cancer cells and a xenograft model Is overcome by inhibition of nuclear factor-kB activation. *Ca Res* 2000; 60, 2323-30.

30. Sclabas G, Fujioka S, Schmidt C. Restoring apoptosis in pancreatic cancer cells by targeting the nuclear factor-Kb signaling pathway with the anti-epidermal growth factor antibody IMC-C225. *J Gastrointest Surg* 2003; 7: 37-43.
31. Bandyopadhyay D, Mandal M, Adam L, *et al.* Physical interaction between epidermal growth factor receptor and DNA-dependent protein kinase in mammalian cells. *J Biol Chem* 1998; 273(3): 1568-73.
32. Maughan TS, James RD, Kerr DJ, *et al.* Comparison of intermittent and continuous palliative chemotherapy for advanced colorectal cancer: a multicentre randomised trial. *Lancet* 2003; 361(9356): 457-64.
33. Cassidy J, Scheithauer W, McKendrick J, *et al.* Capecitabine (X) vs bolus 5-FU/leucovorin (LV) as adjuvant therapy for colon cancer (the X-ACT study): efficacy results of a phase III trial. ASCO Annual Meeting, 2004.

PART II: FRONTIERS IN IBD

Chapter 12

Adjuvant treatment after Crohn's resection

Emma R Greig PhD MRCP, Consultant Gastroenterologist
Taunton and Somerset NHS Trust, UK

What is the problem?

Crohn's disease is a chronic relapsing and remitting illness. It is thought to result from a genetically-determined, inappropriately severe and/or prolonged mucosal inflammatory response to (as yet) unidentified enteric microbial or environmental factor(s) [1]. The challenge of managing Crohn's disease is to maximise periods of symptom-free remission thus allowing patients to lead a normal life with minimal disease activity and few medication-related side effects. As Crohn's disease may affect any part of the gastrointestinal tract, medical treatment is used whenever possible to avoid significant loss of intestinal length and function. However, for some patients, surgery for conditions such as recurrent intestinal obstruction, fistula and/or abscess formation, acute or chronic gastrointestinal bleeding, or growth failure in children may allow remission and reduce chronic ill health [2]. The evidence for maintaining remission differs, depending on whether it is achieved by medical or surgical means. This chapter will concentrate on evidence for using therapies following surgically-achieved remission but will contrast these with differences in management following medically-achieved remission.

Risks of disease recurrence following resection

Surgery in Crohn's disease aims to overcome complications; it is never a cure. Crohn's disease is made up of a heterogeneous series of disease entities, such as ileocolonic, exclusively small bowel, gastroduodenal, oral or peri-anal disease. Within these disease patterns, patients may exhibit stricturing or perforating disease characteristics, with perforating disease being fistula and/or abscess formation. The site of disease has a significant effect on the need for surgery and risk of postoperative recurrence: both are greater in ileocolonic disease than in purely small bowel Crohn's [3]. Disease phenotype is also important: the average interval to second operation is 5 years for perforating and 9 years for non-perforating disease [3]. Patients younger than 20 years at diagnosis are more likely to need surgery [4], while patients over 40 years tend to have a more benign disease course and lower probability of surgery [4]. A modern study of the natural history of the disease would be beneficial, incorporating up-to-date thinking about minimising surgical resection margins together with advances in disease modification using immunosuppressives and biological therapies.

Table 1. Maintenance of remission in Crohn's disease.	
All patients	Stop smoking
Remission achieved medically	Azathioprine / 6-mercaptopurine or methotrexate for refractory disease Infliximab
Remission achieved surgically	Aminosalicylates (Pentasa for ileal disease) Metronidazole (3 months only) Azathioprine or 6-mercaptopurine

Postoperative recurrence following a resection for Crohn's disease is an ever present concern. Long-term studies of disease progression suggest that the majority of patients will require surgery at some point, with older studies suggesting that 90% will undergo surgery by 30 years after onset [5]. Even a limited right hemicolectomy for terminal ileal and caecal disease is associated with approximately 50% clinical relapse at 5 years with half of these patients requiring a further operation by 10 years [6]. Because malabsorption of minerals, vitamins and bile salts becomes increasingly likely with successive resections, it is important to minimise the length of bowel resected to maintain gastrointestinal function. The end result of multiple resections of small and large intestine may be intestinal failure, where absorption is sufficiently limited that macronutrients, water and electrolyte supplements are needed to maintain health and/or growth [7]. This may result from an insufficient length of bowel, with or without active intestinal inflammation, fistula formation or prolonged ileus. Trials of adjuvant therapies following resection may use differing definitions of disease recurrence. Endoscopic and symptomatic recurrences represent different disease states and trial data must be interpreted cautiously. From the patients' perspective, reducing the rate of symptomatic recurrence is a more important clinical endpoint. Unfortunately, endoscopic recurrence is more often used as an endpoint in clinical trials.

Where are we now?

Some basic interventions are proven to prolong symptomatic remission after surgery. Stopping smoking is probably the single most important intervention with the best supporting evidence. As time to relapse is unpredictable, controlled trial data for pharmacological therapies are limited. The evidence for 5-aminosalicylates, corticosteroids, thiopurines and other immunosuppressives, infliximab and using nutrition is discussed below.

Stopping smoking

The most effective measure to prevent relapse in patients who smoke is to stop: the risk of relapse in ex-smokers at 5 years is reduced by approximately 40% [8, 9]. This is the case whether remission has been achieved by medical or surgical means [8, 9]. A prospective interventional trial has confirmed that cessation of smoking improves the natural history of disease, particularly in women [10]. Risk of relapse in non-smokers and those who had stopped smoking was significantly reduced at 2 years compared with continuing smokers [10]. The need for corticosteroids, immunosuppressives and surgery was increased in continuing smokers and particularly in women [10]. Crohn's patients have the same willingness to quit as the rest of the population [11], with factors increasing this likelihood including their particular physician, previous intestinal surgery, high socio-economic status and use of oral contraceptives [10].

Drug prophylaxis

Unfortunately, there are few data to support the use of drugs to reduce the rate of symptomatic as opposed to endoscopic postoperative recurrence in patients with Crohn's disease [12]. The heterogeneity of disease presentations and the varying natural history of each type make comparison between drugs difficult. Finally, there is variation in efficacy of treatments which depend upon whether remission is achieved by medical or surgical means. These data are summarised in Table 1. An advised regimen for toxicity monitoring is given in Table 2.

12 Adjuvant treatment after Crohn's resection

Table 2. Toxicity monitoring for pharmacological therapies in Crohn's disease.

Pharmacological agent	Prior to starting treatment	During treatment	Complications necessitating stopping treatment
Aminosalicylates (ASA)	Renal function, liver function tests, folate (sulphasalazine only)	**Sulphasalazine** - Renal function 3-6 monthly with additional full blood count, liver function tests and folate **Other ASA** - renal function 6-12 monthly	Interstitial nephritis Hepatitis
Azathioprine/ 6-mercaptopurine	Liver function tests, full blood count, TPMT activity or genotype (if available)	Full blood count and liver function tests fortnightly for 2 months, then every 2-3 months	Pancreatitis, opportunistic infection, bone marrow depression, lymphoma
Methotrexate	Liver function tests, full blood count	Full blood count and liver function tests fortnightly for 2 months, then every 2-3 months. Lung function tests and CXR if patient breathless Liver biopsy particularly at cumulative dose of 5g/or if transaminases rise	Hepatoxicity, pneumonitis, opportunistic infection, bone marrow depression, teratogenic so cannot be used by either partner within 6 months of planned pregnancy
Infliximab	Tuberculosis skin test, chest X-ray	None	Opportunistic infection, severe infusion reaction
Corticosteroids	Blood pressure, serum glucose, serum sodium or potassium levels	Sodium and potassium levels 3-6 monthly, bone densitometry scanning	

Aminosalicylates

A recent re-analysis [13, 14] of a previous meta-analysis [15] suggested that long-term mesalazine slightly reduced the risk of symptomatic relapse after surgery (risk reduction of 8% with a number needed to treat [NNT] of 12). The older meta-analysis [15] had included a non-blinded and non-placebo controlled study [16]. This re-analysis was based on four studies [17-20] and included a placebo-controlled European study [20] which showed no advantage for Pentasa (at 4g/day) except in isolated ileal disease when the clinical relapse rate at 18 months was 22% on Pentasa and 40% on placebo. The re-analysis was considerably less favourable than the initial meta-analysis and the NNT too high to support the use of aminosalicylates except in isolated ileal disease [13, 14]. Similar data suggest that olsalazine and sulphasalazine play no part in maintaining remission [21]. Patients rarely need to stop aminosalicylates as a result of side effects, especially using the newer aminosalicylates such as mesalazine or balsalazide [22].

Nitroimidazole antibiotics

Oral metronidazole given at 20mg/kg per day for 3 months after surgery reduces both symptomatic and endoscopic recurrence 1 year after surgery with the benefit over placebo being lost with longer follow-up [23]. The side effects of metronidazole vary from nausea, rashes, vomiting and an "Antabuse" effect with alcohol, to a potentially irreversible sensory peripheral neuropathy [24]. The risk of neuropathy limits the duration of treatment to 3 months [24]. Ornidazole, another nitroimidazole antibiotic, given at 1g/day for a year, reduces clinical and endoscopic relapse at 1 year, but is no better tolerated than metronidazole and cannot therefore be recommended for long-term postoperative prophylaxis [25]. The effects of metronidazole may be enhanced by the co-administration of ciprofloxacin in ileocolonic and colonic disease [26, 27], but adequate controlled data are lacking.

Corticosteroids

Prednisolone has no prophylactic role in preventing postoperative recurrence [28]. Budesonide (a controlled-release preparation designed to allow drug release in the ileum) at 6mg/day, halved postoperative endoscopic recurrence at 1 year for inflammatory but not fibrostenotic disease. However, the rate of clinical relapse was the same as for patients in the placebo arm [29]. Once again, there is little to recommend this therapy in the longer term.

Thiopurines

Although the thiopurines are not licensed in the UK for this purpose, there is strong evidence that azathioprine (a pro-drug) and its metabolite 6-mercaptopurine are effective steroid-sparing agents in active Crohn's disease with a role in maintaining remission in the longer term [30-32]. In addition, as azathioprine allows mucosal healing, it is conceivable that this could alter the natural history of disease [33]. Specific studies within the medical literature provide limited data for using thiopurines to maintain a surgically-achieved remission. One controlled study in children showed that 6-mercaptopurine at 1mg/kg for 2 years was more effective in preventing postoperative recurrence than aminosalicylates or no medication [34]. However, the number of patients in this study was small and it is difficult to draw significant conclusions. A study in adults using low-dose 6-mercaptopurine (at 50mg/day) showed it to be better than placebo and aminosalicylates in preventing clinical, endoscopic and radiological recurrence after surgery [35]. Even so, the relapse rate while taking 6-mercaptopurine was 53%, while for placebo this was 70% [35]. Thus, a larger study of 6-mercaptopurine (1-1.5mg/kg/day) or azathioprine (2-2.5mg/kg/day) would be beneficial to establish the actual benefit in reducing postoperative recurrence.

Although thiopurines probably represent the best option for patients with steroid-dependent disease or for those who have undergone several resections, the range of side effects is significant, regular toxicity monitoring is required and thiopurines are not universally effective. Approximately 10-20% of patients need to stop azathioprine as a result of side effects such as headache, abdominal pain, nausea or arthralgia which are often attributed to the imidazole group [36]. Switching to 6-mercaptopurine may alleviate these symptoms in 50% of those affected and allow continued therapy [37, 38]. There is little published evidence for using thiopurines beyond 4 years. The most recent multicentre study of duration of therapy, only published in abstract form, showed that in Crohn's patients with a remission time of greater than 42 months, azathioprine withdrawal resulted in a relapse rate of 21% at 18 months compared with 8% of those continuing azathioprine [39]. This result needs to be considered alongside the risks of long-term therapy such as lymphoma, and patients require careful counselling until more evidence is available.

There has been considerable interest in genetic susceptibility to the side effects of azathioprine. Azathioprine is converted to 6-mercaptopurine in the liver by glutathione transferase, then to 6-thioguanine nucleotides (6-TGN) by three main enzymes in the liver and gut. These 6-thioguanine nucleotides are thought to be the therapeutically active components, and also to cause leucopenia and/or pancytopenia. The breakdown pathway of thiopurines is shown in Figure 1 [40]. Homozygosity or heterozygosity for deficiency of thiopurine methyl transferase (TPMT) occurs in 0.2 and 10% of the population respectively and predisposes to bone marrow depression [22]. However, this does not represent the whole picture, with low TMPT levels causing an increase in intracellular 6-TGN in lymphocytes and apparently improving the clinical efficacy of thiopurines [41]. Assays of TMPT genotype or activity, and of erythrocyte 6-thioguanine nucleotides levels, are not widely available yet, nor is it clear how measurements may help dose selection [41]. However, if a patient is homozygous for TMPT deficiency, thiopurines should be avoided [22]. This does not eliminate the need for regular toxicity monitoring as problems may be encountered even in patients with normal TMPT levels [41]. This necessitates fortnightly full blood counts and liver function tests for the first 2 weeks, then every 2-3 months for the duration of prescription of the drug [42]. Finally, mesalazine is known to reversibly inhibit TPMT and thus increase 6-thioguanine nucleotide levels with the risk of myelotoxicity [43, 44].

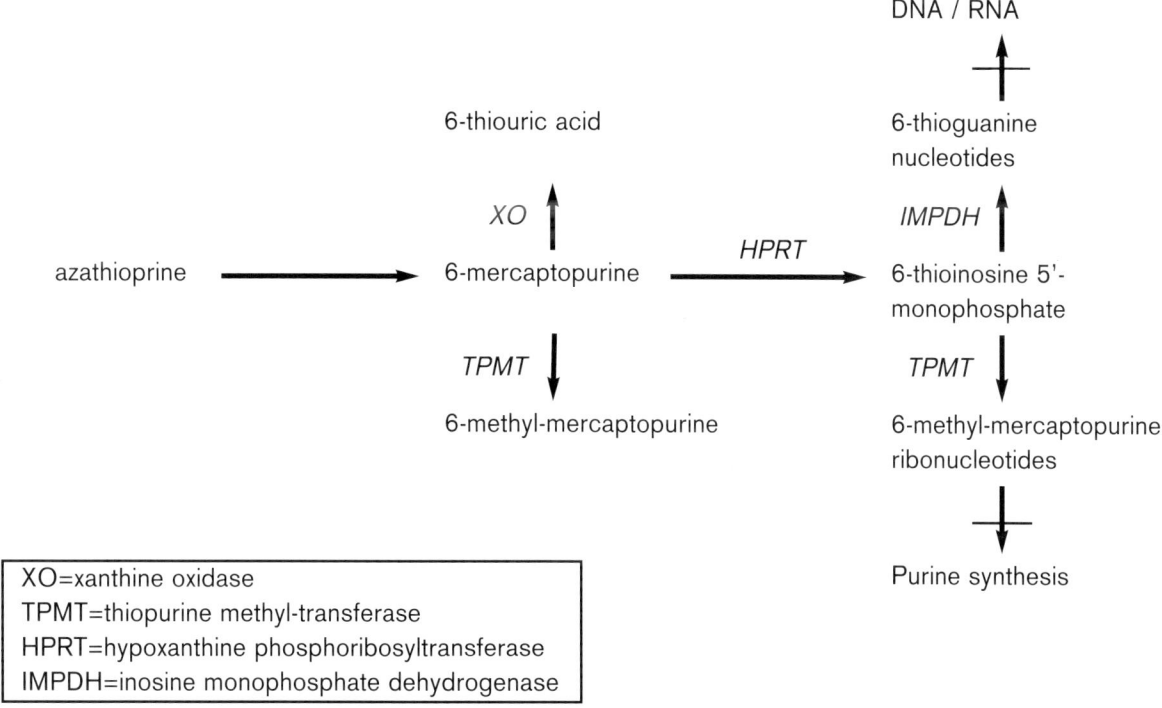

Figure 1. Breakdown of thiopurine drugs. Dubinsky MC et al, 2001 [40]. Reproduced with permission from the American Gastroenterological Association, © 2000.

Methotrexate

Methotrexate is proven to achieve remission at doses of 25mg/week and to maintain remission at 15mg/week when both are given intramuscularly [45, 46]. Remission rates at 40 weeks were 65% compared with 39% using placebo [46]. This regimen is difficult to provide in clinical practice and the oral preparation is used more commonly in the UK. Side effects and contra-indications are significant with methotrexate [47], and necessitate drug cessation in 20% of patients [48]. These risks are greater and necessitate stopping treatment more often than equivalent doses of thiopurines. Unfortunately, there are no published data showing that methotrexate can maintain remission if this is achieved using surgery or another pharmacological therapy than methotrexate itself.

Infliximab

Infliximab is the first biological therapy which has been licensed for chronic refractory and fistulising Crohn's disease [49, 50, 51]. The dosage regimen of 5mg/kg given at 0, 2 and 6 weeks allows treatment of relapse, while a maintenance regimen of 5mg/kg every 8 weeks aims to prolong remission in those patients with chronic steroid- and immunosuppressive-refractory disease [51, 52, 53]. Long-term remission seems likely in 25% of this group; however, efficacy is more likely in non-smokers, in patients receiving concomitant immunosuppressives, and in patients with raised C-reactive protein levels [54]. At present, there are no data to suggest that maintenance infliximab may be used following surgically-induced remission and further research is required.

Newer medical therapies

Advances in our understanding of the immune response and inflammatory process have led to the development of a wide range of new agents designed to act at specific pathophysiological targets. Many of these new agents are at the clinical trial stage and have not yet been evaluated as maintenance therapies. Gut luminal flora are thought to play a pivotal role in driving the mucosal immune and inflammatory response [55]. Thus modification of microbial flora for therapeutic gain has led to feeding patients with probiotic ("friendly") bacteria thought to have a protective or anti-inflammatory role [56].

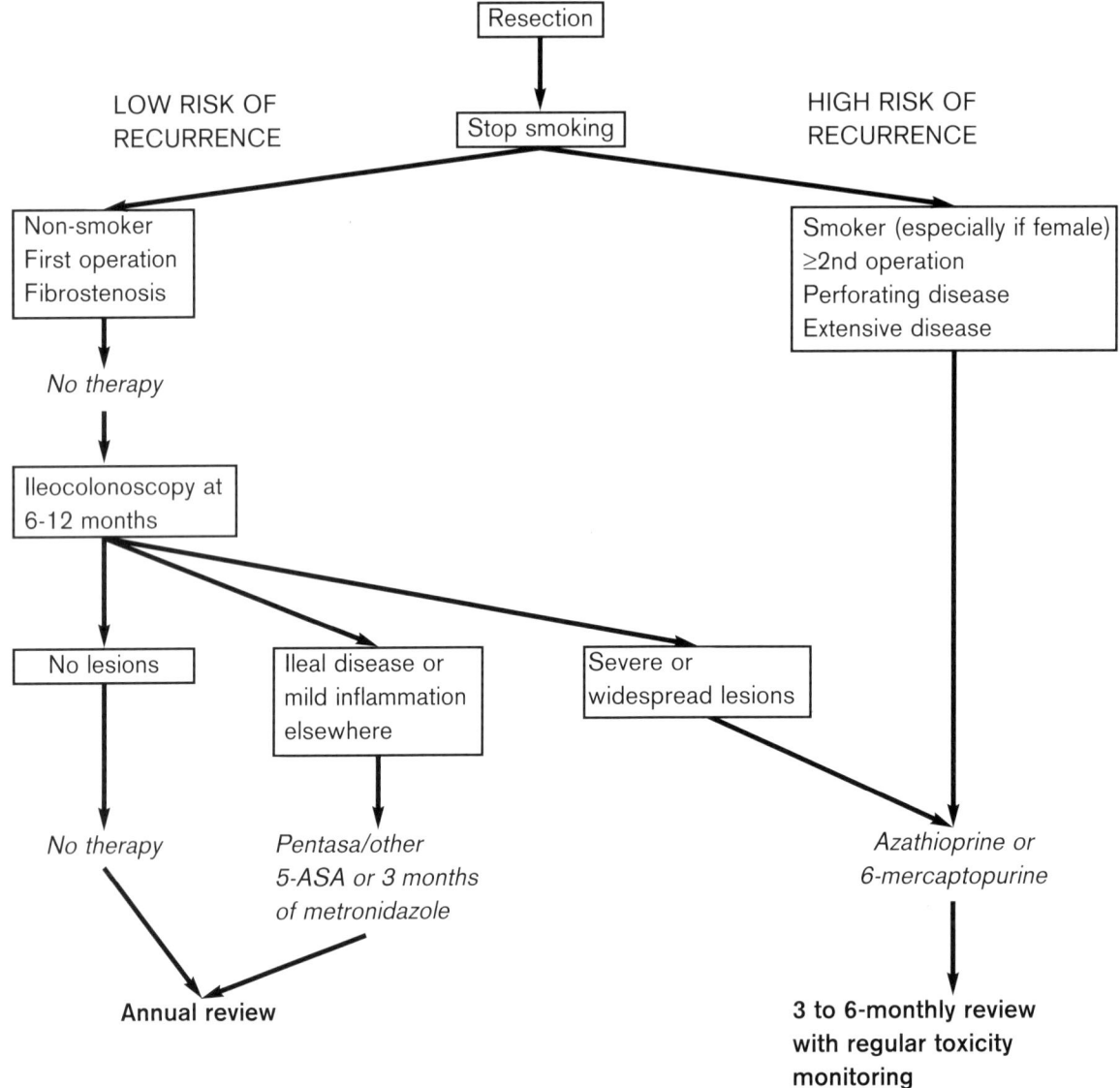

Figure 2. Prophylaxis after resection for ileocolonic Crohn's disease. Adapted from Rutgeerts PJ, 2002 [64]. Reproduced with permission from the BMJ Publishing Group.

Unfortunately, a trial of probiotic *Lactobacillus GG* proved to be no more effective than placebo in maintaining remission following resection [56].

Interleukin-10 is a regulatory cytokine which inhibits antigen presentation and release of pro-inflammatory cytokines and was thought to have substantial therapeutic potential [57]. Unfortunately, this has not been substantiated in practice for either inducing remission in active Crohn's disease or maintaining endoscopic or clinical remission after surgical resection at 1 year [57, 58]. The results of current clinical trials are awaited for other new therapies.

Nutritional therapies

Enteral diets may be used as sole nutrition to treat relapse, when efficacy approaches that for corticosteroids [59, 60]. Proposed mechanisms of action include reduction in epithelial permeability, mucosal secretion and exposure to food antigens, together with changes in gut flora and mucosal immunity [61]. However, patients may relapse in the months after starting food and at present there is no evidence for the role of enteral diet to maintain remission following surgical resection [62]. Adults find that keeping to this restricted diet is difficult; however, children can benefit from its use as adjuvant therapy in the longer term both to maintain remission and allow growth [61].

Summary

In summary, time to relapse after surgically-induced remission is highly variable. Endoscopic recurrence often predicts later symptomatic recurrence with endoscopic severity predicting future disease activity [12, 63, 64]. The most effective intervention according to the current evidence base is stopping smoking. Patients with uncomplicated disease may be advised that there is little benefit from any of the available pharmacological interventions at the present time. However, in patients with exclusively ileal disease, Pentasa at 4g/day is a reasonable choice with minimal side effects [20]. For patients with aggressive, perforating or extensive disease, or those undergoing a second or subsequent resection, a thiopurine such as azathioprine (2-2.5mg/kg/day) or 6-mercaptopurine (1-1.5mg/kg/day) is probably a reasonable choice despite the lack of controlled data using these doses [64, 65]. Sadly, at present, it is impossible to reassure patients that any medication will reduce their risk of disease recurrence in the longer-term. A suggested algorithm for using adjuvant therapies is shown in Figure 2.

Where are we going?

As our knowledge and understanding of the pathophysiology of Crohn's disease increases, targeted biological therapies are likely to become available. At present, few have reached clinical trials, although the first of these therapies, infliximab, plays an established role in treating relapse and subsequently maintaining remission. Overall, these drugs should increase the therapeutic arsenal and improve patient outcomes. Improvements in the evidence base for older therapies, combined with multicentre trials guiding dosage and treatment duration will benefit patients. Thiopurines have become a mainstay of treatment for maintaining remission in steroid-dependent disease, but their safety profile and effectiveness beyond 4 years remains unknown.

Identification of particular subgroups of patients with certain genotypic or phenotypic disease may define likelihood of response or toxicity from particular agents. Our understanding of the genetic determinants of Crohn's disease is increasing rapidly, with certain disease phenotypes appearing to have a genetic background [1]. This is of particular interest when considering the new area of pharmacogenetics. Genotype may determine individual response to drugs such as thiopurines, steroids, methotrexate and infliximab [1, 41, 66]. Unrecognised genotypic differences between patients are likely to explain much of the variability of response in clinical trials and probably represent the next wave of advances in therapy for Crohn's disease.

References

1. Ahmad T, Pesi C, Jewell D, Colombel J-F. Clinical relevance of advances in genetics and pharmacogenetics of IBD. *Gastroenterology* 2004; 126: 1533-49.
2. Lock MR, Farmer RG, Fazio VW, *et al*. Recurrence and reoperation for Crohn's disease: the role of disease location in prognosis. *N Engl J Med* 1981; 304: 1586-8.
3. Farmer RG, Whelan G, Fazio VW. Long-term follow-up of patients with Crohn's disease. Relationship between clinical pattern and prognosis. *Gastroenterology* 1985; 88: 1818-25.
4. Polito JM, Childs B, Mellits ED, *et al*. Crohn's disease: influence of age at diagnosis on site and clinical type of disease. *Gastroenterology* 1996; 111: 580-6.
5. Mekhijan HS, Sweitz DM, Watts HD, *et al*. National cooperative Crohn's disease study: factors determining recurrence of Crohn's disease after surgery. *Gastroenterology* 1979; 77: 907-13.
6. Moum B, Ekbom A, Vatn MH, *et al*. Clinical course during the 1st year after diagnosis in ulcerative colitis and Crohn's disease. *Scand J Gastroenterol* 1997; 32: 1005-12.
7. Nightingale JM. The short-bowel syndrome. *Eur J Gastroenterol Hepatol* 1995; 6. 514-20.

8. Sutherland LR, Ramcharan S, Bryant H, et al. Effect of cigarette smoking on recurrence of Crohn's disease. Gastroenterology 1990; 98: 1123-8.
9. Cottone M, Rosselli M, Orlando A, et al. Smoking habits and recurrence in Crohn's disease. Gastroenterology 1994; 106: 643-8.
10. Cosnes J, Beaugerie L, Carbonnel F, et al. Smoking cessation and the course of Crohn's disease: an intervention study. Gastroenterology 2001; 120: 1093-9.
11. Hilsden RJ, Hodgins D, Czechowsky D, et al. Attitudes toward smoking and smoking behaviours of patients with Crohn's disease. Am J Gastroenterol 2001; 96: 1849-53.
12. Rutgeerts P, Geboes K, Vantrappen G, et al. Predictability of the postoperative course of Crohn's disease. Gastroenterology 1990; 99: 956-63.
13. Sutherland LR. Mesalamine for the prevention of postoperative recurrence: is nearly there the same as being there? Gastroenterology 2000; 118: 436-8.
14. Sutherland LR. Mesalamine and relapse prevention in Crohn's disease. Gastroenterology 2000; 118: 597.
15. Cammá C, Giunta M, Rosselli M, et al. Mesalazine in the maintenance treatment of Crohn's disease: a meta-analysis adjusted for confounding variables. Gastroenterology 1997; 113: 1465-73.
16. Caprilli R, Andreoli A, Capurso L, et al. Oral mesalazine (5-aminosalicylic acid; Asacol) for the prevention of post-operative recurrence of Crohn's disease. Aliment Pharmacol Ther 1994; 8: 35-43.
17. Brignola C, Cottone M, Pera A, et al. Mesalamine in the prevention of endoscopic recurrence after intestinal resection for Crohn's disease. Italian Cooperative Study Group. Gastroenterology 1995; 108: 345-9.
18. McLeod RS, Wolff BG, Steinhart AH, et al. Prophylactic mesalamine treatment decreases postoperative recurrence of Crohn's disease. Gastroenterology 1995; 109: 404-13.
19. Sutherland LR, Martin F, Bailey RJ, et al. A randomized, placebo-controlled, double-blind trial of mesalamine in the maintenance of remission of Crohn's disease. The Canadian Mesalamine for Remission of Crohn's disease Study group. Gastroenterology 1997; 112: 1069-77.
20. Lochs H, Mayer M, Fleig WE, et al. Prophylaxis of postoperative relapse in Crohn's disease with mesalamine: European Cooperative Crohn's disease Study VI. Gastroenterology 2000; 118: 264-73.
21. Mahmud N, Kamm MA, Dupas JL, Jewell DP, O'Morain CA, Weir DG, Kelleher D. Olsalazine is not superior to placebo in maintaining remission of inactive Crohn's colitis and ileocolitis: a double-blind, parallel randomised, multicientre study. Gut 2001; 49: 552-6.
22. Rampton DS. Medical management: how can efficacy and safety be maximised? In: Inflammatory Bowel Disease, Clinical Diagnosis and Management. Rampton DS, Ed. Martin Dunitz Ltd, London, UK, 2000: 143-84.
23. Rutgeerts P, Hiele M, Geboes K, et al. Controlled trial of metronidazole treatment for prevention of Crohn's recurrence after ileal resection. Gastroenterology 1995; 108: 1617-21.
24. Duffy LF, Daum F, Fisher SE, et al. Peripheral neuropathy in Crohn's disease patients treated with metronidazole. Gastroenterology 1985; 88: 681-4.
25. Rutgeerts PJ, van Assche G, D'Haens G, et al. Ornidazol for prophylaxis of post-operative Crohn's disease: final results of a placebo-controlled trial. Gastroenterology 2002; 122: A135.
26. Prantera C, Zannoni F, Scribano ML, et al. An antibiotic regime for the treatment of active Crohn's disease: a randomized controlled clinical trial of metronidazole plus ciprofloxacin. Am J Gastroenterol 1996; 91: 328-32.
27. Greenbloom SL, Steinhart AH, Greenberg GR. Combination ciprofloxacin and metronidazole for active Crohn's disease. Can J Gastroenterol 1998; 12: 53-6.
28. Steinhart AH, Ewe K, Griffiths AM, et al. Corticosteroids for maintaining remission of Crohn's disease. Cochrane Database Syst Rev 2001; CD000301.
29. Hellers G, Cortot A, Jewell D, et al. Oral budesonide for prevention of postsurgical recurrence in Crohn's disease. The IOIBD Budesonide Study Group. Gastroenterology 1999; 116: 294-300.
30. Candy S, Wright J, Gerber M, et al. A controlled double blind study of azathioprine in the management of Crohn's disease. Gut 1995; 37: 674-8.
31. Pearson DC, May GR, Fick GH, et al. Azathioprine and 6-mercaptopurine in Crohn's disease: a meta-analysis. Ann Intern Med 1995; 122: 132-42.
32. Pearson DC, May GR, Fick G, et al. Azathioprine for maintaining remission of Crohn's disease. In: The Cochrane Library. The Cochrane Collaboration, Oxford, 1999; Update software; issue 2.
33. D'Haens G, Geboes K, Ponette E, et al. Healing of severe recurrent ileitis with azathioprine therapy in patients with Crohn's disease. Gastroenterology 1997; 112: 1475-81.
34. Kader HA, Raynor SC, Young R, et al. Introduction of 6-mercaptopurine in Crohn's disease patients during the perioperative period: a preliminary evaluation of recurrence of disease. J Paediatr Gastroenterol Nutr 1997; 25: 93-7.
35. Korelitz B, Hanauer S, Rutgeerts P, et al. Post-operative prophylaxis with 6-MP, 5-ASA or placebo in Crohn's disease: a two year multi-centre trial. Gastroenterology 1998; 114: G4141.
36. McGovern DPB, Travis SPL, Duley J, et al. Azathioprine intolerance in patients with IBD may be imidazole-related and is independent of TPMT activity. Gastroenterology 2002; 122: 838-9.
37. Boulton-Jones JR, Pritchard K, Mahmoud AA. The use of 6-mercaptopurine in patients with inflammatory bowel disease after failure of azathioprine therapy. Aliment Pharmacol Ther 2000; 14: 1561-5.
38. Bowen DG, Selby WS. Use of 6-mercaptopurine in patients with inflammatory bowel disease previously intolerant of azathioprine. Dig Dis Sci 2000; 45: 1810-3.
39. Lemann M, Bouhnik Y, Columbel JF, Duclos B, Soule JC, Lerebours E, Mary JY, Modigliani R. Randomized double blind placebo-controlled multicenter azathioprine withdrawal trial in Crohn's disease. Gastroenterology 2002; 122: A174.

40. Dubinsky MC, Lamothe S, Yang HY, et al. Pharmacogenomics and metabolite measurement for 6-mercaptopurine therapy in inflammatory bowel disease. *Gastroenterology* 2000; 118: 705-13
41. Lennard L. TPMT in the treatment of Crohn's disease with azathioprine. *Gut* 2002; 51: 143-6.
42. Connell WR, Kamm MA, Ritchie JK, et al. Bone marrow toxicity caused by azathioprine in inflammatory bowel disease. *Gut* 1993; 34: 1081-5.
43. Dewit O, Vanheurverzwyn R, Desager JP, et al. Interaction between azathioprine and aminosalicylates: an *in vivo* study in patients with Crohn's disease. *Aliment Pharmacol Ther* 2002; 16: 79-85.
44. Lowry PW, Franklin CL, Weaver AL, et al. Leucopenia resulting from a drug interaction between azathioprine or 6-mercaptopurine and mesalamine, sulphasalazine, or balsalazide. *Gut* 2001; 49: 656-64.
45. Feagan BG, Rochon J, Fedorak RN, et al. Methotrexate for the treatment of Crohn's disease. The North American Crohn's Study Group Investigators. *N Engl J Med* 1995; 332: 292-7.
46. Feagan BG, Fedorak RN, Irvine EJ, et al. A comparison of methotrexate with placebo for the maintenance of remission in Crohn's disease. North American Crohn's Study Group Investigators. *N Engl J Med* 2000; 342: 1664-6.
47. Kremer JM, Alarcon GS, Lightfoot RW, et al. Methotrexate for rheumatoid arthritis: suggested guidelines for monitoring liver toxicity: American College of Rheumatology. *Arthritis and Rheumatism* 1994; 37: 316-28.
48. Arora S, Katkov W, Cooley J, et al. Methotrexate in Crohn's disease: results of a randomised, double-blind, placebo-controlled trial. *Hepatogastroenterology* 1999; 46: 1724-9.
49. Targan SR, Hanauer SB, van Deventer SJH, et al. A short-term study of chimeric monoclonal antibody cA2 to tumour necrosis alpha for Crohn's disease. *N Engl J Med* 1999; 337: 1029-35.
50. Present DH, Rutgeerts P, Targan S, et al. Infliximab for the treatment of fistulas in patients with Crohn's disease. *N Engl J Med* 1999; 340: 1398-1405.
51. Sands BE, van Deventer S, Bernstein C, et al. Long-term treatment of fistulizing Crohn's disease: response to infliximab in the ACCENT II trial through 54 weeks. *Gastroenterology* 2002; 122: A136.
52. Rutgeerts P, D'Haens G, Targan S, et al. Efficacy and safety of retreatment with anti-tumor necrosis factor antibody (infliximab) to maintain remission in Crohn's disease. *Gastroenterology* 1999; 117: 761-9.
53. Hanauer SB, Feagan BG, Lichtenstein GR, et al. Maintenance infliximab for Crohn's disease: the ACCENT 1 randomised trial. *Lancet* 2002; 359: 1541-9.
54. Louis E, Vermiere S, Rutgeerts P, et al. A positive response to infliximab in Crohn's disease: association with a higher systemic inflammation before treatment but not with -308 TNF polymorphism. *Scand J Gastroenterol* 2002; 37: 818-24.
55. Shanahan F. Inflammatory bowel disease: immunodiagnostics, immunotherapeutics, and ecotherapeutics. *Gastroenterology* 2001; 120: 622-35.
56. Prantera C, Scribano ML, Falasco G, et al. Ineffectiveness of probiotics in preventing recurrence after curative resection for Crohn's disease: a randomised controlled trial with Lactobacillus GG. *Gut* 2002; 51: 405-9.
57. Lindsay JO, Hodgson HJ. Review article: the immunoregulatory cytokine interleukin-10 - a therapy for Crohn's disease? *Aliment Pharmacol Ther* 2001; 15: 1709-16.
58. Colombel JF, Rutgeerts P, Malchow H, et al. Interleukin-10 (Tenovil) in the prevention of postoperative recurrence of Crohn's disease. *Gut* 2001; 49: 42-6.
59. Fernandez-Benares F, Cabre E, Esteve-Comas M, et al. How effective is enteral nutrition in inducing clinical remission in Crohn's disease? A meta-analysis of the randomised clinical results. *J Parenter Enteral Nutr* 1995; 19: 356-64.
60. Griffiths AM, Ohlsson A, Scherman PM, et al. Meta-analysis of enteral nutrition as a primary treatment of active Crohn's disease. *Gastroenterology* 1995; 108: 1056-67.
61. Russell RI. Nutritional management: central importance in Crohn's disease but peripheral role in ulcerative colitis? In: *Inflammatory Bowel Disease, Clinical Diagnosis and Management*. Rampton DS, Ed. Martin Dunitz Ltd, London, UK, 2000: 185-207.
62. Gorard DA, Hunt JB, Payne-James JJ, et al. Initial response and subsequent course of Crohn's disease treated with elemental diet or prednisolone. *Gut* 1993; 34: 1198-1202.
63. Olaison G, Smedh K, Sjodahl R. Natural course of Crohn's disease after ileocolic resection: endoscopically visualised ileal ulcers preceding symptoms. *Gut* 1992; 33: 331-5.
64. Rutgeerts PJ. Crohn's disease recurrence can be prevented after ileal resection. *Gut* 2002; 51: 152-3.
65. Egan LJ, Sandborn WJ. Advances in the treatment of Crohn's disease. *Gastroenterology* 2004; 126: 1574-81.
66. Farrell RJ, Murphy A, Long A, et al. High multidrug resistance (P-glycoprotein 170) expression in inflammatory bowel disease who fail medical therapy. *Gastroenterology* 2000; 118: 279-88.

Chapter 13

New pharmacology

Anton Emmanuel MD FRCP, Senior Lecturer Gastrointestinal Physiology and
Honorary Consultant Gastroenterologist
St. Mark's Hospital, Harrow, Middlesex, UK

What is the issue?

The inflammatory bowel diseases (IBD) are chronic inflammatory conditions caused by an exaggerated immune response to commensal gut flora or other luminal antigens in a genetically susceptible host [1]. This chapter will initially focus on the current gold standards of management of IBD. Recent advances in our understanding of aetio-pathogenesis suggests that there is a complex relationship between genetic, bacterial and environmental factors (such as smoking and stress). These result in persistent activation of the mucosal immune system which in turn damages intestinal barrier function, allowing further release of immune factors. The consequence of this is persistent inflammation culminating in tissue destruction. The latter part of this chapter will deal with the therapeutic directions being taken specifically to target individual steps in this process through the use of biological agents and probiotics.

The current dogma of therapy for IBD is long-term drug treatment, surgery being reserved for refractory disease and acute and chronic complications. Treatment is directed towards either inducing or maintaining remission, using anti-inflammatory agents or immunosuppressants. The standard for induction of remission in mild or moderate ulcerative colitis (UC) is aminosalicylates (approximately 75% efficacy), with corticosteroids being reserved for more severe colitis (approximately 80% efficacy) [2]. Steroids are ineffective maintenance agents, with high rates of relapse and toxicity. In refractory cases, cyclosporine may be used, although this should be reserved for use in experienced centres with monitoring facilities [3]. Aminosalicylates are considerably less effective in mild Crohn's disease (CD) and therapy for a severe flare-up of CD would be with steroids (approximately 75% efficacy). Methotrexate is of proven efficacy in inducing remission in CD, and has a role in maintenance too [4]. Toxicity, however, is common and potentially serious, and needs careful monitoring. Immunomodulators are the gold standard in maintenance of remission in both UC and CD, although again careful monitoring is required [2]. What is clear is that these limitations in the safety and efficacy of current therapy have prompted a dramatic increase in studies of potential new therapies in IBD.

The current conventional drug approaches discussed above are effective through modification of the immune system in a non-specific fashion. Advances in understanding of the aetio-pathogenesis of IBD in the 1990s have opened up new, more specific, immune system targets in the early part of the 21st Century.

A major advance in recent years has been the identification of the CARD15/NOD 2 gene as a susceptibility locus for Crohn's disease. Three major mutations of this gene have been identified, accounting for approximately one-quarter of cases of Crohn's disease in the Caucasian population. As yet, however, recognition of the patient's genotype has no proven place in the individualisation of disease management [5]. This gene acts as a receptor for bacterial factors, and thus represents a link between IBD and immune tolerance [5]. The potential for exploiting this knowledge in terms of the use of probiotics (viable micro-organisms with beneficial physiological effects) will be discussed in detail.

Where are we now?

The mucosal immune system of the gut, as the key activator of intestinal inflammation, forms the target for almost all drug therapy of IBD. Recent developments have seen improvement in our understanding of how to use conventional therapies, such as immuno-modulators like azathioprine. Emerging therapies are directed towards suppression of pro-inflammatory factors or stimulation of anti-inflammatory ones.

Conventional therapy

Azathioprine and 6-mercaptopurine (6-MP) are long-proven mainstays of maintenance therapy for both UC and CD, acting by altering protein synthesis and hence inhibiting cell growth. Azathioprine is a pro-drug which is rapidly metabolised to active 6-MP, which is in turn degraded through three different enzyme pathways. There is a genetic polymorphism in the activity of one of these enzymes, thiopurine methyl-transferase (TPMT) [6]. This enzyme is absent in 0.3% of the population, and heterozygously low in 11% [6]. TPMT enzyme activity can be measured, and has potential implications in predicting both potential for development of adverse effects and potential efficacy through permitting up-titration of the dose. The convention for azathioprine use in IBD has been to aim for a dose of 2mg/kg/day. Up-titration to a dose of up to 2.5mg/kg/day is associated with significant benefit in UC and CD patients who have not responded to 2mg/kg/day [7]. Dose escalation above 2.5mg/kg/day is less likely to be effective, and is associated with a substantial risk of leucopoenia and intolerance [7].

Understanding of the metabolism of azathioprine has resulted in the potential for looking at metabolites of this pro-drug which may be more effective than the parent compound. For example, over 50% of patients who are unable to take azathioprine due to nausea will tolerate 6-MP at a dose of 1mg/kg/day [8]. Additionally, 6-thioguanine (a thiopurine closely related to azathioprine) is an emerging alternative in patients who are hypersensitive to both azathioprine and 6-MP [9].

Emerging therapies

Suppressing pro-inflammatory cytokines

Targeting tumour necrosis factor

Tumour necrosis factor-alpha (TNF) is expressed in large quantities from the T-cells in biopsies of patient with CD, and levels of TNF correlate with disease activity [10]. These observations led to the development of a chimeric (75% human, 25% murine) IgG monoclonal antibody against TNF, infliximab. The first randomised placebo-controlled study of infliximab showed that a single infusion resulted in a 65% response rate compared to a 17% placebo response [11]. The highest response rate, 81%, was with the 5mg/kg dose [11]. Since it soon became obvious that the effect of these single infusions was not maintained in over one third of patients [12], subsequent studies have focused on the efficacy of multiple dosing as a maintenance strategy [12,13]. What can be concluded from these studies is that with infusions approximately every 8 weeks (after an initial set of three infusions at 0, 2 and 6 weeks), remission is maintained in approximately one third of patients on infliximab, compared to 20% on placebo. This remission with infliximab only (and not placebo) is associated with endoscopic and histological healing of Crohn's lesions [14]. In addition to these studies of infliximab in refractory intestinal CD, the drug has also been investigated for fistulising disease. Using a regimen of three 5mg/kg infusions at 0, 2 and 6 weeks, response (closure of more than 50% of fistulae) is seen in two thirds of patients, with a median duration of response of 3 months [15-17]. The unequivocal efficacy of infliximab in CD has led to investigation of its effect in severe acute steroid-refractory UC with promising results in open-label studies [18,19]. Formal placebo-controlled blinded trials are in progress in both acute severe UC and medically refractory acute-on-chronic UC.

Use of infliximab is associated with the development of human anti-chimeric antibodies. This results in acute infusion reactions, delayed hypersensitivity and loss of efficacy. Accordingly, less immunogenic, more humanised antibodies have been developed, of which the most studied is CDP571 (95% human, 5% murine). Studies to date suggest that the effect on luminal inflammatory CD is approximately 40% (compared to a placebo effect of 20%) [20,21]. Subgroup analysis suggests that patients with an elevated CRP have particular benefit. CDP571 may have a modest steroid-sparing effect in patients intolerant of infliximab. Both infliximab and CDP571 are associated with an increased risk of systemic infection, including tuberculosis; there is also a theoretical increased risk of malignancy, although this has not been observed to a significantly greater rate in CD patients (in contrast to rheumatoid arthritis patients who have received these antibodies).

An alternative strategy to antagonising TNF is to block the receptor through which it acts to exert its pro-inflammatory action. Etanercept is a human protein which binds this receptor. Unfortunately, in contrast to its proven efficacy in rheumatoid arthritis, the drug has not shown any effect in moderate to severe CD [22].

TNF can also be inhibited by blocking the effect of mitogen-activated protein kinases, which are enzymes that regulate cell proliferation. Specific inhibitors of these enzymes, such as CNI-1493, have been studied in CD patients who have failed to respond to infliximab [23]. Clinical and endoscopic response has been observed in more than two thirds of this severe CD population [23].

The controversial drug thalidomide, which was originally pioneered in the 1950s and 1960s as a sedative and hypnotic, also has anti-TNF activity through the degradation of TNF messenger RNA. Thalidomide has been shown to be effective in open-label studies of refractory Crohn's disease and UC, but caution with regard to teratogenic and neuropathic side effects may limit the use of this agent [24,25]. It has been suggested that the drug may have a place in maintaining remission induced by infliximab.

Targeting interleukin-6
Interleukin-6 (IL-6) is a pro-inflammatory cytokine whose levels are strongly positively correlated to disease activity in CD. A humanised monoclonal antibody to the IL-6 receptor has recently been studied in active CD [26]. Response rates of 80% (versus 31% with placebo) and remission rates of 20% (versus 0% placebo) were reported with a bi-weekly infusion regimen. No significant adverse effects were noted in this initial study [26].

Enhancing anti-inflammatory cytokines

Targeting interleukin-10
Interleukin-10 (IL-10) suppresses the production of a range of pro-inflammatory proteins and IL-10 knock-out mice develop enterocolitis. As such, it was a disappointment that clinical trials of IL-10 proved ineffective in both acute and chronic active CD and also UC [27,28]. The postulated reason for the lack of effect is poor tissue penetration of the infused IL-10. Subsequent animal studies have focused on incorporating the cytokine into microbial vectors that result in better delivery to the mucosa.

Targeting interleukin-11
Subcutaneous administration of recombinant human interleukin-11 (IL-11) given bi-weekly is effective in over one third of patients with active CD (compared to a placebo response of about 5%) [29,30]. There is concern about the potential development of adverse effects, in particular thrombocytosis (of concern in a pro-thrombotic condition such as CD).

Preventing leucocyte adhesion and recruitment

Adhesion of white blood cells to the endothelium at sites of mucosal inflammation results in up-regulation of pro-inflammatory cytokines. This adhesion is mediated by specific molecules which can be selectively blocked.

Natalizumab is a humanised monoclonal antibody (-mab) that blocks leucocyte aggregation. Placebo-controlled studies in active CD have shown response rates of 71% (versus 38% with placebo) with two infusions of 3mg/kg given 4 weeks apart [31,32]. The placebo response in these studies was surprisingly high, but nevertheless the effect of this well-tolerated therapy is similar to the early studies with infliximab. Optimism about this line of therapy needs however to be tempered by the observation that controlled studies with other anti-adhesion molecules has not shown efficacy in CD [33,34]. One of these molecules, MLN-02, has shown efficacy in a placebo-controlled study in acute UC [35]. Another, ISIS 2302, has also shown efficacy when used as an enema for 6 weeks in patients with chronic pouchitis [36].

Preventing T-cell differentiation

The immunopathogenesis of CD suggests that the differentiation of T-lymphocytes down the T-helper 1 (Th-1) pathway is of central importance. Inhibition of this Th-1 polarisation is a novel strategy that has shown some promise in trials of moderate and severe CD. Anti-interferon-gamma therapy with a monoclonal antibody, HuZaf, has shown a dose-dependent effect on inducing response and remission [37].

Inhibitors of T-cell proliferation

It is thought that one of the major reasons that cyclosporine is effective in acute UC is that the drug inhibits interleukin-2 (IL-2) which is involved in T-lymphocyte proliferation. Antibodies to the IL-2 receptor have been developed and investigated in open-label studies of steroid-resistant UC. Of these, basiliximab in single-dose infusion is effective in inducing remission symptomatically and histologically [38]. Open-label studies have increasingly sought mucosal healing (endoscopic and/or histologic) as an endpoint, in an attempt to maximise the objective efficacy of the drug under study.

Tacrolimus is a macrolide antibiotic which inhibits IL-2 in a similar manner to cyclosporine. Oral tacrolimus has been the subject of a placebo-controlled trial in fistulating (enterocutaneous and peri-anal) Crohn's disease [39]. Reduction of fistula drainage occurred in 43% of patients compared to a placebo response of 8%. However 38% of tacrolimus recipients developed significantly elevated creatinine levels whilst on treatment [39]. A paediatric study of topical tacrolimus in Crohn's disease suggested that low-dose tacrolimus ointment was effective in healing peri-anal disease without systemic absorption [40].

Miscellaneous combination immune therapies

Broad-spectrum stimulation of the immune system with granulocyte-macrophage stimulating factor (sagramostim) has been shown to induce clinical remission in 80% of subjects in an open-label study of active and fistulising CD [41]. The extension of this study to maintenance therapy showed much less impressive efficacy [42].

Epidermal growth factor (EGF) has been studied in active UC due to its ability to maintain barrier function of the inflamed colon. In active left-sided UC, 14 days of EGF enemas induced remission in 83% of patients compared to an 8% placebo response [43]. The positive data from this small positive study need to be reproduced in larger studies, and caution needs to be retained in view of the theoretical potential for malignant transformation (due to EGF-induced up-regulation of oncogenes in a potentially pre-malignant condition such as UC).

An alternative strategy that has begun to be investigated is the use of growth hormone to induce mucosal healing, by stimulating collagen synthesis. In a 4-month trial of subcutaneous growth hormone in moderate-to-severe CD, a significant response was observed with no major adverse effects [44].

RDP58 is a novel oral therapy with a combination of immune effects. It blocks production of TNF and a variety of other pro-inflammatory cytokines. In a placebo-controlled study of mild-to-moderate UC, remission was induced in 70% (versus a placebo-response of 40%) [45]. Since RDP58 is not absorbed systemically, there is no toxicity.

Mycophenolate mofetil suppresses lymphocyte proliferation and reduces interferon production by T-cells. In chronic active CD, it has similar efficacy to azathioprine, but is more rapidly effective [46]. The drug may have a role in those patients with frequent relapsing CD who are intolerant of azathioprine.

Miscellaneous non-immune therapies

Heparin and related compounds are commonly prescribed in hospitalised patients with acute exacerbations of disease. In addition, vasculitis is a not uncommon phenomenon in inflammatory bowel disease. Thus, the use of heparin has been proposed as potentially of direct benefit in patients with acute disease. The results of controlled trials with heparin have been conflicting. When co-prescribed with aminosalicylates in severe UC, heparin is as effective as intravenous steroids [47]. By contrast, monotherapy with heparin is less effective than steroids in moderate to severe UC [48].

Epidemiologic studies have suggested that discontinuation of smoking is of aetiological significance in the onset of symptoms in some patients with UC. A placebo-controlled trial of transdermal nicotine patches in acute UC has suggested that nicotine doses of 15-25mg per day are effective and well tolerated [49]. However, the drug is not effective in maintaining remission, and disappointing results from nicotine enema studies suggest that the compound has no real role in treating IBD [50].

The evolving notion that the central nervous system and stress response influences gut immune function in functional gastrointestinal disorders has led to the suggestion that neuromodulatory agents may have a role in the treatment of IBD. An open-label study of lignocaine gel in a heterogenous group of patients with UC showed a remission rate with treatment of 10% [51]. Relapse on withdrawal was high. Oral and transdermal preparations of clonidine, an alpha-2 adrenoceptor agonist, have been shown to be effective in mild to moderate left-sided UC [52]. However, the effect of both these neuromodulatory agents is weak, and their role is likely to be limited.

Antibiotics in IBD

Commensal gut flora are undoubtedly implicated in the aetiopathogenesis of some forms of inflammatory bowel disease, most notably Crohn's colitis and pouchitis. The use of metronidazole and ciprofloxacin (in combination or individually) as an adjunct to aminosalicylates, steroids or immunosuppressants is supported by clinical trial data in Crohn's colitis, ileo-colitis and peri-anal disease [53,54]. Use of antibiotics as monotherapy or as combination therapy in small bowel CD is not supported; the same is true for UC. In pouchitis, use of broad spectrum antibiotics for up to 2 weeks is supported by the limited available clinical data [55,56].

Probiotics in IBD

Probiotics are live micro-organisms that are capable of altering the microbial environment and so exert a beneficial health effect. Probiotic preparations were originally derived from cultured milks, and have generated much interest due to patients' enthusiasm for such "natural" products.

Probiotic use in pouchitis

The most extensive investigation of the effect of probiotics in IBD is in both the treatment and prophylaxis of pouchitis. The particular agent to be best studied, VSL#3, is a combination probiotic, comprising four strains of *Lactobacilli*, three strains of *Bifidobacter* and one of *S. salivarium*, with a total of 9 x 10^{11} bacteria per daily dose. The recurrence of pouchitis can be prevented, once remission with antibiotics has been induced, with 85% of patients still in remission at 1 year compared to a placebo rate of 6% [57]. Furthermore, treating a pouch patient with VSL#3 from the time of ileostomy closure results in a 10% 1-year occurrence of pouchitis, compared to 40% on placebo [58].

Probiotic use in UC and CD

Open-label use of VSL#3 induced remission in 87% of patients with mild to moderate UC [59]. A more controversial uncontrolled study of six patients with steroid-refractory colitis showed that all six patients improved after translocation of bacteria via faecal enemas from healthy subjects [60]. In terms of maintenance of remission, a non-pathogenic strain of *E. coli* (*E. coli* Nissle 1917) has been shown to be as effective as low-dose aminosalicylate in UC [61].

By contrast, studies in Crohn's disease have shown no beneficial effect of probiotics. The most studied preparation has been a strain of *Lactobacillus*, *Lactobacillus GG*, which has no effect in terms of inducing or maintaining remission in CD and also no effect in terms of preventing postoperative relapse after ileal or ileocaecal resection [62,63].

Where are we going?

The consequences of the successful first use of infliximab in Crohn's disease in 1997 have been as dramatic as the initial impact of glucocorticoids in inflammatory bowel disease 50 years ago. The beneficial effects of infliximab, coupled with advances in the understanding of the aetiopathogenesis of IBD, have resulted in the accelerated development of a range of new biological agents for both ulcerative colitis and Crohn's disease. These agents are the subject of progressively improving clinical trial design, aimed at not only producing improvement in symptoms, but also at inducing mucosal healing. The critical issue with all these agents is to define their individual place in the algorithm of management. It may be possible in time to define the individual subgroups capable of responding to specific biological therapies. This may be true in terms of not only inducing and maintaining response, but also in the prophylaxis of these chronic conditions.

In addition to these biological therapies aimed at altering immunopathogenesis, a major future direction in IBD research is the understanding and exploitation of the commensal flora in IBD. These non-toxic probiotics are doubly appealing to patients. What remains to be determined is the composition, dose and duration of probiotic therapy for each IBD indication. It is likely that individualisation of probiotic species will need to be considered, in relation to host factors and disease factors, since to date combination preparations (such as VSL#3) have had more beneficial effects than single strains. A final critical factor will be the elucidation of therapy for these chronic inflammatory conditions. It may be that "prebiotics" (namely, dietary substances that stimulate the growth of beneficial commensal gut bacteria) will offer a more attractive "dietary" therapy that patients can adhere to.

References

1. Podolsky DK. Inflammatory bowel disease. *N Engl J Med* 2002; 347: 417-29.
2. Stein RB, Hanauer SB. Medical therapy for inflammatory bowel disease. *Gastroenterol Clin North Am* 1999; 28: 297-321.
3. Lichtiger S, Present DH, Kornbluth A, *et al*. Cyclosporine in severe ulcerative colitis refractory to steroid therapy. *N Engl J Med* 1994; 330: 1841-5.
4. Feagan BG, Alfadhli A. Methotrexate in inflammatory bowel disease. *Gastroenterol Clin North Am* 2004; 33: 407-20.
5. Ahmad T, Tamboli CP, Jewell D, *et al*. Clinical relevance of advances in genetics and pharmacogenetics of inflammatory bowel disease. *Gastroenterology* 2004; 126: 1533-49.
6. Lennard L. TPMT in the treatment of Crohn's disease with azathioprine. *Gut* 2002; 51: 143-6.
7. Rayner CK, Hart AL, Hayward CM, Emmanuel AV, Kamm MA. Azathioprine dose escalation in inflammatory bowel disease. *Aliment Pharmacol Ther* 2004; 20: 65-71.
8. Su C and Lichtenstein GR. Treatment of inflammatory bowel disease with azathioprine and 6-mercaptopurine. *Gastroenterol Clin North Am* 2004; 33: 209-34.
9. Dubinsky MC, Feldman EJ, Abreu MT, *et al*. Thioguanine: a potential alternate thiopurine for IBD patients allergic to 6-mercaptopurine or azathioprine. *Am J Gastroenterol* 2003; 98: 1058-63.
10. Braegger CP, Nicholls S, Murch SH, *et al*. Tumour necrosis factor alpha in stool as a marker of intestinal inflammation. *Lancet* 1992; 339: 89-91.
11. Targan SR, Hanauer SB, van Deventer SJ, *et al*. A short-term study of chimeric monoclonal antibody cA2 to tumour necrosis factor α for Crohn's disease. *N Engl J Med* 1997; 337: 1029-35.
12. Rutgeerts P, D'Haens G, Targan S, *et al*. Efficacy and safety of retreatment with anti tumour necrosis factor antibody (infliximab) to maintain remission in Crohn's disease. *Gastroenterology* 1999; 117: 761-9.
13. Hanauer SB, Feagan BG, Lichtenstein GR, *et al*. Maintenance infliximab for Crohn's disease: the ACCENT I randomised trial. *Lancet* 2002; 359: 1541-9.
14. D'Haens G, van Deventer SJ, van Hogezand R, *et al*. Endoscopic and histological healing with infliximab anti tumour necrosis factor antibodies in Crohn's disease: a European multicenter trial. *Gastroenterology* 1999; 116: 1029-34.
15. Present DH, Rutgeerts P, Targan S, *et al*. Infliximab for the treatment of fistulas in patients with Crohn's disease. *N Engl J Med* 1999; 340: 1398-1405.
16. Ricart E, Panaccione R, Loftus EV, *et al*. Infliximab for Crohn's disease in clinical practice at the Mayo Clinic: the first 100 patients. *Am J Gastroenterol* 2001; 96: 722-9.
17. Ardizzone S, Colombo E, Maconi G, *et al*. Infliximab in treatment of Crohn's disease: the Milan experience. *Digest Liver Dis* 2002; 34: 411-8.

18. Sands BE, Tremaine WJ, Sandborn WJ, et al. Infliximab in the treatment of severe steroid-refractory ulcerative colitis: a pilot study. *Inflamm Bowel Dis* 2001; 7: 83-8.
19. Chey WY, Hussain A, Ryan C, et al. Infliximab for refractory ulcerative colitis. *Am J Gastroenterol* 2001; 96: 2373-81.
20. Stack WA, Mann SD, Roy AJ, et al. Randomised controlled trial of CDP571 antibody to tumour necrosis factor-alpha in Crohn's disease. *Lancet* 1997; 349: 521-4.
21. Sandborn WJ, Feagan BG, Hanauer SB, et al. An engineered human antibody to TNF (CDP571) for active Crohn's disease: a randomised double-blind placebo-controlled trial. *Gastroenterology* 2001; 120: 1330-8.
22. Sandborn WJ, Hanauer SB, Katz S, et al. Etanercept for active Crohn's disease: a randomised double-blind, placebo-controlled trial. *Gastroenterology* 2001; 121: 1088-94.
23. Hommes D, Van Den Blink B, Plasse B, et al. Inhibition of stress-activated MAP kinases induces clinical improvement in moderate to severe Crohn's disease. *Gastroenterology* 2002; 122: 7-14.
24. Ehrenpreis ED, Kane SV, Cohen LB, et al. Thalidomide therapy for patients with refractory Crohn's disease: an open-label trial. *Gastroenterology* 1999; 117: 1271-7.
25. Kam LY, Vasilauskas EA, Abreu MT, et al. Open-label pilot study of thalidomide as a novel therapy for medically resistant ulcerative colitis. *Gastroenterology* 2000; 118: A582.
26. Ito H, Takazoe M, Fukuda Y, et al. Effective treatment of active Crohn's disease with humanised monoclonal antibody MRA to interleukin-6 receptor: a randomised placebo-controlled trial. *Gastroenterology* 2003; 124: A25.
27. Fedorak RN, Gangl A, Elson CO, et al. Recombinant human interleukin 10 in the treatment of patients with mild to moderate Crohn's disease: the interleukin-10 inflammatory bowel disease cooperative study group. *Gastroenterology* 2000; 119: 1473-82.
28. Schreiber S, Fedorak RN, Nielsen OH, et al. Safety and efficacy of recombinant interleukin-10 in chronic active Crohn's disease: the interleukin-10 inflammatory bowel disease cooperative study group. *Gastroenterology* 2000; 119: 1461-72.
29. Sands BE, Bank S, Sninsky CA, et al. Preliminary evaluation of safety and activity of recombinant human interleukin-11 in patients with active Crohn's disease. *Gastroenterology* 1999; 117: 58-64.
30. Sands BE, Winston BD, Salzberg B, et al. Randomised, controlled trial of recombinant human interleukin-11 in patients with active Crohn's disease. *Aliment Pharmacol Ther* 2002; 16: 399-406.
31. Gordon FH, Lai CW, Hamilton MI, et al. A randomised placebo-controlled trial of a humanised monoclonal antibody to alpha4 integrin in active Crohn's disease. *Gastroenterology* 2001; 121: 268-74.
32. Ghosh S, Goldin E, Gordon FH, et al. Natalizumab for Crohn's disease. *N Engl J Med* 2003; 348: 24-32.
33. Yacyshyn BR, Chey WY, Goff J, et al. Double blind placebo controlled trial of the remission-inducing and steroid-sparing properties of an ICAM-1 antisense oligodeoxynucleotide, alicaforsen (ISIS 2302) in active steroid-dependent Crohn's disease. *Gut* 2002; 51: 30-6
34. Feagan BG, Greenberg G, Wild G, et al. Efficacy and safety of a humanised alpha4 beta7 antibody in active Crohn's disease. *Gastroenterology* 2003; 124: A25.
35. Feagan B, Greenberg G, Wild G, et al. A randomised controlled trial of a humanised alpha4 beta7 antibody in ulcerative colitis. *Am J Gastroenterol* 2003; 98: S248-249.
36. Miner PB, Bane B, Bradley JD, et al. ICAM-1 antisense inhibition by enema improves pouchitis and suggests long-term mucosal healing in patients with chronic unremitting disease. *Am J Gastroenterol* 2003; 98: S246-247.
37. Rutgeerts P, Reinisch W, Colombel JF, et al. Preliminary results of a phase I/II study of HuZaf, an anti-IFN-monoclonal antibody, in patients with moderate to severe active Crohn's disease. *Gastroenterology* 2002; 122: A61.
38. Creed TJ, Norman MR, Probert CS, et al. Basiliximab (anti-CD25) in combination with steroids may be an effective new treatment for steroid-resistant ulcerative colitis. *Aliment Pharmacol Ther* 2003; 18: 65-75.
39. Sandborn WJ, Present DH, Isaacs KL, et al. Tacrolimus (FK506) for the treatment of perianal and enterocutaneous fistulas in patients with Crohn's disease: a randomised double-blind placebo-controlled trial. *Gastroenterology* 2003; 125: 380-8.
40. Casson DH, Eltumi M, Tomlin S, et al. Topical tacrolimus may be effective in the treatment of oral and perianal Crohn's disease. *Gut* 2000; 47: 436-40.
41. Dieckegraefe BK, Korzenik JR. Treatment of active Crohn's disease with recombinant human granulocyte-macrophage stimulating factor. *Lancet* 2000; 360: 1478-80.
42. Korzenik J, Pittler A, Dieckegraefe B. Immunostimulation in Crohn's disease: retreatment and maintenance therapy with GM-CSF. *Gastroenterology* 2002; 122: A423.
43. Sinha A, Nightingale J, West KP, et al. Epidermal growth factor enemas with oral mesalamine for mild-to-moderate left-sided ulcerative colitis or proctitis. *N Engl J Med* 2003; 349: 350-7.
44. Slonim AE, Bulone L, Damore MB, et al. A preliminary study of growth hormone therapy for Crohn's disease. *N Engl J Med* 2000; 342: 1633-7.
45. Travis SPL, Yap LM, Hawkey CM, et al. RDP-58: novel and effective therapy for ulcerative colitis: results of parallel, prospective, placebo-controlled trials. *Am J Gastroenterol* 2003; 98: S239.
46. Neurath MF, Wanitschke R, Peters M, et al. Randomised trial of mycophenolate mofetil versus azathioprine for treatment of chronic active Crohn's disease. *Gut* 1999; 44: 625-8.
47. Ang YS, Mahmud N, White B, et al. Randomised comparison of unfractioned heparin with corticosteroids in severe active inflammatory bowel disease. *Aliment Pharmacol Ther* 2000; 14: 1015-22.
48. Panes J, Esteve M, Cabre E, et al. Comparison of heparin and steroids in the treatment of moderate and severe ulcerative colitis. *Gastroenterology* 2000; 119: 903-8.
49. Pullan RD, Rhodes J, Ganesh S, et al. Transdermal nicotine for active ulcerative colitis. *N Engl J Med* 1994; 330: 811-815.
50. Thomas GAO, Rhodes J, Mani V, et al. Transdermal nicotine as maintenance therapy for ulcerative colitis. *N Engl J Med* 1995; 332: 988-92.

51. Bjorsk S, Dahlstrom A, Johansson L, et al. Treatment of the mucosa with local anaesthetics in ulcerative colitis. *Agents Action* 1992; Special Conference Issue: C60-72.
52. Ardizzone S, Bollani S, Manzionna G, et al. Efficacy of transdermal clonidine for mild to moderate active left-sided ulcerative colitis: a pilot study. *Gastroenterology* 1999; 116: G2892.
53. Prantera C, Zannoni F, Scribano ML, et al. An antibiotic regimen for the treatment of active Crohn's disease: a randomised controlled trial of metronidazole plus ciprofloxacin. *Am J Gastroenterol* 1996; 91: 328-32.
54. Arnold GL, Beaves MR, Pryjdun VO, et al. Preliminary study of ciprofloxacin in active Crohn's disease. *Inflamm Bowel Dis* 2002; 8: 10-5.
55. Madden MV, McIntyre AS, Nicholls RJ. Double-blind cross-over trial of metronidazole versus placebo in chronic unremitting pouchitis. *Dig Dis Sci* 1994; 39: 1193-6.
56. Shen B, Achkar JP, Lashner BA, et al. A randomised clinical trial of ciprofloxacin and metronidazole to treat active pouchitis. *Inflamm Bowel Dis* 2001; 7: 301-5.
57. Mimura T, Rizzello F, Helwig U, et al. Once daily high dose probiotic therapy (VSL#3) for maintaining remission in recurrent or refractory pouchitis. *Gut* 2004; 53: 108-14.
58. Gionchetti P, Rizzello F, Helwig U, et al. Prophylaxis of pouchitis onset with probiotic therapy: a double-blind placebo controlled trial. *Gastroenterology* 2003; 124: 1202-9.
59. Fedorak RN, Gionchetti P, Campieri M, et al. VSL3 probiotic mixture induces remission in patients with active ulcerative colitis. *Gastroenterology* 2003; 124: A377.
60. Borody TJ, Warren EF, leis S, et al. Treatment of ulcerative colitis using fecal bacteriotherapy. *J Clin Gastroenterol* 2003; 37: 42-7.
61. Rembacken BJ, Snelling AM, Hawkey PM, et al. Non pathogenic *Escherichia coli* versus mesalazine for the treatment of ulcerative colitis: a randomised trial. *Lancet* 1999; 354: 635-9.
62. Prantera C, Scribano ML, Falasco G, et al. Ineffectiveness of probiotics in preventing recurrence after curative resection for Crohn's disease: a randomised controlled trial with *Lactobacillus GG*. *Gut* 2002; 51: 405-9.
63. Schultz M, Timmer A, Herfarth HH, et al. *Lactobacillus GG* in inducing and maintaining remission of Crohn's disease. *BMC Gastroenterol* 2004; 4: 5.

Chapter 14

Management of the devastated perineum

Paul Hollington MB BS PhD FRACS, Consultant Surgeon, Colorectal Surgery
Flinders Medical Centre, Bedford Park SA, Australia

Rajiv Grover BSc MD FRCS (Plast), Consultant Plastic Surgeon
St. Mark's Hospital, Harrow, Middlesex, UK

John MA Northover MS FRCS, Consultant Surgeon
St. Mark's Hospital, Harrow, Middlesex, UK
Professor of Intestinal and Colorectal Disorders, Imperial College, London, UK

What is the problem?

The perineum is an intimate, physiologically complex, and functionally vital part of the anatomy. It can be damaged in anal and pelvic surgery, by radical chemoradiotherapy for anogenital cancer, and by trauma: obstetric, automotive, sexual and ritual. Any patient suffering perineal injury may be "devastated" emotionally, psychologically and/or socially, but for the surgeon the word devastation carries the connotation of a serious degree of anatomical and functional disruption, often requiring an individualised and multidisciplinary approach to attempted remedy.

Perineal devastation may come about through the vicissitudes of medical care:

- Major obstetric injury - "natural" or iatrogenic, or both - leading to so-called cloacal injury.
- Chemoradiotherapy for anal cancer; a large tumour invading the anal sphincters and rectovaginal septum may melt away, resulting in combined sphincter deficiency and rectovaginal fistula. This may result in a cloacal defect; on occasion there is a large fistula with a deficient perineum, comprising little more than a skin bridge. This lesion is best managed as a cloacal defect, dividing the bridge and attempting a composite repair.
- Chronic pelviperineal defects resulting from failed healing after proctectomy for inflammatory bowel disease.

In other cases, the devastation is deliberate, as part of a massive putatively therapeutic intervention. Major surgery to treat anal cancer (today usually after failed chemoradiotherapy) or recurrent pelvic cancer, may result in a large dead space in the pelvis and a large defect in the perineum, often in a radiation field. Wide excision of superficial peri- and intra-anal disease may be sufficient to require the use of plastic surgical techniques, and therefore might be seen as falling within the bracket of perineal devastation.

Where are we now?

Plastic surgical techniques are increasingly being employed in the management of both benign and malignant colorectal conditions involving the perineum and pelvis.

Repair of major perineal and pelvic disruption demands a multidisciplinary approach, usually including the expertise of a plastic surgeon; the authors feel strongly that, although there are some plastic techniques that can be used perfectly satisfactorily by an experienced colorectal surgeon, there should nevertheless be a low threshold for involving "the real thing". Others involved may include a urologist, gynaecologist, orthopaedic surgeon, or any combination of these; in the main, the details of their involvement are beyond the remit of this chapter [1,2]. Rather, we will concentrate on the combined efforts of the colorectal and plastic surgeons in trying to put the patient - and in particular, their perineum - back together.

Reconstructive techniques

The ideal repair provides adequate cosmesis and functional restoration, requiring skin cover and volume replacement. Healthy replacement tissue is needed to fill defects and/or to promote healing, particularly in areas affected by radiotherapy [3]. Loss limited to skin should be replaced with skin, whilst composite defects are repaired using myocutaneous flaps, and remote or complex defects with free tissue transfer.

A variety of techniques is available for pelviperineal reconstruction. Healthy tissue may be transposed by free grafting or the raising of flaps [4]. Grafts recruit a local blood supply, whereas flaps bring their supply with them, either via a pedicle, or as free flaps perfused via their own vessels anastomosed to arteries and veins adjacent to the recipient site, such as the femoral or gluteal vessels [5]. The design of specific flaps relies on axial perfusion, whereby flap length is constrained only by the territory of its axial blood supply [6].

Skin grafts are used to replace tissue loss limited to superficial structures, and may comprise split or full thickness skin [4]. Graft thickness is determined by the size of the defect, the underlying vascularity, the required degree of cosmetic recovery, and recipient site contour, taking into consideration the degree of mobility of underlying structures.

The perineum usually requires at least medium-thickness split skin grafts in order to achieve durable wound cover. If the degree of tissue loss is greater, or if recipient site vascularity is likely to be insufficient to support a graft, local advancement flap reconstruction is preferred. This is dependent upon the availability of mobile tissue adjacent to the defect. If local tissue cannot be used, it must be recruited from elsewhere, comprising muscle alone, or muscle with overlying skin (myocutaneous), or deep fascia and overlying skin alone based on a perforating vessel (fasciocutaneous). Myocutaneous flaps can fill large spaces as well as providing skin replacement [1,7]. Muscle flaps alone, particularly the rectus abdominis, can be used for interposition after separation of visceral fistulae, for the exclusion of the small intestine from the pelvis, and for pelvic floor reconstruction [8].

Once established, flaps can be further modified to improve their cosmesis or function, most frequently involving flap thinning by liposuction.

Careful flap planning is important. The donor tissue must be transposable and inset without tension or compromise of its blood supply. Vascular inflow is critical; duplex ultrasound scanning of feeding vessels may be useful to confirm their position, size, and patency. Such examination of the inferior epigastric artery should be used in patients being considered for a rectus-based flap who have undergone appendicectomy or stoma closure. Outflow is also critical, and it is important to ensure that the pedicle of a flap is not kinked or twisted resulting in venous obstruction. Factors resulting in vessel spasm, such as smoking, may also compromise viability. Pedicled flaps are more likely to survive than free flaps.

Reconstructive options

Superficial perineal wounds

Large superficial perineal wounds result from excision of widespread, severe anal intra-epithelial neoplasia, Paget's disease, or early invasive squamous cell carcinoma.

Extensive circumferential defects can be repaired very satisfactorily using split skin grafts, even when involving the anal canal. A defunctioning colostomy is fashioned immediately before the perineal procedure, and an indwelling urinary catheter placed. After excision in the prone position, the posterior thigh is an accessible donor site during perineal surgery. For excisions extending into the anal canal, four truncated pyramids of skin graft are fashioned, two wide ones at the sides and two narrow anteriorly and posteriorly. The apical end of each (1-2cm wide) is sutured to the dentate line to ensure circumferential cover to the dentate line (Figure 1a). It greatly simplifies the procedure if the split skin is first placed onto tullegras and the split skin/tullegras combination cut and

14 Management of the devastated perineum

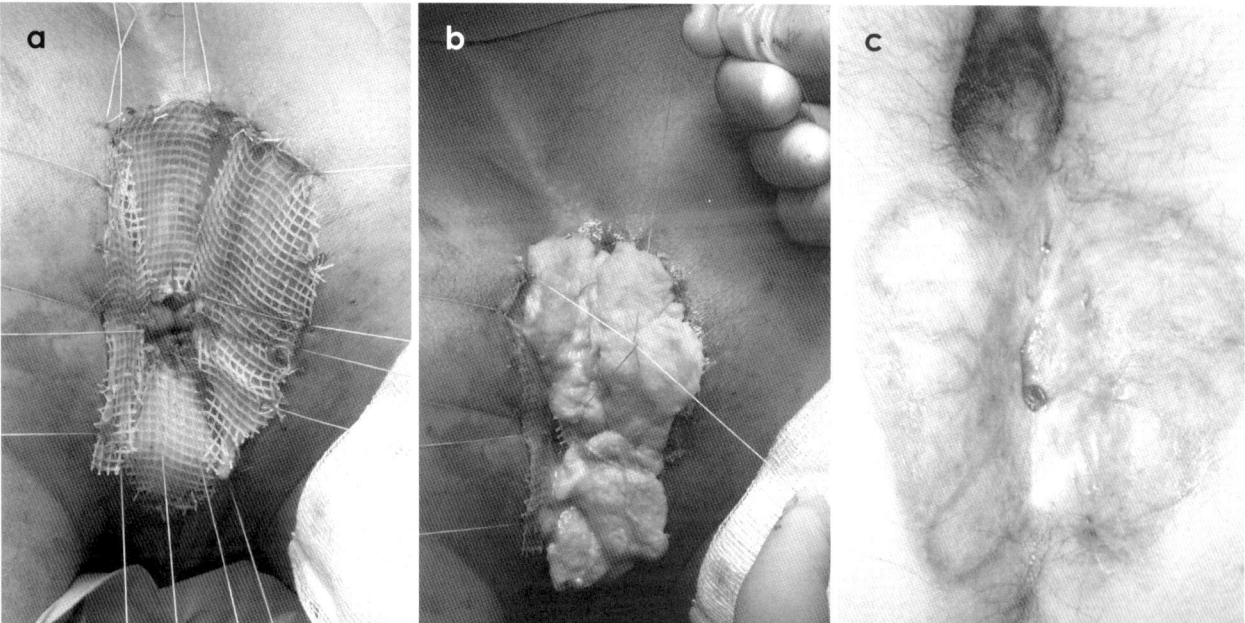

Figure 1. a) Four split skin graft truncated pyramids *in situ* prior to dressing with tie-over proflavine cotton wool boluses. b) Proflavine dressings being cross-tied in place using sutures applied to four corners of the truncated pyramid graft. c) Split skin graft 5 weeks after surgery.

sutured. When the sutures dissolve the tullegras backing falls away leaving the grafted anal canal. The large number of sutures required at the periphery of the graft are best controlled during placement by sticking them to the surrounding drapes in radial fashion using very small amounts of fresh lubricant gel. A tie-over bolus (proflavine cotton wool) dressing is applied to each of the four grafted segments to maintain apposition (Figure 1b); these should remain in place for 5-7 days, with the patient on strict bed rest in the prone and lateral positions. High rates of graft survival have been observed adopting these measures, and the medium and long-term outcome is very good (Figure 1c).

Smaller asymmetric anal excision wounds can be repaired using local island advancement flaps (where the pedicle comprises subcutaneous tissue only), such as the "house" flap, so-called because of its shape (Figure 2). This is also useful to correct gutter deformities resulting from surgery for fistula-in-ano; up to one third of the circumference of the anal verge can

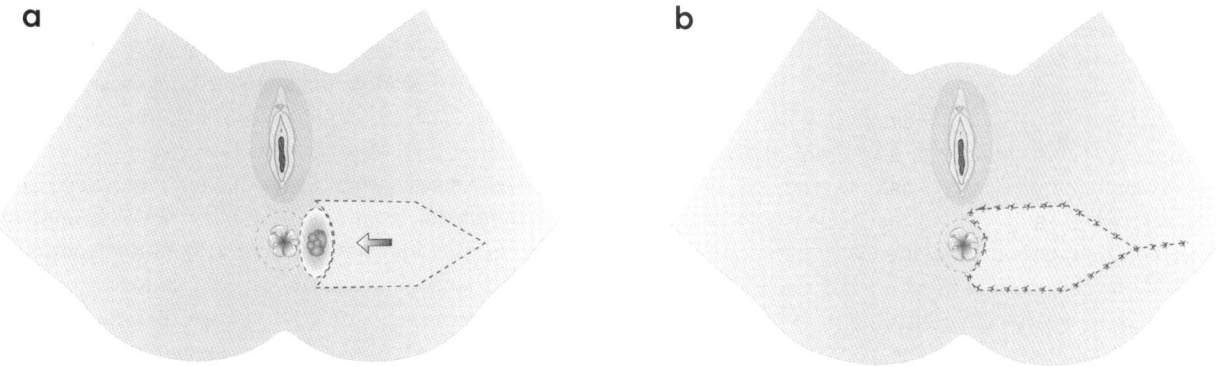

Figure 2. a) House advancement flap. The dimensions are marked out pre-operatively. b) The flap mobilized to allow primary closure of the donor site.

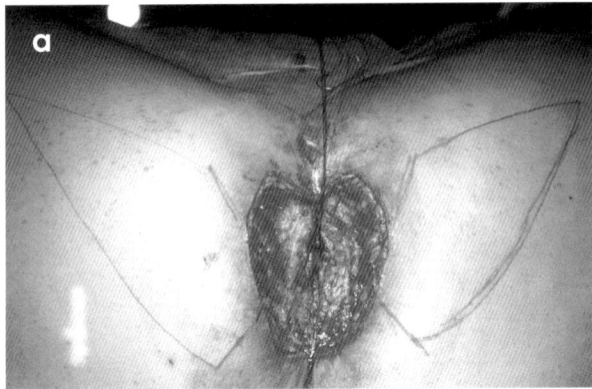
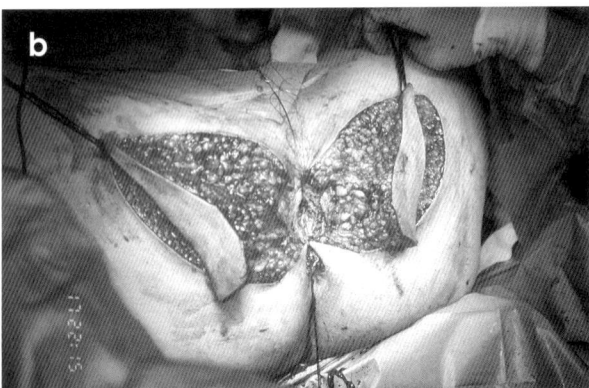
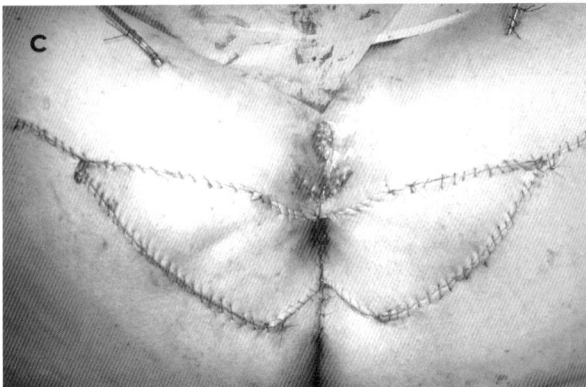

Figure 3. a) Skin markings prior to bilateral V-Y advancement flap mobilisation. b) Completed mobilisation to show fatty pedicle. c) Completed V-Y advancement repair.

technique borrows "spare" tissue from either side of the defect, to be moved as island flaps, providing the most robust method for peri-anal defects, with the benefit of primary wound healing (Figure 3). Each flap can be advanced approximately 3-4cm. The procedure is best performed in the prone position and, as with all of these perineal procedures, judicious use of the Lone Star retractor can facilitate dissection and suturing inside the anal canal.

Cloacal defects

The great majority of cloacal defects are due to obstetric injury, and do not require tissue replacement, as there has been no tissue loss - it is merely in the wrong place! (Figure 4a). These defects involve the introitus, anal canal, rectovaginal septum and anal sphincters. Repair is achieved simply by returning all displaced tissues to their normal anatomical position; this is facilitated by careful and accurate apposition of the main landmarks: the posterior fourchette, dentate line and anal verge. There is no need to try to reconstitute the "perineal body", a non-existent structure; repair of the sphincters is all that is necessary to restore anatomical and cosmetic normality. Following repair the cosmetic and functional outcome is usually very satisfactory (Figure 4b). Cloacal defects with tissue loss (after trauma or chemoradiotherapy for anterior invasive anal cancer) are more difficult to repair, and may require skin and subcutaneous tissue replacement after attempted primary repair of the sphincters. Local options include bilateral V-Y advancement flaps for limited defects [14-17]. In some, myocutaneous transfers, based on the gracilis muscle or even the rectus abdominis muscle, may be required [18] (for technical details, see below). High rates of rectus-based flap survival and wound healing have been reported, as well as low rates of donor site morbidity [19]. As the vagina usually has sufficient redundant skin, sometimes only muscle transfer is required as a bulking agent over which the skin can be closed.

be replaced using the house flap [9]. Mobilisation is performed down to the fascia of the underlying gluteus maximus muscle; the house has high "walls" to ensure a large enough pedicle, and a high pitched "roof" to facilitate donor site closure. Care must be taken to avoid tension at the flap corners.

Alternatively, bilateral V-Y advancement flaps can be used to close larger perineal defects [10-13]. This

The gracilis flap has proven useful in perineal and vaginal reconstruction [20-22] (Figure 5). Advantages include low donor site morbidity due to its limited primary functional role and its accessibility during perineal operations; it also avoids the laparotomy required for fashioning of a rectus flap. It does have limitations, including a higher risk of flap loss compared to rectus flaps, and its mobility is limited by

14 Management of the devastated perineum

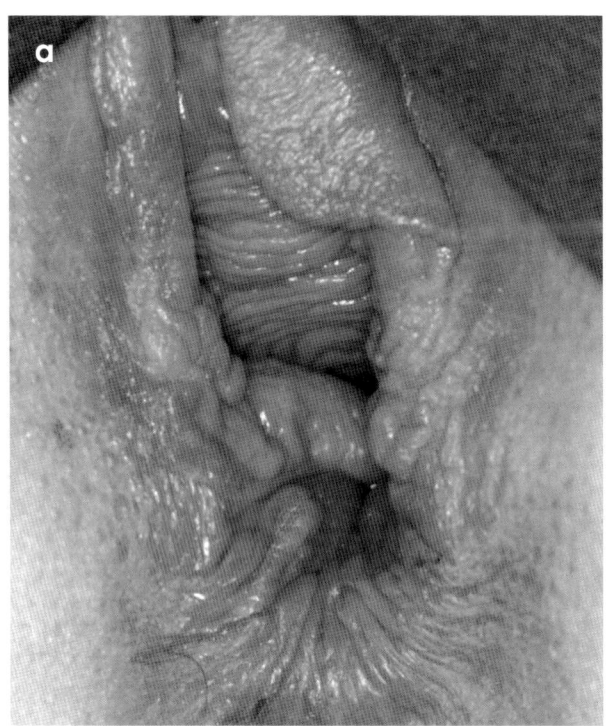

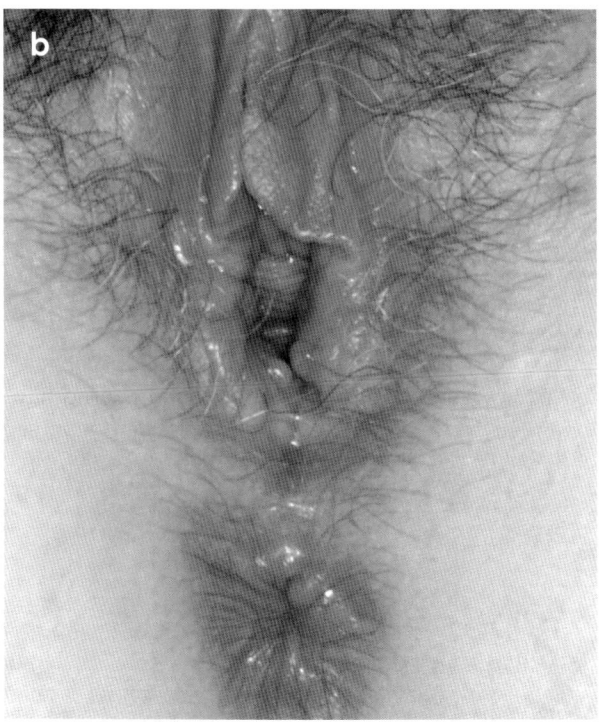

Figure 4. a) Cloacal injury prior to repair. b) Mature result following cloacal injury repair. As here, often the scars of repair are hardly apparent.

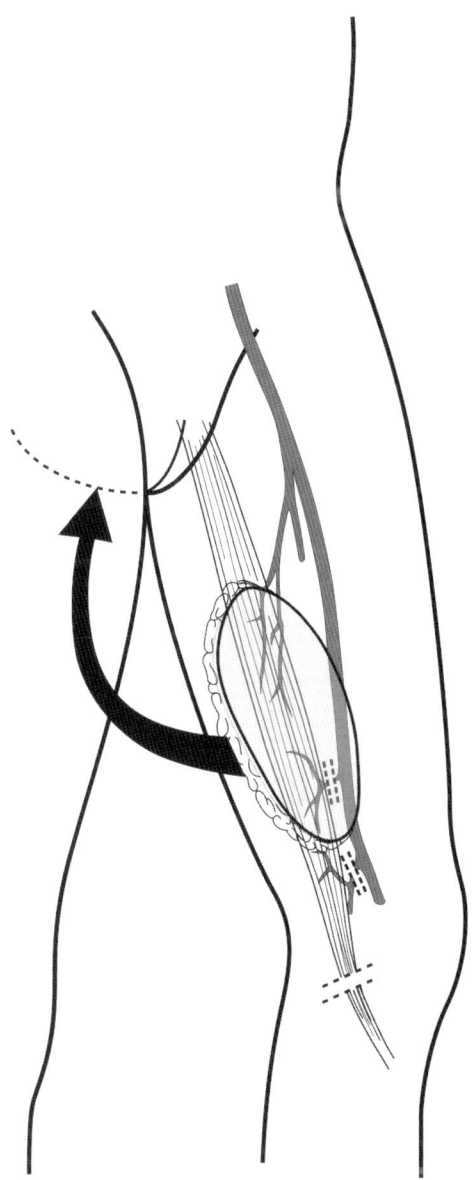

Figure 5. Gracilis flap. The femoral circumflex perforator vessels act as a pivot point allowing transfer of the muscle with or without an overlying skin paddle.

the point of entry of the femoral circumflex perforator, which supplies the muscle and also acts as its pivot point [23,24]. As it is a thin muscle, careful pre-operative localisation is imperative, and care must be taken to design the skin paddle, which must comprise tissue lying directly over the muscle in order to include myocutaneous perforating vessels. This flap should be used with caution in patients who smoke,

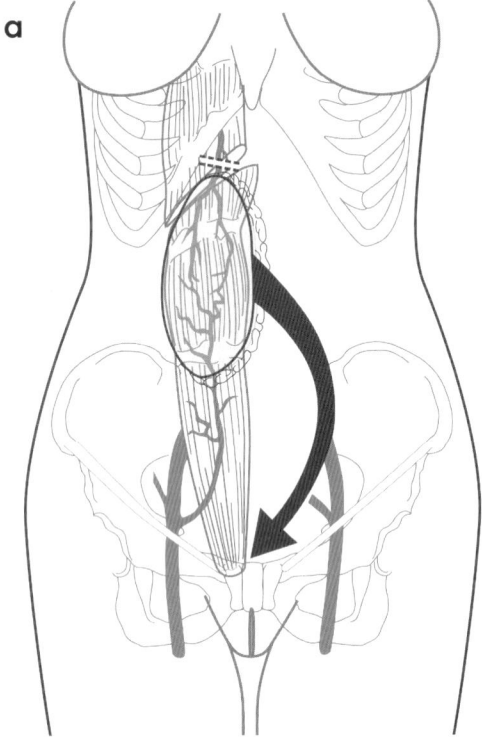
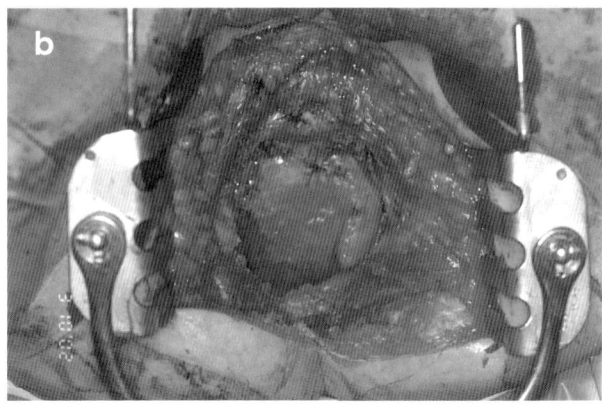
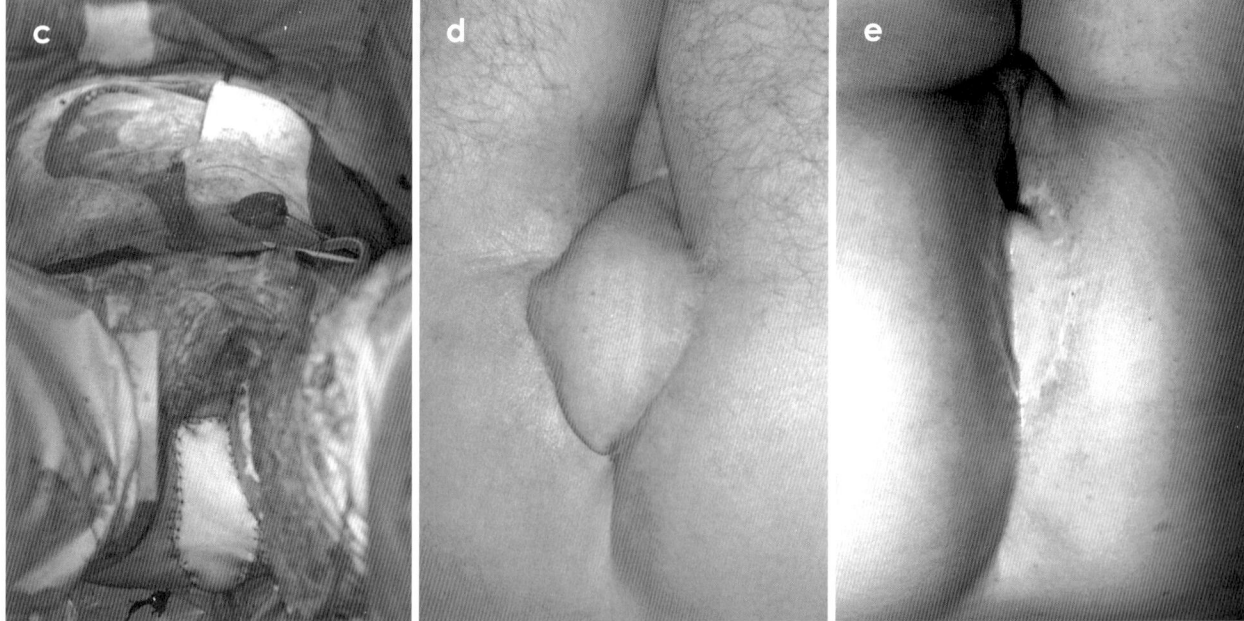

Figure 6. a) Rectus abdominis flap. The inferior epigastric vascular bundle acts as a pivot point allowing transfer of the muscle with or without an overlying skin paddle. b) Extensive perineal defect following wide excision and proctectomy for recurrence of anal cancer following failed primary chemoradiotherapy. c) Rectus myocutaneous flap in place, showing also the myocutaneous abdominal defect prior to wound closure. d) Mature healing of the rectus flap skin paddle, showing bulge due to excess subcutaneous fat. e) Same, but following liposuction to improve contour.

particularly if the muscle is narrow, rendering the skin paddle less reliable. Partial flap necrosis limited to the skin and subcutaneous tissue may be salvaged using split skin grafting. It is important to anchor the muscle at the recipient site to prevent muscle retraction if skin and subcutaneous necrosis occur.

Posterior thigh fasciocutaneous flaps have also been employed to replace perineal skin and subcutaneous tissue, and are useful in providing skin for vaginal reconstruction [25-27]. Harvest is easier in the lithotomy position; the inferior gluteal artery upon which it is based should be located and marked using duplex ultrasound pre-operatively. The donor tissue is tunnelled subcutaneously to reach the perineum.

Postoperative pelviperineal defects

Although suction dressings have been shown to aid closure of persisting perineal cavities, the vacuum pressure of 125mm Hg required can damage nearby structures such as pelvic side wall vessels and the small bowel. In the irradiated pelvis, this method of management is less effective.

Large pelviperineal wounds following radical excisions that might include rectum, uterus, bladder and sacrum require reconstruction using composite tissue transfer, usually the rectus flap (see below) [28]. The use of regional or distant flaps for reconstruction greatly increases the likelihood of primary healing, particularly in patients who have undergone radiotherapy [7,29]. The gluteus flap (comprising the gluteus maximus and its overlying fascia and skin, being supplied by the superior gluteal pedicle) is suitable for closing some perineal defects after abdominoperineal excision, resection of pelvic tumours, and especially after *en bloc* sacral resection [30,31]. It is important to note that, if the constituent tissue of this flap has been in a radiotherapy field, viability and mobility of tissue may be compromised. The gluteus flap can be fashioned and placed in either the prone or lithotomy position. Very large defects can be covered by transposing tissue from both sides by superiorly-based rotation on one side and inferiorly-based rotation on the other. A disadvantage is its inadequacy for filling the pelvic space, permitting the small bowel to descend, potentially resulting in later morbidity. The use of an omental plug based on the left or (preferentially) the right gastro-epiploic vessels can at least partially reduce the pelvic dead space in these circumstances [32,33].

The rectus myocutaneous flap, with or without a skin paddle, is supplied by the inferior epigastric pedicle. It is a very useful technique for filling dead space and facilitating rapid healing with low morbidity [34-41]. The overlying skin and fascia are supplied by multiple perforators from the epigastric vessels, allowing the muscle belly to be divided and raised with a paddle of overlying skin and subcutaneous tissue, which can then be transposed via the abdominopelvic cavity to reach the pelviperineal defect (Figures 6a-c). The anterior rectus sheath is left *in situ* to allow the donor site to be closed readily without a mesh. The skin can also be used in vaginal reconstruction [42-45]. The muscle invariably shrinks, so it is important to allow for this by tacking it in place with the distal end proud on the perineum. If the skin and subcutaneous tissue are too prominent after mature healing, the graft can be "defatted" at a later date if necessary (Figures 6d & e).

The most ambitious repair technique is the free microvascular myocutaneous flap, usually based on the latissimus dorsi muscle (Figure 7). This procedure is reserved for situations in which no other technique is possible, for instance, when neither rectus muscles are available because they have been transgressed by

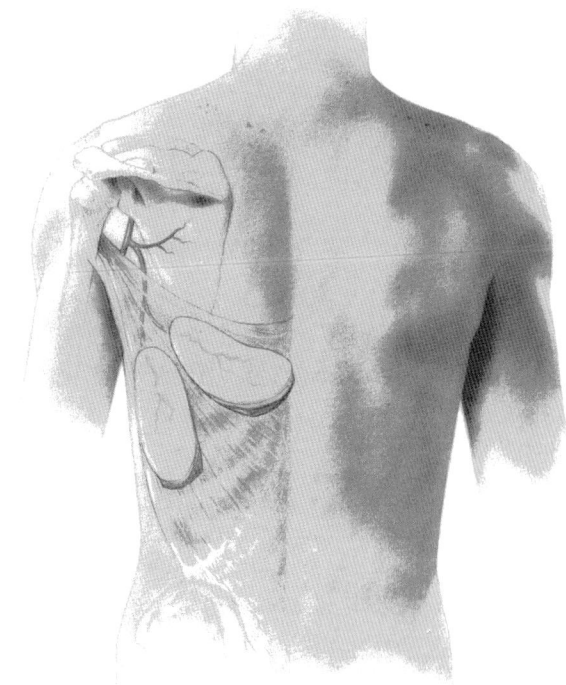

Figure 7. Latissimus dorsi free transfer myocutaneous flap.

an appendicectomy wound or a stoma. The muscle and a suitable skin paddle, together with the circumflex scapular vessels, are removed from their native site, and moved to the perineum and pelvis; the blood supply is secured by microvascular anastomosis to the femoral or gluteal vessels. As might be expected, this formidable operation carries the highest risk of flap failure of all the techniques described, so it should be used only when there is no alternative.

Where are we going?

An extensive reconstructive armamentarium is available for use in patients with a devastated pelvis and/or perineum, ranging from simple and relatively minor procedures performed by the colorectal surgeon to complex composite tissue transfer as part of multidisciplinary team management of those suffering or requiring massive tissue loss. All colorectal surgeons should be aware of these techniques, and be prepared to use them at primary surgery, rather than waiting for failed primary healing before calling in the plastic surgeon.

Acknowledgement

The authors thank Nigel Webb for his drawings.

References

1. McCraw JB, Papp C, Ye Z, Huang V, McMellin A. Reconstruction of the perineum after tumor surgery. *Surg Oncol Clin N Am* 1997; 6(1): 177-89.
2. Temple WJ, Saettler EB. Locally recurrent rectal cancer: role of composite resection of extensive pelvic tumors with strategies for minimizing risk of recurrence. *J Surg Oncol* 2000; 73(1): 47-58.
3. Miller LB, Steele G, Cady B, Wolfort FG, Bothe A, Jr. Resection of tumors in irradiated fields with subsequent immediate reconstruction. *Arch Surg* 1987; 122(4): 461-6.
4. McGregor IA. *Fundamental Techniques of Plastic Surgery and their applications* (8th edition). Churchill Livingstone, London, 1989.
5. Puckett CL, Reinisch JF, Montie JE. Free flap phalloplasty. *J Urol* 1982; 128(2): 294-7.
6. McGregor IA, Morgan G. Axial and random pattern flaps. *Br J Plast Surg* 1973; 26(3): 202-13.
7. Radice E, Nelson H, Mercill S, Farouk R, Petty P, Gunderson L. Primary myocutaneous flap closure following resection of locally advanced pelvic malignancies. *Br J Surg* 1999; 86: 349-54.
8. Kouraklis G. Reconstruction of the pelvic floor using the rectus abdominis muscles after radical pelvic surgery. *Dis Colon Rectum* 2002; 45(6): 836-9.
9. Sentovich SM, Falk PM, Christensen MA, Thorson AG, Blatchford GJ, Pitsch RM. Operative results of house advancement anoplasty. *Br J Surg* 1996; 83(9): 1242-4.
10. Wang TN, Whetzel T, Mathes SJ, Vasconez LO. A fasciocutaneous flap for vaginal and perineal reconstruction. *Plast Reconstr Surg* 1987; 80(1): 95-103.
11. Sagher U, Krausz MM, Peled IJ. V-Y plasty for perianal reconstruction after resection of tumor. *Surg Gynaecol Obstet* 1992; 175(1): 31-2.
12. Tateo A, Tateo S, Bernasconi C, Zara C. Use of V-Y flap for vulvar reconstruction. *Gynecol Oncol* 1996; 62(2): 203-7.
13. Persichetti P, Simone P, Berloco M, Casadei RM, Marangi GF, Cagli B, Di Lella F. Vulvo-perineal reconstruction: medial thigh septo-fascio-cutaneous island flap. *Ann Plast Surg* 2003; 50(1): 85-9.
14. Core GB, Bite U, Pemberton JH, Petty PM. Sliding V-Y perineal island flaps for large perianal defects. *Ann Plast Surg* 1994; 32(3): 328-31.
15. Ricchi E, Fundaro S, Spallanzani A, Carriero A, Farinetti A, Ferrara F, Pezcoller C. Vertical subcutaneous pedicle flaps for posterior perineal reconstruction. Report of three cases. *Dis Colon Rectum* 1996; 39(3): 353-7.
16. Sasaki K, Nozaki M, Kikutchi Y, Yamaki T, Soejima K. Reconstruction of perianal skin defect using a V-Y advancement of bilateral gluteus maximus musculocutaneous flaps: reconstruction considering anal cleft and anal function. *Br J Plast Surg* 1999; 52(6): 471-5.
17. Draganic B, Solomon MJ. Island flap perineoplasty for coverage of perineal skin defects after repair of cloacal deformity. *ANZ J Surg* 2001; 71(8): 487-90.
18. Shukla HS, Hughes LE. The rectus abdominis flap for perineal wounds. *Ann R Coll Surg Engl* 1984; 66(5): 337-9.
19. Tobin GR, Day TG. Vaginal and pelvic reconstruction with distally based rectus abdominis myocutaneous flaps. *Plast Reconstr Surg* 1988; 81(1): 62-73.
20. Burke TW, Morris M, Roh MS, Levenback C, Gershenson DM. Perineal reconstruction using single gracilis myocutaneous flaps. *Gynecol Oncol* 1995; 57: 221-5.
21. Whetzel TP, Lechtman AN. The gracilis myofasciocutaneous flap: vascular anatomy and clinical application. *Plast Reconstr Surg* 1997; 99(6): 1642-52; discussion 1653-5.
22. Shibata D, Hyland W, Busse P, Kim HK, Sentovich SM, Steele G Jr, Bleday R. Immediate reconstruction of the perineal wound with gracilis muscle flaps following abdominoperineal resection and intraoperative radiation

therapy for recurrent carcinoma of the rectum. *Ann Surg Oncol* 1999; 6(1): 33-7.
23. Soper JT, Larson D, Hunter VJ, Berchuck A, Clarke-Pearson DL. Short gracilis myocutaneous flaps for vulvovaginal reconstruction after radical pelvic surgery. *Obstet Gynecol* 1989; 74(5): 823-7.
24. Giordano PA, Abbes M, Pequignot JP. Gracilis blood supply: anatomical and clinical re-evaluation. *Br J Plast Surg* 1990; 43(3): 266-72.
25. Hurwitz DJ, Swartz WM, Mathes SJ. The gluteal thigh flap: a reliable, sensate flap for the closure of buttock and perineal wounds. *Plast Reconstr Surg* 1981; 68(4): 521-32.
26. Achauer BM, Turpin IM, Furnas DW. Gluteal thigh flap in reconstruction of complex pelvic wounds. *Arch Surg* 1983; 118(1): 18-22.
27. Achauer BM, Braly P, Berman ML, DiSaia PJ. Immediate vaginal reconstruction following resection for malignancy using the gluteal thigh flap. *Gynecol Oncol* 1984; 19(1): 79-89.
28. Miles WK, Chang DW, Kroll SS, Miller MJ, Langstein HN, Reece GP, Evans GR, Robb GL. Reconstruction of large sacral defects following total sacrectomy. *Plast Reconstr Surg* 2000; 105(7): 2387-94.
29. Miller LB, Steele G, Cady B, Wolfort FG, Bothe A. Resection of tumors in irradiated fields with subsequent immediate reconstruction. *Arch Surg* 1987; 22(4): 461-6.
30. Baird WL, Hester TR, Nahai F Bostwick J 3rd. Management of perineal wounds following abdominoperineal resection with inferior gluteal flaps. *Arch Surg* 1990; 125(11): 1486-9.
31. Loree TR, Hempling RE, Eltabbakh GH, Recio FO, Piver MS. The inferior gluteal flap in the difficult vulvar and perineal reconstruction. *Gynecol Oncol* 1997; 66(3): 429-34.
32. Ferguson CM. Use of omental pedicle grafts in abdominoperineal resection. *Am Surg* 1990; 56: 310.
33. Nakagoe T, Sawai T, Tuji T, Nanashima A, Yamaguchi H, Yasutake T, Ayabe H. The use of an omental pedicle graft to prevent small-bowel obstruction after restorative proctocolectomy. *Surg Today* 1999; 29(4): 395-7.
34. McCraw J, Kemp G, Given F, Horton CE. Correction of high pelvic defects with the inferiorly based rectus abdominis myocutaneous flap. *Clin Plast Surg* 1988; 15(3): 449-54.
35. Kroll SS, Pollock R, Jessup JM, Ota D. Transpelvic rectus abdominis flap reconstruction of defects following abdominal-perineal resection. *Am Surg* 1989; 55: 632.
36. Skene AI, Gault DT, Woodhouse CRJ, Breach NM, Thomas JM. Perineal, vulval and vaginoperineal reconstruction using the rectus abdominis myocutaneous flap. *Br J Surg* 1990; 77: 635.
37. McAllister E, Wells K, Chaet M, Norman J, Cruse W. Perineal reconstruction after surgical extirpation of pelvic malignancies using the transpelvic transverse rectus abdominal myocutaneous flap. *Ann Surg Oncol* 1994; 1(2): 164-8.
38. Erdmann MW, Waterhouse N. The transpelvic rectus abdominis flap: its use in the reconstruction of extensive perineal defects. *Ann R Coll Surg Engl* 1995; 77(3): 229-32.
39. Loessin SJ, Meland NB, Devine RM, Wolff BG, Nelson H, Zincke H. Management of sacral and perineal defects following abdominoperineal resection and radiation with transpelvic muscle flaps. *Dis Colon Rectum* 1995; 38(9): 940-5.
40. Jain AK, DeFranzo AJ, Marks MW, Loggie BW, Lentz S. Reconstruction of pelvic exenterative wounds with transpelvic rectus abdominis flaps: a case series. *Ann Plast Surg* 1997; 38(2): 115-22; discussion 122-3.
41. Tei TM, Stolzenburg T, Buntzen S, Laurberg S, Kjeldsen H. Use of transpelvic rectus abdominis musculocutaneous flap for anal cancer salvage surgery. *Br J Surg* 2003; 90(5): 575-80.
42. Tobin GR, Pursell SH, Day TG Jr. Refinements in vaginal reconstruction using rectus abdominis flaps. *Clin Plast Surg* 1990; 17(4): 705-12.
43. de Haas WG, Miller MJ, Temple WJ, Kroll SS, Schusterman MA, Reece GP, Skibber JM. Perineal wound closure with the rectus abdominis musculocutaneous flap after tumor ablation. *Ann Surg Oncol* 1995; 2(5): 400-6.
44. Smith HO, Genesen MC, Runowicz CD, Goldberg GL. The rectus abdominis myocutaneous flap: modifications, complications, and sexual function. *Cancer* 1998; 83(3): 510-20.
45. Small T, Friedman DJ, Sultan M. Reconstructive surgery of the pelvis after surgery for rectal cancer. *Semin Surg Oncol* 2000; 18(3): 259-64.

Chapter 15

Ulcerative colitis surveillance

Matt Rutter MD FRCP, Consultant Gastroenterologist
University Hospital of North Tees, Stockton-on-Tees, Cleveland, UK

What is the problem?

Cancer risk in ulcerative colitis

Colon cancer in ulcerative colitis was first noted by Crohn and Rosenberg in 1925, and it is now well established that patients with ulcerative colitis are at increased risk of developing colorectal cancer. However, the magnitude of increased risk has proved difficult to quantify. Most studies have been hospital-based and of surveillance populations and hence susceptible to selection bias. Interpretation is also hampered as patients may undergo colectomy for dysplasia prior to the development of colorectal cancer, thus removing the risk of cancer development. In general, studies report the relative colorectal cancer risk in ulcerative colitis as being between three and twenty times that of the general population [1, 2]. However, a Danish study has reported no increased risk of colorectal cancer in patients with extensive colitis after 25 years, perhaps explained by a high colectomy rate of 32% [3]. The most reliable data probably come from a population-based study from Sweden, which reported a standardised incidence ratio of 5.7 for all patients with ulcerative colitis [4].

In patients with colitis, colorectal cancer tends to occur at a younger age than in the general population [5], and may carry a worse prognosis.

Management strategies for excess cancer risk

Clinicians have three potential management strategies to address the excess cancer risk in ulcerative colitis. The first option is to wait until patients develop a symptomatic cancer, by which time many cancers will be beyond cure. Secondly, a prophylactic panproctocolectomy can be performed when the risk of cancer first develops. However, the majority of these patients will be young and asymptomatic, and only a minority would ever have progressed to colorectal cancer. Thirdly, surveillance can be performed on patients at increased cancer risk.

Following the advent of colonoscopy in the early 1970s, this has become the preferred surveillance modality in ulcerative colitis. Colonoscopic surveillance relies on the detection of premalignant dysplastic tissue, with colectomy being performed

> **Table 1. Historical St. Mark's ulcerative colitis surveillance programme.**
>
> **Inclusion criteria:**
>
> - Histologically proven ulcerative colitis
> - Macroscopic inflammation extending proximal to the splenic flexure
> - At least 8 years' colitic symptom duration
>
> **Surveillance protocol:**
>
> - Biennial colonoscopic surveillance
> - Any suspicious areas of mucosa are biopsied
> - Segmental non-targeted mucosal biopsies are also taken (approximately 10-12 per examination)
> - Patients undergo clinical assessment in the intervening year, at which time rigid sigmoidoscopy and rectal biopsy is performed
>
> **Dysplasia management:**
>
> - Any biopsy showing dysplasia is independently reported by two experienced pathologists
> - Where either low or high-grade dysplasia is confirmed, the patient is strongly advised to have a colectomy
> - Patients with dysplasia who decline surgery are placed on a more frequent colonoscopic surveillance protocol

once dysplasia occurs (Table 1). It was assumed that such targeted colectomies would reduce morbidity and mortality, both from cancer and from unnecessary surgery. However, no controlled trial was performed to corroborate this supposition.

Where are we now?

Dysplasia

Dysplasia is an unequivocal neoplastic change of the colonic epithelium without invasion into the lamina propria, and is a premalignant state. The data supporting the use of colonic dysplasia as a marker for cancer risk are more compelling than for any other test to date [6].

Despite a standardised classification for dysplasia in ulcerative colitis [7], there remain problems in interpreting dysplasia, especially in the presence of inflammation when it can be difficult to distinguish from reactive epithelial changes. It remains imperative that all diagnoses of dysplasia are reviewed and confirmed by an experienced histopathologist.

High-grade dysplasia

Bernstein's analysis of ten prospective studies of ulcerative colitis surveillance determined that the risk of cancer at immediate colectomy performed for high-grade dysplasia was 42% [8]. In patients not undergoing immediate colectomy, high-grade dysplasia progressed to colorectal cancer in 33%.

Low-grade dysplasia

Several studies have shown that low-grade dysplasia also carries a high risk of rapid progression to (or synchronous) high-grade dysplasia or cancer. Bernstein's analysis showed the risk of cancer at colectomy for low-grade dysplasia was 19%, and that 16-29% of patients with low-grade dysplasia not undergoing surgery progress to advanced neoplasia [8]. Two other studies have demonstrated a 53-54% rate of progression of untreated patients with low-grade dysplasia to advanced neoplasia within 5 years [9, 10]. Conversely, other studies have shown cancer rates following low-grade dysplasia detection as low as 10% after 10 years [11]. It is likely that the variability in reported rates of low-grade dysplasia incidence and progression are due to the difficulty in histological discrimination of dysplasia from regenerative mucosal changes.

Thus, although the correlation between dysplasia and cancer is high, not all patients with dysplasia will develop colorectal cancer [5, 8]. Nevertheless, because we cannot predict which patients with dysplasia will develop cancer, and because the risk is felt by many to be too high and to outweigh the additional unnecessary colectomies incurred, most centres advocate colectomy following the detection of high-grade dysplasia, and many centres now consider low-grade dysplasia an indication for colectomy [8, 9].

Dysplasia-associated lesions/masses and sporadic adenomas

The term DALM (dysplasia-associated lesion or mass) is used to describe areas of raised dysplasia in ulcerative colitis (Figure 1) [12]. Bernstein's review determined that the risk of cancer at immediate colectomy following the discovery of a DALM was 43% [8]. It has become widely accepted that the detection of a DALM is an indication for immediate colectomy.

Sporadic adenomatous polyps can also develop in ulcerative colitis, both proximal to and within an area of inflammation. Unlike DALMs, studies suggest that both sessile and pedunculated adenomas can be removed safely by endoscopic polypectomy, and prolonged follow-up indicates no excess cancer risk [9, 13-18].

However, although the distinction between a DALM and a polyp has been felt to be crucial in light of their markedly different prognoses, there is no clear-cut endoscopic, histological or immunohistochemical distinction. Indeed, the definition of a DALM varies from study to study, providing little help for the clinician. In clinical terms the categorisation of dysplastic lesions into DALMs and adenomatous polyps is probably unimportant. The key factor is probably whether a lesion can safely be removed endoscopically [19]. If endoscopic resection is complete, the prognosis is excellent. If the lesion is not endoscopically resectable, surgery is mandatory, due to the high risk of cancer within that lesion.

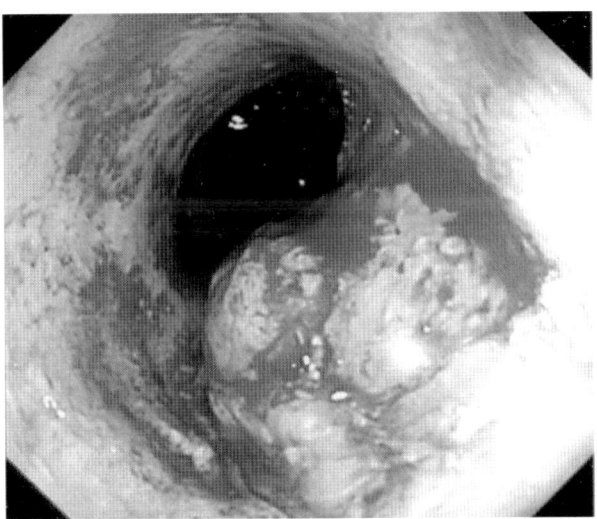

Figure 1. Dysplasia-associated lesion/mass (DALM).

Non-targeted biopsies

Early studies demonstrated that dysplasia usually occurred in flat mucosa and was often widespread [20, 21]. In light of this, most surveillance protocols recommend taking multiple non-targeted colonic biopsies. Rubin et al calculated that 33 biopsies per procedure were required to detect dysplasia with 90% confidence [22]. Because of this, American and UK guidelines recommend taking two to four non-targeted mucosal biopsies at 10cm intervals along the colorectum [23, 24]. In practice this number of specimens is rarely achieved [9, 25].

With modern video-endoscopic equipment and improved detection techniques such as pan-colonic dye spraying, the proportion of dysplastic lesions that are discovered macroscopically is increasing. A recent retrospective series of 14 years of dysplasia detection in ulcerative colitis at St. Mark's Hospital, showed that at least three quarters of surveillance-detected dysplasia came from colonoscopically visible lesions [19]. As macroscopically invisible lesions are in the minority, the value of non-targeted colorectal biopsies may be lower than previously assumed. Indeed, a recent prospective colonoscopic dye spraying study, again from St. Mark's Hospital, reported no episode of dysplasia detected from over 2900 non-targeted biopsies [26].

Surveillance interval

The optimal surveillance interval in ulcerative colitis has yet to be determined. The more frequent the examination, the greater the probability of detecting dysplasia, but the higher the cost, workload, risk of complications and inconvenience to patients. Each successive interval reduction will have a diminishing return in terms of additional dysplasia detection. Therefore, the optimal surveillance interval is a balance of these factors. As these variables will not be the same in all geographical areas, the optimal surveillance interval may alter according to local considerations.

Does surveillance work?

With no randomised controlled trial, it is difficult to know whether surveillance programmes reduce cancer morbidity and mortality. Although many centres have reported a favourable outcome from their surveillance programmes [9, 13-16, 27-37], others express doubts. Lynch et al reported that only one of nine cancers detected during their study period had been detected as a result of the surveillance programme [38]. Disappointingly, many studies have also reported the development of advanced malignancy during surveillance [9, 34-36].

Data from surveillance-detected cancers at St. Mark's Hospital show 5-year survival rates of 90.6% for Dukes' A tumours, 87.8% for Dukes' B, and 28.3% for Dukes' C tumours and 0% for disseminated malignancy [39]. These data support the view that early diagnosis improves survival.

Several studies suggest that patients not undergoing surveillance have a worse outcome [13, 31, 32, 38, 40, 41]. One study calculated the overall 5-year survival rate for those who had cancers diagnosed during surveillance was 87%, compared with 55% for those who did not participate in surveillance (p=0.024) [39]. Other studies report 5-year survival rates of 31-55% following surgery for symptomatic colorectal cancer in ulcerative colitis [39, 42-46]. However, comparison between surveillance and non-surveillance detected cancers are fraught with biases, as the populations are unmatched, and a surveillance diagnosis might simply shift the time of diagnosis forward, rather than shifting the time of death backward (lead-time bias) [47].

Three decision analyses have been published aiming to assess how best to manage colorectal cancer risk in ulcerative colitis. The first suggested colonic surveillance for dysplasia was superior to colectomy [48], the second favoured prophylactic colectomy at 10 years [49], and the most recent could not demonstrate colonoscopic surveillance effectiveness [50]. These studies, with differing conclusions, are limited by their reliance on assumptions of risk for multiple variables – small inaccuracies in any variable can markedly alter the conclusion.

More recently, a nested population-based case control study indicated that ulcerative colitis surveillance may be associated with a decreased risk of dying from colorectal cancer (relative risk 0.29), although this did not reach statistical significance [51].

Workload

Surveillance requires considerable clinical and administrative effort. Connell et al determined that 66 surveillance colonoscopies were required per benefit [9]. Axon's review of 12 studies, using strict criteria by excluding the initial 10-year colonoscopy from the analysis, calculated that 3807 colonoscopies had been performed to detect eight Dukes' A or B cancers, equating to one cancer per 476 examinations [52]. On the basis of these figures, the cost-benefit of ulcerative colitis surveillance has been questioned.

Risk factors for cancer in colitis

Chronic inflammation

It is widely believed that the excess colorectal cancer risk in ulcerative colitis is acquired secondary to chronic inflammation. A hypothesis also exists that there might be a genetic factor influencing both ulcerative colitis and colorectal cancer risk in an individual [53]. Were this true, there should be an increased risk of colorectal cancer in relatives of patients with inflammatory bowel disease, but a recent population-based study concluded that this was not the case [54]. Thus, it is probable that chronic inflammation is indeed the main cause of the increased risk.

Anatomical extent of colonic inflammation

The macroscopic extent of colonic inflammation is a key risk factor for colorectal cancer development. A population-based study from Sweden gives perhaps the best quantification of this risk, demonstrating standardised incidence ratios compared to the general population of 14.8 for extensive colitis (95% CI 11.4-18.9), 2.8 for left-sided colitis (CI 1.6-4.4), and 1.7 for proctitis (95% CI 0.8-3.2; not significant) [4]. Similar ratios were found by two other studies [55, 56]. However, a Danish study found no difference between cancer rates for extensive and left-sided disease, although in this series colectomy rates were much higher for extensive colitis, reaching 31% at 18 years of disease [57]. The relevance of microscopic inflammation proximal to the macroscopic extent of disease involvement remains unclear.

Disease duration

The risk of a patient with ulcerative colitis developing colorectal cancer within 8-10 years of diagnosis is low, after which it increases by approximately 0.5-1% per annum in extensive colitis [49, 58, 59]. The risk in patients with left-sided colitis may also start to increase after 20 years' duration [4, 60]. Reported cancer incidences in extensive colitis range from 5-13.8% at 20 years, 16.5-25% at 30 years, [4, 32, 55, 56, 60, 61] and up to 43% at 35 years [62]. Meta-analysis suggests cumulative incidences of 2% at 10 years, 8% at 20 years and 18% at 30 years [63].

Severity of inflammation

In 1964, Edwards and Truelove reported an increased cancer risk in patients with chronic continuous symptoms, and in those with a severe first attack of colitis [64]. More recently, two modest case control studies have failed to find an association between severity of symptoms and cancer risk [65, 66]. However, it is recognised that clinical disease activity indices correlate only modestly with colonoscopic and histological inflammation [67].

A recent case control study from St. Mark's Hospital based on prospectively collected endoscopic data has demonstrated a clear and significant association between increasing severity of colonic inflammation and an increase in the rate of colorectal neoplasia [68].

Family history of colorectal cancer

In the general population, a family history of colorectal cancer approximately doubles the individual's colorectal cancer risk. A similar increase is also seen in ulcerative colitis patients with a first degree relative with colorectal carcinoma, according to a large population-based cohort study (relative risk 2.5; 95% CI 1.4-4.4) [2]. The risk is further increased if the relative's cancer occurred before the age of 50 (relative risk 9.2; CI 3.7-23) equivalent to an absolute risk of 29% at 54 years of age.

Primary sclerosing cholangitis

Up to 80% of patients with primary sclerosing cholangitis (PSC) have ulcerative colitis, which tends to be both mild and extensive. About 5% of patients with extensive colitis have PSC, and 0.5% of those with distal disease [69]. An increased prevalence of PSC in colitis patients with aneuploidy, dysplasia or colorectal cancer has been noted [70].

Differing study methodologies and confounding factors make analysis of reports on PSC difficult. A well-matched Swedish case control series showed the cumulative incidence of dysplasia or carcinoma in patients with PSC and colitis to be 9%, 31%, and 50% at 10, 20, and 25 years of disease duration, compared with 2%, 5%, and 10% in patients with ulcerative colitis but no PSC (p<0.001) [71]. Three other studies also indicated a three-fold relative risk of cancer or dysplasia in patients with PSC [72-74], but two large studies showed no additional risk [75, 76], and two others were inconclusive [77, 78].

There is now a consensus that the risk of colorectal cancer is higher in patients with PSC. However, the reason for this is unclear. Hypotheses include a shared underlying genetic abnormality, or an alteration in the bile salt pool. It is also possible that the excess risk is related to a longer than appreciated duration of colonic inflammation, as colonic inflammation in PSC is often mild, and may be subclinical for many years. However, as patients with mild colonic inflammation are in fact at lower risk than those with more severe inflammation [68], it is perhaps more likely that PSC is an independent risk factor.

Backwash ileitis

Backwash ileitis is the term used for the finding of mucosal inflammation proximal to the ileocaecal valve in patients with extensive colitis. It is reported to occur in 10-20% of cases, and is probably the result of reflux through disease-related incompetence of the ileocaecal valve (Figure 2), although it is also possibly a primary ileal inflammatory process [59, 79, 80].

A retrospective study of colectomy specimens showed a strong association between backwash ileitis and colorectal carcinoma in extensive colitis [59]. The study has, however, been criticised for methodological biases, and it may be that backwash ileitis simply represents a surrogate marker for active total colitis, rather than being an independent risk factor.

5-aminosalicylic acid drugs

Sulfasalazine competitively inhibits folate absorption, and contributes to the decreased folate levels often seen in patients with ulcerative colitis. Thus, theoretically, sulfasalazine might predispose to colorectal cancer, although this has not been borne out in the literature [81]. Conversely, it is recognised that aspirin and non-steroidal anti-inflammatory drugs reduce the development of sporadic colorectal adenomas and cancer, hence 5-aminosalicylates may potentially protect against colorectal neoplasia. One case control study reported that a minimum of 3 months' amino-salicylate therapy was associated with a relative risk of colorectal cancer of 0.38 (95% CI 0.20-0.69) [66]. Another study found a cumulative cancer risk of 3% in those on long-term sulfasalazine, but 31% in those

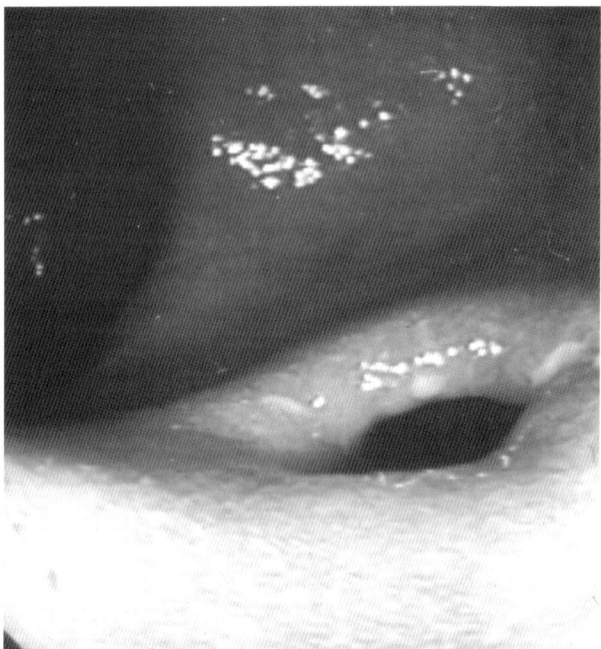

Figure 2. Patulous ileocaecal valve in chronic total ulcerative colitis.

whose treatment had been discontinued or who were non-compliant (p<0.001) [82]. A further case control study reported an adjusted odds ratio of 0.19 (CI 0.06-0.61; p=0.006) for patients taking at least 1.2g of mesalazine a day [65]. This paper and another case control study [68] found no significant effect from sulfasalazine, and the latter report found no effect from mesalazine at any dose. Thus, on balance, it appears that 5-aminosalicylates, but perhaps less so sulfasalazine, are protective against colorectal cancer.

Folate deficiency

Folate deficiency is associated with dysplasia in cancer models, and supplementation may reduce cancer risk. Two case control studies from the same centre showed a possible reduction in colorectal neoplasia in colitis patients receiving folate supplementation [81], and a significant risk reduction of 18% for each 10ng/mL rise in red cell folate level [83]. A recent historical cohort study has also suggested a reduced cancer risk in patients with ulcerative colitis taking folate supplements [84].

Age at onset of ulcerative colitis

Some reports have suggested that patients with an early age of onset of ulcerative colitis have a higher risk of cancer [4, 62, 85, 86]. However other series have not; indeed, some data suggest the opposite may be true [19, 60]. Even if there is an increased risk in this cohort, there is further uncertainty as to whether this is an independent risk factor, perhaps due to a genetic predisposition, or simply a marker of those patients who have the propensity for a longer disease duration, and hence cancer risk [55, 60, 87]. A further confounding factor to account for these discrepancies is the tendency for children to have more extensive colitis.

Smoking

The epidemiological link between ulcerative colitis and non-smoking is well known (relative risks from 0.13-0.7) [88-91]. It is also recognised that smoking promotes colorectal adenoma and cancer development in the non-colitic population.

Two studies have suggested a modest reduction of colorectal neoplasia in patients with ulcerative colitis who smoke cigarettes [66, 68], but neither reached statistical significance. Data from one of the studies were re-analysed to examine patients who had smoked since the onset of their colitis (assessing any possible anti-inflammatory effect of smoking on their colitis); this revealed no obvious trend towards any association between smoking and cancer risk.

Risk factors are summarised in Table 2.

Reducing incidence over time

Current data from St. Mark's Hospital demonstrate that there has been a significant decrease in cancer incidence over time, which appears to be due to a reduction in proximal cancers. Other studies have reported a similar reduction in colorectal cancer over time [92]. This is possibly due to a combination of the effect of the surveillance programme, and a more general reduction in cancer incidence within the colitic population, perhaps brought about by increased use of long-term anti-inflammatory drugs.

Table 2. Risk factors for colorectal cancer in ulcerative colitis.

Known risk factors:

- Anatomical extent of inflammation
- Duration of colitis
- Severity of colonic inflammation
- Family history of colorectal cancer
- Primary sclerosing cholangitis
- 5-aminosalicylic acid therapy (protective)

Possible risk factors:

- Backwash ileitis
- Early age of onset of ulcerative colitis
- Folate deficiency
- Smoking (protective?)

Considered not to be a risk factor:

- Family history of inflammatory bowel disease

Where are we going?

Colonoscopic surveillance probably has a modest protective effect against colorectal cancer. However, in its current form it is undoubtedly imperfect. There are several potential areas for improvement. Firstly, there can be better selection of patients at higher risk of developing colorectal cancer; secondly, there can be an improvement in dysplasia detection, or even the delineation of a more reliable and reproducible premalignant marker; and thirdly, there can be improved therapy for premalignant lesions. There is also potential to reduce the incidence of colorectal cancer in ulcerative colitis *per se*.

Primary prevention

Without prophylactic surgery, there is no absolute means to prevent colitic cancers. However, by minimising colonic inflammation, there should be a reduction of colorectal cancer risk. Thus, an asymptomatic patient who attends for colonoscopic surveillance and is found to have active inflammation should be advised to increase their anti-inflammatory medication, aiming for macroscopic and preferably microscopic disease quiescence.

Patients who are folate deficient should be placed on folate supplements, particularly if they are on maintenance sulfasalazine therapy.

Improved patient selection

Genetic screening

With current advances in genetic screening for cancer susceptibility, it may soon be possible to perform a screen of all patients with ulcerative colitis, to determine those with an underlying genetic predisposition to colorectal cancer development, thus delineating a high risk cohort of patients for whom surveillance can be intensified.

Stool DNA screening

An exciting development in colorectal cancer screening is the use of multiple assay DNA-based stool tests. Cells from adenomas and cancers are constantly shed into the colonic lumen. Neoplasia-specific DNA alterations can be amplified more than a billion-fold by polymerase chain reaction. Assays for a series of different mutations, such as K-ras, APC, p53, Bat26 (a marker of microsatellite instability) and long (non-apoptotic) DNA provide a sensitive and highly specific screening test [93, 94]. Large, multicentre comparative studies of stool-based DNA testing in the general population are in progress.

This form of screening is non-invasive, requires no bowel preparation or dietary restriction and can be performed at home and mailed to the screening centre. Samples can be assayed by automated procedures, making it suitable for large-scale screening. If ongoing studies are favourable, it might be possible to use such a test as a frequent, non-invasive first-line surveillance procedure, with colonoscopic examinations being reserved for those patients who test positive.

Severity of inflammation

Given the data now available, it should be possible to adjust a patient's surveillance frequency according to the severity of active inflammation and to the appearance of chronic colonoscopic features. Thus, if a colonoscopy shows no active inflammation, and no features indicative of previous severe inflammation (such as post-inflammatory polyps and strictures), the cancer risk is no higher than that of the general UK population over a 5-year follow-up period, and in these patients it might be appropriate to reduce the surveillance frequency to every 5 years, or even, in the absence of other risk factors, discontinue surveillance altogether. Conversely, clinicians should consider intensifying surveillance for those with active inflammation.

Better colonoscopic dysplasia detection

Colonoscopic examination technique

With the current generation of video-endoscopes and improved endoscopic techniques, previously undiagnosed dysplastic lesions may now be colonoscopically detectable. Careful mucosal inspection performed by an experienced colonoscopist is imperative for all surveillance procedures, especially in ulcerative colitis where changes can be particularly subtle. Multiple positional shifts of the patient, mucosal washing, suction of fluid pools and intravenous antispasmodic medication should be used. Any suspicious area of mucosa should be biopsied or removed.

Dye spraying

There are now two studies that demonstrate an increased dysplasia yield with dye spraying in ulcerative colitis surveillance (Figure 3) [26, 95]. The technique is simple, safe and cheap. Dye spraying takes about the same amount of time as taking quadrantic biopsies along the length of the colorectum, yet the dysplasia yield is higher. It seems likely that colonoscopic surveillance procedures will in future be performed with the aid of dye spray, or possibly after the ingestion of a dye capsule taken with the bowel preparation. These techniques may remove the need for taking multiple random biopsies.

15 Ulcerative colitis surveillance

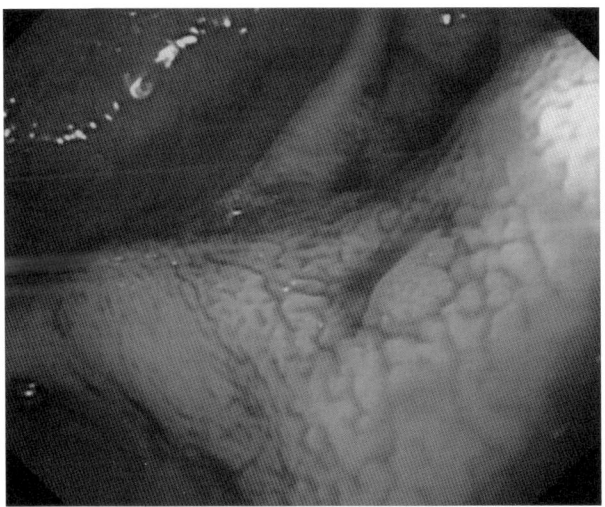

Figure 3. Small dysplastic lesion highlighted by indigo carmine.

Finding a colonoscopic dye spray specific for colonic dysplasia is an exciting prospect. Current dye sprays are relatively non-specific: indigo carmine highlights surface contours only, whereas methylene blue is preferentially absorbed by non-dysplastic and non-inflamed mucosa. Endoscopic fluorescence, by which the colonic mucosa is first photosensitised with an oral dose of 5-aminolevulinic acid, then fluoresced with a blue endoscopic light, is a more specific technique for dysplasia detection. However, this technique is currently limited by false positive fluorescence from endogenous porphyrins in bowel mucosal secretions and inflammation.

Dysplasia *in vivo* diagnosis

Once a mucosal abnormality is detected at colonoscopy, it would be preferable to be able to confirm immediately whether that area is dysplastic. One technique currently under assessment is magnification endoscopy, whereby the endoscopist can examine the mucosa in fine detail, permitting a more accurate characterisation of a lesion. Perhaps even more promising is laser-induced fluorescence (LIF) spectroscopy ("optical biopsying"). This quantitative technique uses a low energy laser to excite endogenous tissue fluorophores [96]. To enhance tumour demarcation, a tumour-seeking exogenous fluorophore can also be used. The resultant fluorescence is detected by a spectrophotometer. This technique can be performed endoscopically. The intensity and pattern of the returned signal defines a characteristic tissue signature. If LIF spectroscopy can differentiate between inflamed mucosa and dysplasia *in vivo*, it could provide an instantaneous assessment of the mucosa, permitting greater sampling of the colorectal mucosa, and allowing the colonoscopist to map out a dysplastic area or confidently remove the lesion endoscopically in its entirety.

Better markers of pre-malignancy

One problem with ulcerative colitis surveillance is the significant histopathologist inter-observer variation in the qualitative reporting of dysplasia. It would be a major advance if a quantitative method could be found to assess pre-malignancy. Potential methods include DNA aneuploidy, and stereological assessment of biopsy specimens.

Endoscopic resection of dysplastic lesions

With improved endoscopic detection and delineation of colorectal dysplasia, and with rapid advances in endoscopic resection techniques, it is now quite realistic to expect that a significant proportion of patients who would previously have undergone a panproctocolectomy will in future be treated by primary endoscopic resection of the lesion, avoiding major surgery and its associated morbidity and mortality. Further endoscopic advances on the horizon may also permit endoscopic full thickness resections of early cancers, with formal surgery being reserved for those with advanced malignancy, or where dysplasia is widespread.

In summary, patients with ulcerative colitis are at increased risk of developing colorectal cancer, although the excess risk is probably reducing. Current colonoscopic surveillance programmes are imperfect, but with improved disease control, patient selection and surveillance techniques, there is potential to reduce both colorectal cancer mortality and incidence, whilst also reducing the need for panproctocolectomy.

References

1. Ekbom A, Helmick CG, Zack M, Holmberg L, Adami HO. Survival and causes of death in patients with inflammatory bowel disease: a population-based study. *Gastroenterology* 1992; 103: 954-60.
2. Askling J, Dickman PW, Karlen P, Brostrom O, Lapidus A, Lofberg R, et al. Family history as a risk factor for colorectal cancer in inflammatory bowel disease. *Gastroenterology* 2001; 120: 1356-62.
3. Langholz E, Munkholm P, Davidsen M, Binder V. Colorectal cancer risk and mortality in patients with ulcerative colitis [see comments]. *Gastroenterology* 1992; 103: 1444-51.
4. Ekbom A, Helmick C, Zack M, Adami HO. Ulcerative colitis and colorectal cancer. A population-based study. *New Engl J Med* 1990; 323: 1228-33.
5. Jonsson B, Ahsgren L, Andersson LO, Stenling R, Rutegard J. Colorectal cancer surveillance in patients with ulcerative colitis. *Br J Surg* 1994; 81: 689-91.
6. Balducci G, Petrocca S, Meli L, Ziparo V. [Colorectal neoplasms in patients with ulcerative rectocolitis. Their surgical treatment and follow-up]. [Italian]. *Chirurgia Italiana* 1999; 51: 271-5.
7. Riddell RH, Goldman H, Ransohoff DF, Appelman HD, Fenoglio CM, Haggitt RC, et al. Dysplasia in inflammatory bowel disease: standardized classification with provisional clinical applications. *Human Pathology* 1983; 14: 931-68.
8. Bernstein CN, Shanahan F, Weinstein WM. Are we telling patients the truth about surveillance colonoscopy in ulcerative colitis? [see comments]. *Lancet* 1994; 343: 71-4.
9. Connell WR, Lennard-Jones JE, Williams CB, Talbot IC, Price AB, Wilkinson KH. Factors affecting the outcome of endoscopic surveillance for cancer in ulcerative colitis [see comments]. *Gastroenterology* 1994; 107: 934-44.
10. Ullman T, Croog V, Harpaz N, Sachar D, Itzkowitz S. Progression of flat low-grade dysplasia to advanced neoplasia in patients with ulcerative colitis. *Gastroenterology* 2003; 125: 1311-9.
11. Lim CH, Dixon MF, Vail A, Forman D, Lynch DA, Axon AT. Ten-year follow-up of ulcerative colitis patients with and without low grade dysplasia. *Gut* 2003; 52: 1127-32.
12. Blackstone MO, Riddell RH, Rogers BH, Levin B. Dysplasia-associated lesion or mass (DALM) detected by colonoscopy in long-standing ulcerative colitis: an indication for colectomy. *Gastroenterology* 1981; 80: 366-74.
13. Biasco G, Brandi G, Paganelli GM, Rossini FP, Santucci R, Di F, et al. Colorectal cancer in patients with ulcerative colitis. A prospective cohort study in Italy. *Cancer* 1995; 75: 2045-50.
14. Lofberg R, Brostrom O, Karlen P, Tribukait B, Ost A. Colonoscopic surveillance in longstanding total ulcerative colitis - a 15-year follow-up study. *Gastroenterology* 1990; 99: 1021-31.
15. Rozen P, Baratz M, Fefer F, Gilat T. Low incidence of significant dysplasia in a successful endoscopic surveillance program of patients with ulcerative colitis [see comments]. *Gastroenterology* 1995; 108: 1361-70.
16. Woolrich AJ, DaSilva MD, Korelitz BI. Surveillance in the routine management of ulcerative colitis: the predictive value of low-grade dysplasia [see comments]. *Gastroenterology* 1992; 103: 431-8.
17. Rubin PH, Friedman S, Harpaz N, Goldstein E, Weiser J, Schiller J, et al. Colonoscopic polypectomy in chronic colitis: conservative management after endoscopic resection of dysplastic polyps. *Gastroenterology* 1999; 117: 1295-300.
18. Engelsgjerd M, Farraye FA, Odze RD. Polypectomy may be adequate treatment for adenoma-like dysplastic lesions in chronic ulcerative colitis [see comments]. *Gastroenterology* 1999; 117: 1288-94 discussion.
19. Rutter MD, Saunders BP, Wilkinson KH, et al. Most dysplasia in ulcerative colitis is visible at colonoscopy. *Gastrointest Endosc* 2004; 60: 334-9.
20. Morson BC, Pang LS. Rectal biopsy as an aid to cancer control in ulcerative colitis. *Gut* 1967; 8: 423-34.
21. Hulten L, Kewenter J, Ahren C. Precancer and carcinoma in chronic ulcerative colitis. A histopathological and clinical investigation. *Scand J Gastroenterology* 1972; 7: 663-9.
22. Rubin CE, Haggitt RC, Burmer GC, Brentnall TA, Stevens AC, Levine DS, et al. DNA aneuploidy in colonic biopsies predicts future development of dysplasia in ulcerative colitis. *Gastroenterology* 1992; 103: 1611-20.
23. Eaden JA, Mayberry JF. Guidelines for screening and surveillance of asymptomatic colorectal cancer in patients with inflammatory bowel disease. *Gut* 2002; 51 Suppl 5: V10-V12.
24. The role of colonoscopy in the management of patients with inflammatory bowel disease. American Society for Gastrointestinal Endoscopy. *Gastrointest Endosc* 1998; 48: 689-90.
25. Eaden JA, Ward BA, Mayberry JF. How gastroenterologists screen for colonic cancer in ulcerative colitis: an analysis of performance [see comments]. *Gastrointest Endosc* 2000; 51: 123-8.
26. Rutter MD, Saunders BP, Schofield G, Forbes A, Price AB, Talbot IC. Pancolonic indigo carmine dye spraying for the detection of dysplasia in ulcerative colitis. *Gut* 2004; 53: 256-60.
27. Brostrom O, Lofberg R, Ost A, Reichard H. Cancer surveillance of patients with longstanding ulcerative colitis: a clinical, endoscopical, and histological study. *Gut* 1986; 27: 1408-13.
28. Lennard-Jones JE, Morson BC, Ritchie JK, Williams CB. Cancer surveillance in ulcerative colitis. Experience over 15 years. *Lancet* 1983; 2: 149-52.
29. Fuson JA, Farmer RG, Hawk A, Sullivan BH. Endoscopic surveillance for cancer in chronic ulcerative colitis. *Am J Gastroenterol* 1980; 73: 120-6.
30. Leidenius M, Kellokumpu I, Husa A, Riihela M, Sipponen P. Dysplasia and carcinoma in longstanding ulcerative colitis: an endoscopic and histological surveillance programme. *Gut* 1991; 32: 1521-5.
31. Lindberg B, Persson B, Veress B, Ingelman-Sundberg H, Granqvist S. Twenty years' colonoscopic surveillance of patients with ulcerative colitis. Detection of dysplastic and malignant transformation. *Scand J Gastroenterology* 1996; 31: 1195-204.

32. Lennard-Jones JE, Melville DM, Morson BC, Ritchie JK, Williams CB. Precancer and cancer in extensive ulcerative colitis: findings among 401 patients over 22 years. *Gut* 1990; 31: 800-6.
33. Nugent FW, Haggitt RC. Long-term follow-up, including cancer surveillance, for patients with ulcerative colitis. *Clinics in Gastroenterology* 1980; 9: 459-68.
34. Lashner BA, Kane SV, Hanauer SB. Colon cancer surveillance in chronic ulcerative colitis: historical cohort study. *Am J Gastroenterol* 1990; 85: 1083-7.
35. Nugent FW, Haggitt RC, Gilpin PA. Cancer surveillance in ulcerative colitis [see comments]. *Gastroenterology* 1991; 100: 1241-8.
36. Rosenstock E, Farmer RG, Petras R, Sivak MVJ, Rankin GB, Sullivan BH. Surveillance for colonic carcinoma in ulcerative colitis. *Gastroenterology* 1985; 89: 1342-6.
37. Rutegard J, Ahsgren L, Stenling R, Janunger KG. Ulcerative colitis. Cancer surveillance in an unselected population. *Scand J Gastroenterology* 1988; 23: 139-45.
38. Lynch DA, Lobo AJ, Sobala GM, Dixon MF, Axon AT. Failure of colonoscopic surveillance in ulcerative colitis [see comments]. *Gut* 1993; 34: 1075-80.
39. Connell WR, Talbot IC, Harpaz N, Britto N, Wilkinson KH, Kamm MA, et al. Clinicopathological characteristics of colorectal carcinoma complicating ulcerative colitis. *Gut* 1994; 35: 1419-23.
40. Jones HW, Grogono J, Hoare AM. Surveillance in ulcerative colitis: burdens and benefit. *Gut* 1988; 29: 325-31.
41. Choi PM, Nugent FW, Schoetz DJJ, Silverman ML, Haggitt RC. Colonoscopic surveillance reduces mortality from colorectal cancer in ulcerative colitis [see comments]. *Gastroenterology* 1993; 105: 418-24.
42. Gyde SN, Prior P, Thompson H, Waterhouse JA, Allan RN. Survival of patients with colorectal cancer complicating ulcerative colitis. *Gut* 1984; 25: 228-31.
43. Hughes RG, Hall TJ, Block GE, Levin B, Moossa AR. The prognosis of carcinoma of the colon and rectum complicating ulcerative colitis. *Surgery, Gynecology & Obstetrics* 1978; 146: 46-8.
44. Lavery IC, Chiulli RA, Jagelman DG, Fazio VW, Weakley FL. Survival with carcinoma arising in mucosal ulcerative colitis. *Ann Surg* 1982; 195: 508-12.
45. Ohman U. Colorectal carcinoma in patients with ulcerative colitis. *Am J Surg* 1982; 144: 344-9.
46. van Heerden JA, Beart RW, Jr. Carcinoma of the colon and rectum complicating chronic ulcerative colitis. *Dis Colon Rectum* 1980; 23: 155-9.
47. Lennard-Jones JE. Cancer risk in ulcerative colitis: surveillance or surgery. *Br J Surg* 1985; 72 Suppl: S84-S86.
48. Gage TP. Managing the cancer risk in chronic ulcerative colitis. A decision-analytic approach. *J Clin Gastroenterology* 1986; 8: 50-7.
49. Provenzale D, Kowdley KV, Arora S, Wong JB. Prophylactic colectomy or surveillance for chronic ulcerative colitis? A decision analysis [see comments]. *Gastroenterology* 1995; 109: 1188-96.
50. Delco F, Sonnenberg A. A decision analysis of surveillance for colorectal cancer in ulcerative colitis. *Gut* 2000; 46: 500-6.
51. Karlen P, Kornfeld D, Brostrom O, Lofberg R, Persson PG, Ekbom A. Is colonoscopic surveillance reducing colorectal cancer mortality in ulcerative colitis? A population-based case control study [see comments]. *Gut* 1998; 42: 711-4.
52. Axon AT. Cancer surveillance in ulcerative colitis - a time for reappraisal [see comments]. *Gut* 1994; 35: 587-9.
53. Rhodes JM. Unifying hypothesis for inflammatory bowel disease and associated colon cancer: sticking the pieces together with sugar. *Lancet* 1996; 347: 40-4.
54. Askling J, Dickman PW, Karlen P, Brostrom O, Lapidus A, Lofberg R, et al. Colorectal cancer rates among first-degree relatives of patients with inflammatory bowel disease: a population-based cohort study. *Lancet* 2001; 357: 262-6.
55. Gyde SN, Prior P, Allan RN, Stevens A, Jewell DP, Truelove SC, et al. Colorectal cancer in ulcerative colitis: a cohort study of primary referrals from three centres. *Gut* 1988; 29: 206-17.
56. Mir-Madjlessi SH, Farmer RG, Easley KA, Beck GJ. Colorectal and extracolonic malignancy in ulcerative colitis. *Cancer* 1986; 58: 1569-74.
57. Hendriksen C, Kreiner S, Binder V. Long-term prognosis in ulcerative colitis - based on results from a regional patient group from the county of Copenhagen. *Gut* 1985; 26: 158-63.
58. Ransohoff DF. Colon cancer in ulcerative colitis. *Gastroenterology* 1988; 94: 1089-91.
59. Heuschen UA, Hinz U, Allemeyer EH, Stern J, Lucas M, Autschbach F, et al. Backwash ileitis is strongly associated with colorectal carcinoma in ulcerative colitis. *Gastroenterology* 2001; 120: 841-7.
60. Gilat T, Fireman Z, Grossman A, Hacohen D, Kadish U, Ron E, et al. Colorectal cancer in patients with ulcerative colitis. A population study in central Israel. *Gastroenterology* 1988; 94: 870-7.
61. Gillen CD, Walmsley RS, Prior P, Andrews HA, Allan RN. Ulcerative colitis and Crohn's disease: a comparison of the colorectal cancer risk in extensive colitis [see comments]. *Gut* 1994; 35: 1590-2.
62. Devroede GJ, Taylor WF, Sauer WG, Jackman RJ, Stickler GB. Cancer risk and life expectancy of children with ulcerative colitis. *New Engl J Med* 1971; 285: 17-21.
63. Eaden J, Abrams K, McKay H, Denley H, Mayberry J. Inter-observer variation between general and specialist gastrointestinal pathologists when grading dysplasia in ulcerative colitis. *J Pathol* 2001; 194: 152-7.
64. Edwards FC, Truelove SC. The course and prognosis of ulcerative colitis. Part IV: carcinoma of the colon. *Gut* 1964; 5: 15-22.
65. Eaden J, Abrams K, Ekbom A, Jackson E, Mayberry J. Colorectal cancer prevention in ulcerative colitis: a case-control study. *Alimentary Pharmacology & Therapeutics* 2000; 14: 145-53.
66. Pinczowski D, Ekbom A, Baron J, Yuen J, Adami HO. Risk factors for colorectal cancer in patients with ulcerative colitis: a case-control study. *Gastroenterology* 1994; 107: 117-20.
67. Gomes P, du BC, Smith CL, Holdstock G. Relationship between disease activity indices and colonoscopic findings in

patients with colonic inflammatory bowel disease. *Gut* 1986; 27: 92-5.
68. Rutter M, Saunders B, Wilkinson K, Rumbles S, Schofield G, Kamm M, et al. Severity of inflammation is a risk factor for colorectal neoplasia in ulcerative colitis. *Gastroenterology* 2004; 126: 451-9.
69. Olsson R, Danielsson A, Jarnerot G, Lindstrom E, Loof L, Rolny P, et al. Prevalence of primary sclerosing cholangitis in patients with ulcerative colitis. *Gastroenterology* 1991; 100: 1319-23.
70. Broome U, Lindberg G, Lofberg R. Primary sclerosing cholangitis in ulcerative colitis - a risk factor for the development of dysplasia and DNA aneuploidy? [see comments]. *Gastroenterology* 1992; 102: 1877-80.
71. Broome U, Lofberg R, Veress B, Eriksson LS. Primary sclerosing cholangitis and ulcerative colitis: evidence for increased neoplastic potential [see comments]. *Hepatology* 1995; 22: 1404-8.
72. Brentnall TA, Haggitt RC, Rabinovitch PS, Kimmey MB, Bronner MP, Levine DS, et al. Risk and natural history of colonic neoplasia in patients with primary sclerosing cholangitis and ulcerative colitis [see comments]. *Gastroenterology* 1996; 110: 331-8.
73. Shetty K, Rybicki L, Brzezinski A, Carey WD, Lashner BA. The risk for cancer or dysplasia in ulcerative colitis patients with primary sclerosing cholangitis. *Am J Gastroenterol* 1999; 94: 1643-9.
74. Leidenius MH, Farkkila MA, Karkkainen P, Taskinen EI, Kellokumpu IH, Hockerstedt KA. Colorectal dysplasia and carcinoma in patients with ulcerative colitis and primary sclerosing cholangitis. *Scand J Gastroenterology* 1997; 32: 706-11.
75. Loftus EVJ, Sandborn WJ, Tremaine WJ, Mahoney DW, Zinsmeister AR, Offord KP, et al. Risk of colorectal neoplasia in patients with primary sclerosing cholangitis [see comments]. *Gastroenterology* 1996; 110: 432-40.
76. Nuako KW, Ahlquist DA, Sandborn WJ, Mahoney DW, Siems DM, Zinsmeister AR. Primary sclerosing cholangitis and colorectal carcinoma in patients with chronic ulcerative colitis: a case-control study. *Cancer* 1998; 82: 822-6.
77. Gurbuz AK, Giardiello FM, Bayless TM. Colorectal neoplasia in patients with ulcerative colitis and primary sclerosing cholangitis. *Dis Colon Rectum* 1995; 38: 37-41.
78. Choi PM, Nugent FW, Rossi RL. Relationship between colorectal neoplasia and primary sclerosing cholangitis in ulcerative colitis [letter; comment]. *Gastroenterology* 1992; 103: 1707-9.
79. Gustavsson S, Weiland LH, Kelly KA. Relationship of backwash ileitis to ileal pouchitis after ileal pouch-anal anastomosis. *Dis Colon Rectum* 1987; 30: 25-8.
80. Schmidt CM, Lazenby AJ, Hendrickson RJ, Sitzmann JV. Preoperative terminal ileal and colonic resection histopathology predicts risk of pouchitis in patients after ileoanal pull-through procedure. *Ann Surg* 1998; 227: 654-62 discussion.
81. Lashner BA, Heidenreich PA, Su GL, Kane SV, Hanauer SB. Effect of folate supplementation on the incidence of dysplasia and cancer in chronic ulcerative colitis. A case-control study [see comments]. *Gastroenterology* 1989; 97: 255-9.

82. Moody GA, Jayanthi V, Probert CS, Mac K, Mayberry JF. Long-term therapy with sulphasalazine protects against colorectal cancer in ulcerative colitis: a retrospective study of colorectal cancer risk and compliance with treatment in Leicestershire. *Eur J Gastroenterol Hepatol* 1996; 8: 1179-83.
83. Lashner BA. Red blood cell folate is associated with the development of dysplasia and cancer in ulcerative colitis. *J Cancer Res Clin Oncol* 1993; 119: 549-54.
84. Lashner BA, Provencher KS, Seidner DL, Knesebeck A, Brzezinski A. The effect of folic acid supplementation on the risk for cancer or dysplasia in ulcerative colitis. *Gastroenterology* 1997; 112: 29-32.
85. Sugita A, Sachar DB, Bodian C, Ribeiro MB, Aufses AHJ, Greenstein AJ. Colorectal cancer in ulcerative colitis. Influence of anatomical extent and age at onset on colitis-cancer interval. *Gut* 1991; 32: 167-9.
86. Karlen P, Lofberg R, Brostrom O, Leijonmarck CE, Hellers G, Persson PG. Increased risk of cancer in ulcerative colitis: a population-based cohort study. *Am J Gastroenterol* 1999; 94: 1047-52.
87. Greenstein AJ, Sachar DB, Smith H, Pucillo A, Papatestas AE, Kreel I, et al. Cancer in universal and left-sided ulcerative colitis: factors determining risk. *Gastroenterology* 1979; 77: 290-4.
88. Silverstein MD, Lashner BA, Hanauer SB. Cigarette smoking and ulcerative colitis: a case-control study. *Mayo Clin Proc* 1994; 69: 425-9.
89. Lindberg E, Tysk C, Andersson K, Jarnerot G. Smoking and inflammatory bowel disease. A case control study. *Gut* 1988; 29: 352-7.
90. Tobin MV, Logan RF, Langman MJ, McConnell RB, Gilmore IT. Cigarette smoking and inflammatory bowel disease. *Gastroenterology* 1987; 93: 316-21.
91. Samuelsson SM, Ekbom A, Zack M, Helmick CG, Adami HO. Risk factors for extensive ulcerative colitis and ulcerative proctitis: a population-based case-control study. *Gut* 1991; 32: 1526-30.
92. Rubio CA, Befrits R, Ljung T, Jaramillo E, Slezak P. Colorectal carcinoma in ulcerative colitis is decreasing in Scandinavian countries. *Anticancer Res* 2001; 21: 2921-4.
93. Ahlquist DA, Skoletsky JE, Boynton KA, Harrington JJ, Mahoney DW, Pierceall WE, et al. Colorectal cancer screening by detection of altered human DNA in stool: feasibility of a multitarget assay panel. *Gastroenterology* 2000; 119: 1219-27.
94. Traverso G, Shuber A, Olsson L, Levin B, Johnson C, Hamilton SR, et al. Detection of proximal colorectal cancers through analysis of faecal DNA. *Lancet* 2002; 359: 403-4.
95. Kiesslich R, Fritsch J, Holtmann M, Koehler HH, Stolte M, Kanzler S, et al. Methylene blue-aided chromoendoscopy for the detection of intraepithelial neoplasia and colon cancer in ulcerative colitis. *Gastroenterology* 2003; 124: 880-8.
96. Eker C, Montan S, Jaramillo E, Koizumi K, Rubio C, Andersson-Engels S, et al. Clinical spectral characterisation of colonic mucosal lesions using autofluorescence and delta aminolevulinic acid sensitisation. *Gut* 1999; 44: 511-8.

Chapter 16

Laparoscopy at the frontier of colorectal surgery

Timothy A Rockall MD FRCS, Consultant Surgeon
Minimal Access Therapy Training Unit, Royal Surrey County Hospital, Guildford, Surrey, UK

What is the problem?

Laparoscopic colonic and rectal resection has been described for well over a decade with the first laparoscopic assisted segmental colectomies reported in the early 1990s [1,2]. In the UK, the practice is still not widespread with probably less than 1% of all colorectal resections undertaken using laparoscopic techniques. This is a figure in stark contrast to the rapid uptake of laparoscopy for cholecystectomy, first described in 1987 and which is now a day-case procedure in many institutions. Planned cholecystectomy by any other method is now a rare event in any country where the resources and technology are readily available. The discrepancy in the rapidity of uptake of laparoscopic surgery for biliary and colorectal disease is a little surprising as the benefits are potentially even greater to patients avoiding a laparotomy for colorectal resection than to those avoiding an open cholecystectomy. The midline laparotomy represents a significant trauma of access to the patient, which when avoided can lead to a profound impact on early recovery and the avoidance of many of the wound and mobility-related complications.

Why then has laparoscopic colorectal surgery not been widely taken up by the surgical community? There are many reasons but I believe that predominantly it is the fact that laparoscopic colorectal surgery can be technically challenging and many colorectal surgeons do not have a background of training with simpler laparoscopic procedures, most of which are not within the colorectal domain (e.g cholecystectomy, hernia repair, fundoplication etc.). Some of the technical challenges have been considerably eased over the last decade by the advent of new technologies, including ultrasonic dissection devices, new diathermy technology and hand ports.

Importantly, there has also been the debate surrounding the safety of the procedure in malignant disease, in particular port site metastases. This issue has now been broadly resolved with the publication of outcomes from a number of randomised controlled trials. The incidence of wound and port site metastasis in the recently reported Clinical Outcomes of Surgical Therapy trial (COST) [3] was about 1% in both laparoscopic and open arms of the trial. The majority of open colorectal resections in the UK are undertaken for malignancy and in the presence of guidance from the National Institute for Clinical Excellence (NICE) opposing laparoscopic resection for malignancy outside the context of a controlled trial, many surgeons have not been stimulated to develop this technique. This argument obviously does not hold for laparoscopic operations for benign disease, but unfortunately much of the benign disease is actually even more technically challenging than laparoscopic colon cancer surgery.

All described open transabdominal operations on the colon and rectum can and have been performed laparoscopically. There are, of course, limitations, which may be attributable to the disease process, patient factors or the surgeon's skill. Most of the contra-indications are however relative. Adhesions and obesity may make the surgery more challenging; inflammatory masses and fistulation may be impossible to dissect laparoscopically with safety, but this is by no means always the case. When a large laparotomy needs to be made for the purposes of specimen extraction (i.e. in the case of a large inflammatory mass), there seems little benefit in starting the operation laparoscopically. A few patients tolerate a prolonged pneumoperitoneum poorly and this needs to be taken into account when planning surgery.

Issues facing laparoscopic colorectal surgery for inflammatory bowel disease are essentially three-fold:

1. What evidence is there that the patients benefit in the short and long term?
2. How to train surgeons to perform this potentially complex surgery safely and efficiently?
3. What is the cost implication of utilising new technology?

Benefits

Surgical procedures commonly performed in the management of both Crohn's disease and ulcerative colitis are achievable using minimally invasive techniques, including segmental and total colectomy, proctectomy and ileo-anal pouch formation. They may be totally laparoscopic or to a variable extent laparoscopic assisted or may rely on the introduction of a single hand through a hand access system to assist dissection [4]. Other than in circumstances where the specimen is removed through the perineum (e.g. a proctectomy) a small incision is made in the abdominal wall in order to extract the specimen and this may also be used to enable an extra-corporeal anastomosis. Usually this is only 4-5cm in length and appropriately placed to minimise postoperative pain and avoid muscle-cutting incisions.

There is little doubt that patients undergoing laparoscopic colorectal surgery have less post-operative pain, consume less opiate analgesia, mobilise earlier, benefit from earlier return of bowel function and are fit for hospital discharge earlier. Additionally, there is increasing evidence of a lower risk of wound complication, such as infection and incisional hernia and operative blood loss [5-8]. Earlier mobilisation may reduce the risk of deep vein thrombosis and chest infection. FEV1 and other measures of respiratory function are less affected and return to normal faster in patients operated on laparoscopically [9].

All of these are only short-term benefits but they are nonetheless important. They are important to the patient and also to society in terms of reducing the socio-economic impact and potentially the cost to the healthcare system. Many studies have demonstrated very significant reductions in direct hospital costs in laparoscopically operated patients following colonic resection [7, 10, 11]. Others have revealed higher direct hospital costs but similar costs to society in the short to medium term.

Patients may do better following laparoscopic surgery for a number of reasons. The reduction in trauma, pain, disability and earlier return of gut function and mobility are all obvious candidates. It may also be true that there is significant bias in the studies, as none of the surgical trials are blinded and there is likely to be an underlying assumption that the laparoscopic patients will recover more rapidly and so are treated accordingly. It is interesting that most of the large multicentre trials of colonic resection for both malignant and benign disease have not shown the dramatic reduction in hospital stay that other case series have led us to expect. There is accumulating scientific evidence however, that there is a diminution of surgical stress response and a reduced impact on patient immunity following the laparoscopic approach, which could be responsible for some of the benefits that are seen. The evidence is mixed, with some studies showing no changes in measures of immune response (T cells, B cells, CD4:CD8 ratio, Natural Killer Cells, IgG, IgM, IgA, IL6 HLADR expression) [12, 13], whilst others reveal significant effects on cell mediated immunity with less reduction in delayed type hypersensitivity in the laparoscopic group compared to open [14]. IL6, IL10 CRP and Granulocyte elastase have been measured significantly lower in the laparoscopic group in some studies leading the authors to conclude that this was a measure of the reduction in surgical stress [15]. There are also some data which suggest that these very mechanisms may be responsible for improved outcomes in terms of survival and cancer recurrence in colon cancer [16]. Overall, it seems likely that laparoscopic surgery results in a reduced inflammatory response (measured by IL6 and CRP), a reduced immunomodulatory response, improved pulmonary function and reduced hypoxaemia. There are a lack of data on how this impacts on postoperative septic complications, but this may be a mechanism by which infectious complications are reduced in laparoscopic surgery [17].

Training

Training in laparoscopic colorectal surgery is not formalised within the speciality in the UK. Surgeons wishing to undertake laparoscopic colonic resection in the UK have been for the most part self-taught on a background of laparoscopic skills attained within other sub-specialities of general surgery. Courses are available in Europe which allow tuition and practice on models and live animals. Courses with live surgery are also available in the UK. However, there has so far been little emphasis on one-to-one tuition in live cases and many surgeons remain essentially self-taught. Studies looking at the learning curve in laparoscopic surgery suggest that at least 30 cases may be required in the training surgeon [18] and as many as 70 to 80 cases in the self-educated are required before a surgeon reaches a steady state [19]. Additionally, and not surprisingly, there is evidence of lower intra-operative and postoperative complications in the high volume compared to the low volume surgeon [20]. Currently, the availability to learn laparoscopic colorectal surgery in the UK is very limited. Fellowships are available in the UK and abroad but are very limited in number at the present time.

Cost

There are several aspects to cost and cost-benefit analysis. There is no doubt that new technology is generally more expensive, at least in the short term. Initial investment in hardware, maintenance costs, disposable equipment, increased operating times and surgical training all add to the overall cost of introducing the technology. As well as the standard laparoscopic equipment, other new technologies such as ultrasonic dissectors (Ultracision™, Harmonic scalpel™) and advanced diathermy technology (Ligasure™) have become very important, and some would say indispensible, tools in laparoscopic colorectal surgery and all require significant investment in generators and disposable parts. Some studies show that there is an increased direct cost to the healthcare system for the surgical procedure when compared to open surgery. This is however, very variable depending on the use of new technologies and disposable items in both techniques. The costs of laparoscopic surgery can be dramatically affected by the judicious use of disposables and equally the cost of open surgery can rise dramatically for similar reasons.

However, laparoscopic surgery is associated with a number of cost savings. Reduced hospital stay is the most obvious, but equally, reduced utilisation of HDU and ITU facilities, reduced transfusion requirements, reduced wound and respiratory complications and reduced analgesia requirements all reduce direct hospital costs. In the longer term it may be that a reduction in re-operation for adhesion-related complications, such as small bowel obstruction, incisional hernia and chronic pain, will also reduce the overall cost to the healthcare system. The individual benefits of earlier return to normal function and work have an economic impact which is hard to measure. In Crohn's disease specifically, several studies from the USA reveal a significant economic advantage for laparoscopic ileocaecal resection with direct costs reduced by as much as 40-50% [7, 10, 11, 21].

In malignant disease, economic analysis of patients randomised in the COLOR trial reveals no difference in total cost to society at 12 weeks post-operation, but a higher cost to the healthcare system for the laparoscopic approach with a difference of mean cost of 2244 Euros [22].

Where are we now?

Only a small proportion of all colorectal resections in the UK are undertaken laparoscopically and because of issues of definition it is likely that a proportion of the laparoscopically assisted procedures will differ very little from a laparotomy in terms of the size of the ultimate incision. In any event very few surgeons in the UK undertake laparoscopic resection routinely or at all. Europe and America are undoubtedly ahead of the UK but even there the proportion of cases undertaken laparoscopically is low. We are at a stage however, that it is quite clear that the majority of resectional procedures undertaken for inflammatory bowel disease are safely amenable to the laparoscopic approach. In Crohn's disease, ileocaecal resection, small bowel resection, strictureplasty, colectomy and proctectomy are all potentially suitable operations. Large series of ileocaecal resections have been published revealing similar operating times and reduced hospital stay and access-related complications. A variety of approaches are described with either intra- or extracorporeal anastomosis. There is probably no benefit in performing the anastomosis intracorporeally unless the incision that is made for specimen retrieval is significantly smaller than that which would be necessary for the extracorporeal anastomosis. For most thin Crohn's patients this is not the case.

Crohn's disease

For many authors and investigators, the laparoscopic approach to ileocaecal resection is the preferred approach. For uncomplicated disease it is relatively simple with a very low conversion rate. Randomised controlled trials of laparoscopic versus open ileocolic resection for refractory Crohn's disease revealed a reduction in median incision length, reduced blood loss, improved FEV1, earlier return of bowel function, earlier discharge and fewer complications [23]. Long-term follow-up in another study has revealed lower 5-year small bowel obstruction rates despite a similar anastomotic recurrence rate [24]. Operating on patients with recurrent and complicated disease is also very feasible but undoubtedly requires more laparoscopic skill and experience. Patients with enteric fistulae can be challenging and inevitably have a higher conversion rate but this has been reported as low as 4.1%, despite the fact that 40% had prior surgery and 30% multiple fistulae [25]. Other authors also report good results [26, 27]. Hasegawa [28] reported a series of recurrent disease with longer operating times but similar postoperative complication rates and hospital stay.

Predicting conversion is possible in as much as the bulk of conversions occur in patients with recurrent disease and abdominal masses [29]. As in all laparoscopic surgery, obesity and adhesions make surgery more difficult.

Children also benefit from the laparoscopic approach with reductions in hospital stay, narcotic use and ileus following ileocolic resection [30-32].

Colectomy and pouch surgery

One-stage ileo-anal pouch reconstruction has been described laparoscopically [33]. It appears feasible, safe and effective with equal results to the open operation. In a case-matched study [34] on patients undergoing pouch surgery for UC and FAP, the operating time was increased significantly and the patients had similar complication rates, but bowel function returned earlier and there was a reduction in hospital stay, most marked in the diverted patients. In patients undergoing total colectomy, the same advantage of reduced hospital stay was accompanied by a reduction in postoperative complications and a significant reduction in wound complications and respiratory complications to zero. Long-term complications of impotence, incisional hernia and ileostomy problems were reduced from 60% to 20% in the laparoscopic group. In the same study however, patients undergoing proctocolectomy derived no specific benefit.

Where are we going?

There is little doubt that a laparoscopic approach to colorectal disease is now firmly established and surgeons are able to undertake this type of surgery for the whole range of colonic and rectal procedures and for both benign and malignant disease with a low case exclusion rate and a low conversion rate. As experience, techniques and technology advance it is likely that these will reduce even further. Technology continues to advance and this will result in more complex procedures becoming easier to achieve using minimally invasive techniques and will allow a greater uptake of minimally invasive techniques amongst the surgical community. New technologies currently in use are likely to reduce in cost. Expensive new technologies, such as robotics, are being evaluated but are as yet unproven and their contribution to surgery uncertain. Robotic technologies have been utilised in laparoscopic colorectal procedures and the operations are undoubtedly feasible [35-37]. The advantages of increased laparoscopic dexterity and improved three-dimensional vision have yet to be shown to translate into improvements in outcome for patients.

The oncological argument against laparoscopic surgery for malignant disease is now much diminished with the publication of data from a variety of large randomised studies. The arguments against its deployment for benign disease are even more difficult to uphold with increasing evidence of advantages in recovery times and reduced complication rates. In experienced hands the operations are not significantly longer and although they may be initially more expensive this is likely to be more than made up for by the reduction in hospital stay, reduced utilisation of high dependency units and reduced risk of requiring district nurse care after discharge. The true advantage in hospital stay is yet to be exactly established and has to be compared with open surgery in an equal accelerated recovery protocol [17]. However, there is little doubt amongst the converted that the advantage will be significant. It seems inconceivable that patients could be discharged as little as 36 hours after their anaesthetic following an open anterior resection, but this can be achieved with the laparoscopic approach. There are many reasons why large multicentre trials have so far not demonstrated this advantage and it is important to look at individual case series to see what can be achieved.

Accelerated recovery programmes combined with the laparoscopic approach are likely to be the way forward in patient care. The relative importance of the anaesthetic regimen, analgesia, postoperative mobilisation and enteral nutrition are yet to be fully established. Laparoscopic surgery has the potential for allowing opiate-free surgery which may have a very significant impact on restoration of bowel function, which is often the factor delaying discharge.

The biggest hurdle to the uptake of laparoscopic surgery is the lack of trained colorectal surgeons undertaking the procedures. Like several other specialties, such as urology, pure coloproctology has not incorporated laparoscopy in many of its procedures or its training. It suffers from the fact that none of the colorectal procedures that can be performed laparoscopically can be considered basic training procedures. Laparoscopic colonic resection has therefore been mostly taken up by surgeons with training and a practice that includes laparoscopic cholecystectomy, hernia repair and fundoplication. The move from open surgery to laparoscopic resection is therefore often difficult. It is important however, that the problems seen with the increase in bile duct injury following the introduction of laparoscopic cholecystectomy are not repeated with colorectal resection. To this end the development of training programmes, fellowship training and preceptorship are of paramount importance. Guidelines for training are being developed with proposals for the number of cases to be seen, assist with and perform under supervision before independent practice in an effort to reduce the complications and problems that are seen on the learning curve. It will not be long however before the body of colorectal surgeons practising laparoscopic resection increases with an associated beneficial impact on trainees in surgery. For many colorectal diseases, benign and malignant, I would propose that laparoscopic resection is now the method of choice.

References

1. Fowler DL, White SA. Laparoscopy-assisted sigmoid resection. *Surg Laparosc Endosc* 1991; 1(3): 183-8.
2. Jacobs M, Verdeja JC, Goldstein HS. Minimally invasive colon resection (laparoscopic colectomy). *Surg Laparosc Endosc* 1991; 1(3): 144-50.
3. A comparison of laparoscopically assisted and open colectomy for colon cancer. *N Engl J Med* 2004; 350(20): 2050-9.
4. Litwin DE, Darzi A, Jakimowicz J, Kelly JJ, Arvidsson D, Hansen P, *et al*. Hand-assisted laparoscopic surgery (HALS) with the HandPort system: initial experience with 68 patients. *Ann Surg* 2000; 231(5): 715-23.
5. Gonzalez R, Smith CD, Mattar SG, Venkatesh KR, Mason E, Duncan T, *et al*. Laparoscopic vs open resection for the treatment of diverticular disease. *Surg Endosc* 2004; 18(2): 276-80.
6. Kiran RP, Delaney CP, Senagore AJ, Millward BL, Fazio VW. Operative blood loss and use of blood products after

6. laparoscopic and conventional open colorectal operations. *Arch Surg* 2004; 139(1): 39-42.
7. Shore G, Gonzalez QH, Bondora A, Vickers SM. Laparoscopic vs conventional ileocolectomy for primary Crohn disease. *Arch Surg* 2003; 138(1): 76-9.
8. Seshadri PA, Poulin EC, Schlachta CM, Cadeddu MO, Mamazza J. Does a laparoscopic approach to total abdominal colectomy and proctocolectomy offer advantages? *Surg Endosc* 2001; 15(8): 837-42.
9. Milsom JW, Hammerhofer KA, Bohm B, Marcello P, Elson P, Fazio VW. Prospective, randomized trial comparing laparoscopic vs. conventional surgery for refractory ileocolic Crohn's disease. *Dis Colon Rectum* 2001; 44(1): 1-8; discussion 8-9.
10. Duepree HJ, Senagore AJ, Delaney CP, Brady KM, Fazio VW. Advantages of laparoscopic resection for ileocecal Crohn's disease. *Dis Colon Rectum* 2002; 45(5): 605-10.
11. Msika S, Iannelli A, Deroide G, Jouet P, Soule JC, Kianmanesh R, et al. Can laparoscopy reduce hospital stay in the treatment of Crohn's disease? *Dis Colon Rectum* 2001; 44(11): 1661-6.
12. Dunker MS, Ten Hove T, Bemelman WA, Slors JF, Gouma DJ, Van Deventer SJ. Interleukin-6, C-reactive protein, and expression of human leukocyte antigen-DR on peripheral blood mononuclear cells in patients after laparoscopic vs. conventional bowel resection: a randomized study. *Dis Colon Rectum* 2003; 46(9): 1238-44.
13. Tang CL, Eu KW, Tai BC, Soh JG, MacHin D, Seow-Choen F. Randomized clinical trial of the effect of open versus laparoscopically assisted colectomy on systemic immunity in patients with colorectal cancer. *Br J Surg* 2001; 88(6): 801-7.
14. Kuhry E, Jeekel J, Bonjer HJ. Effect of laparoscopy on the immune system. *Semin Laparosc Surg* 2004; 11(1): 37-44.
15. Hildebrandt U, Kessler K, Plusczyk T, Pistorius G, Vollmar B, Menger MD. Comparison of surgical stress between laparoscopic and open colonic resections. *Surg Endosc* 2003; 17(2): 242-6.
16. Lacy AM, Garcia-Valdecasas JC, Delgado S, Castells A, Taura P, Pique JM, Visa J. Laparoscopy-assisted colectomy versus open colectomy for treatment of non-metastatic colon cancer: a randomised trial. *Lancet* 2002; 359(9325): 2224-9.
17. Kehlet H, Mogensen T. Hospital stay of 2 days after open sigmoidectomy with a multimodal rehabilitation programme. *Br J Surg* 1999; 86(2): 227-30.
18. Schlachta CM, Mamazza J, Seshadri PA, Cadeddu M, Gregoire R, Poulin EC. Defining a learning curve for laparoscopic colorectal resections. *Dis Colon Rectum* 2001; 44(2): 217-22.
19. Bennett CL, Stryker SJ, Ferreira MR, Adams J, Beart RW, Jr. The learning curve for laparoscopic colorectal surgery. Preliminary results from a prospective analysis of 1194 laparoscopic-assisted colectomies. *Arch Surg* 1997; 132(1): 41-4; discussion 45.
20. Agachan F, Joo JS, Weiss EG, Wexner SD. Intraoperative laparoscopic complications. Are we getting better? *Dis Colon Rectum* 1996; 39(10 Suppl): S14-9.
21. Gibson M, Byrd C, Pierce C, Wright F, Norwood W, Gibson T, et al. Laparoscopic colon resections: a five-year retrospective review. *Am Surg* 2000; 66(3): 245-8; discussion 248-9.
22. Janson M, Bjorholt I, Carlsson P, Haglind E, Henriksson M, Lindholm E, et al. Randomized clinical trial of the costs of open and laparoscopic surgery for colonic cancer. *Br J Surg* 2004; 91(4): 409-17.
23. Milsom JW, Hammerhofer KA, Bohm B, Marcello P, Elson P, Fazio VW. Prospective, randomised trial comparing laparoscopic vs. conventional surgery for refractory ileocolic Crohn's disease. *Dis Colon Rectum* 2001; 44(1): 1-8.
24. Bergamaschi R, Pessaux P, Arnaud JP. Comparison of conventional and laparoscopic ileocolic resection for Crohn's disease. *Dis Colon Rectum* 2003; 46(8): 1129-33.
25. Regan JP, Salky BA. Laparoscopic treatment of enteric fistulas. *Surg Endosc* 2004; 18(2): 252-4.
26. Watanabe M, Hasegawa H, Yamamoto S, Hibi T, Kitajima M. Successful application of laparoscopic surgery to the treatment of Crohn's disease with fistulas. *Dis Colon Rectum* 2002; 45(8): 1057-61.
27. Canin-Endres J, Salky B, Gattorno F, Edye M. Laparoscopically assisted intestinal resection in 88 patients with Crohn's disease. *Surg Endosc* 1999; 13(6): 595-9.
28. Hasegawa H, Watanabe M, Nishibori H, Okabayashi K, Hibi T, Kitajima M. Laparoscopic surgery for recurrent Crohn's disease. *Br J Surg* 2003; 90(8): 970-3.
29. Moorthy K, Shaul T, Foley RJ. Factors that predict conversion in patients undergoing laparoscopic surgery for Crohn's disease. *Am J Surg* 2004; 187(1): 47-51.
30. Dutta S, Rothenberg SS, Chang J, Bealer J. Total intracorporeal laparoscopic resection of Crohn's disease. *J Pediatr Surg* 2003; 38(5): 717-9.
31. von Allmen D, Markowitz JE, York A, Mamula P, Shepanski M, Baldassano R. Laparoscopic-assisted bowel resection offers advantages over open surgery for treatment of segmental Crohn's disease in children. *J Pediatr Surg* 2003; 38(6): 963-5.
32. Simon T, Orangio G, Ambroze W, Schertzer M, Armstrong D. Laparoscopic-assisted bowel resection in pediatric/adolescent inflammatory bowel disease: laparoscopic bowel resection in children. *Dis Colon Rectum* 2003; 46(10): 1325-31.
33. Ky AJ, Sonoda T, Milsom JW. One-stage laparoscopic restorative proctocolectomy: an alternative to the conventional approach? *Dis Colon Rectum* 2002; 45(2): 207-10; discussion 210-1.
34. Marcello PW, Milsom JW, Wong SK, Brady K, Goormastic M, Fazio VW. Laparoscopic total colectomy for acute colitis: a case-control study. *Dis Colon Rectum* 2001; 44(10): 1441-5.
35. Delaney CP, Lynch AC, Senagore AJ, Fazio VW. Comparison of robotically performed and traditional laparoscopic colorectal surgery. *Dis Colon Rectum* 2003; 46(12): 1633-9.
36. Hildebrandt U, Plusczyk T, Kessler K, Menger MD. Single-surgeon surgery in laparoscopic colonic resection. *Dis Colon Rectum* 2003; 46(12): 1640-5.
37. Rockall TA, Darzi A. Robot-assisted laparoscopic colorectal surgery. *Surg Clin North Am* 2003; 83(6): 1463-8, xi.

PART III: FRONTIERS AROUND THE ANUS

Chapter 17

Frontiers in fistula

Gordon N Buchanan MSc MD FRCS (Gen), Specialist Registrar in Colorectal Surgery
St. Thomas' Hospital, London, UK

C Richard G Cohen MD FRCS (Gen), Consultant Colorectal Surgeon
St. Mark's Hospital, Harrow, Middlesex, UK

What is the problem?

Fistula-in-ano is a common condition [1] characterised by intermittent pain and discharge, or acute presentation with peri-anal sepsis. Fistula management seeks a balance between sepsis eradication and maintaining function. While most fistulas are simple to define and cure by fistulotomy, surgeons may encounter difficulty, perhaps due to the relationship of the anal sphincter complex, secondary extensions [2], or indeed co-existing conditions such as Crohn's disease or impaired continence. Furthermore, scarring in recurrent disease may impede assessment. This chapter highlights modern strategies for fistula-in-ano, detailing the role of MRI-guided surgery in complex fistula, also discussing infliximab for Crohn's fistula and fibrin sealant therapy.

Where are we now?

Epidemiology

Fistula affects approximately 1:10,000 [3], typically in the fourth decade [4], whilst peri-anal abscess, the acute precursor, presents a couple of years earlier [5]. While males predominate [1], gender differences are not explicable by altered circulating sex hormone levels [6], or differences in anal gland structure or distribution [7]. Other species with human type intramuscular glands, such as dogs, develop fistula-in-ano [7], where again, males predominate.

Over 90% of fistula-in-ano are cryptoglandular, caused by intersphincteric space gland infection. Associated conditions include Crohn's disease [8], tuberculosis [9], which accounts for 15% of fistulas where endemic, and hidradenitis suppurativa [10]. Extrasphincteric fistulas occasionally result from sigmoid diverticular disease or small intestinal fistula [11]. Other rare causes include actinomycosis [12], trauma [13] or foreign body perforation [14]. Although uncommon, carcinoma can develop in a longstanding fistula [15]. Fistulas secondary to presacral dermoids or rectal duplication cysts [16] are extremely rare. Rectovaginal fistula, recto-urethral fistula and pilonidal sinus which must all be differentiated from fistula-in-ano are not discussed further in this chapter.

Aetiology

Cryptoglandular hypothesis

The cryptoglandular theory suggests intersphincteric space gland infection is the initiating event [17,18]. The anal valves, situated at the dentate line between adjacent inferior columns of Morgagni, conceal a sinus, which usually connects via ducts

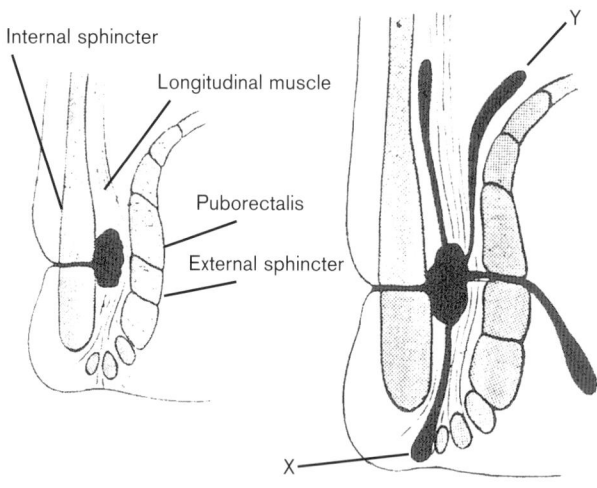

Figure 1. Spread of infection from primary anal gland abscess. The primary anal gland abscess is on the left and the surrounding tissues to the right. The commonest course is that marked X, the most rare Y. Reproduced with permission from the BMJ Publishing Group. Parks AG. Pathogenesis and treatment of fistula-in-ano. *BMJ* 1961; 1: 463-9.

crossing the internal anal sphincter (IAS) to glands [19]. The relationship between anal glands and fistula is long established [20]. Up to ten glands, which seem distinct from scent glands [7], are usually present [18], distributed circumferentially at dentate line level [21]. Glands are usually intersphincteric, although they may penetrate the IAS in up to 50% [7] and sometimes the external anal sphincter (EAS) [21]. Mucus secreted from glands is different to that secreted by the rectum [22].

Eisenhammer believed the IAS impenetrable to sepsis, with the weak point at the anal valves [17], and that spontaneous or incorrect surgical abscess drainage caused fistula. Parks furthered this hypothesis, observing cystic gland dilatation, often relating to an obstructed duct, as a necessary precursor to fistula [18], also describing possible avenues of spread (Figure 1) of sepsis.

Whilst this hypothesis explains most fistula-in-ano, others relate to diseases such as Crohn's or diverticulitis; anal verge fistula with no internal opening probably occur following apocrine gland infection [23].

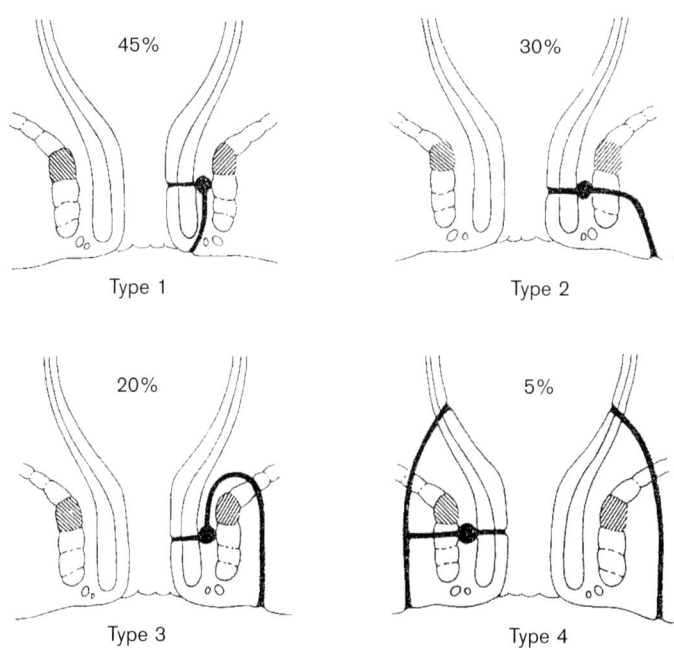

Figure 2. Parks' classification: the four main types of fistula. The external sphincter mass is regarded as the keystone and the terms "trans-", "supra-" and "extra-" refer to it. Type 1: intersphincteric; Type 2: trans-sphincteric; Type 3: suprasphincteric; Type 4: extrasphincteric. Reproduced with permission from John Wiley & Sons Ltd on behalf of the BJSS Ltd. © British Journal of Surgery Society Ltd. Parks AG, Gordon PH, Hardcastle JD. A classification of fistula-in-ano. *Br J Surg* 1976; 63: 1-12.

Microbiological aspects

In acute sepsis, gut organisms help predict an underlying fistula [24,25], while abscesses harbouring skin-derived organisms are rarely associated with fistula. Although culture reports may assist decisions regarding further examination under anaesthetic (EUA) following abscess drainage [23], experienced surgical assessment in the acute setting is actually more accurate [26].

In chronic fistula-in-ano, organisms are hard to culture [27] or demonstrate histologically [28]; therefore, non-specific track epithelialisation is probably the cause for fistula chronicity [29].

Fistula classification

There have been many systems to classify fistula [30-32]. "Simple" or "low" fistula are easy to treat by lay open with little risk to function. Lay open of "complex" or "high" fistula risks major change in continence [33].

Anatomical classification describes fistula tracks relative to anal sphincter anatomy. Parks' classification, in common use today [34], is modified from earlier descriptions [35], and is based upon 400 patients with fistula-in-ano treated at St. Mark's Hospital. Central to this classification is the cryptoglandular hypothesis. The primary track usually has one anal or rectal internal opening, and one external opening. Tracks without internal openings are called sinuses. The four main primary tracks, and their frequencies, are illustrated in Figure 2.

Secondary extensions or abscesses can extend in intersphincteric, ischiorectal or supralevator spaces, either vertically, horizontally or both sides of the internal opening where they are termed horseshoe (Figure 3). Parks emphasised that supralevator sepsis could arise from pelvic disease, upward extension of an intersphincteric fistula, or upward extension of a trans-sphincteric fistula, and stressed the importance of correct diagnosis of fistula origin before drainage [34].

Superficial fistulas, which remain superficial to the sphincters, were later shown to account for 16% of 793 patients studied at St. Mark's [36]. The different proportions of trans-sphincteric and intersphincteric fistulas described in series probably reflect individual interpretations of the lower border of the IAS and EAS [37]. Some believe suprasphincteric fistulas to be

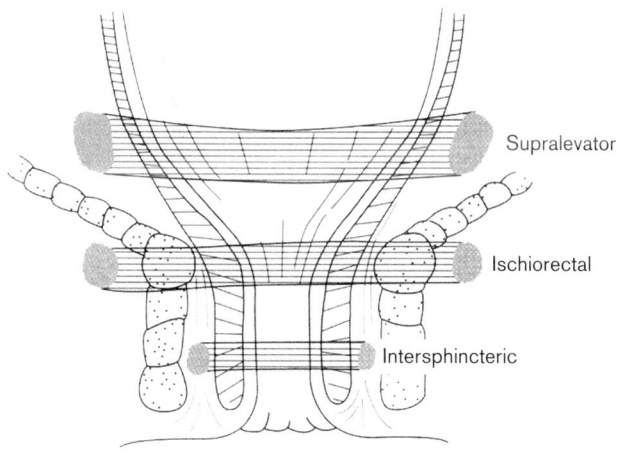

Figure 3. The planes for horseshoe extension. (adapted from: Parks AG, Gordon PH, Hardcastle JD. A classification of fistula-in-ano. Br J Surg 1976; 63: 1-12). Reproduced with permission from John Wiley & Sons Ltd on behalf of the BJSS Ltd. © British Journal of Surgery Society Ltd.

iatrogenic, and created by the general surgeon, as they are rare in other series [37-39] compared to Parks' initial classification [34]; this has subsequently been observed in a later study from St. Mark's Hospital [40].

A reappraisal of fistula anatomy has delineated an important subset of trans-sphincteric fistulas [41], with acutely angulated tracks (<90°) in half of 46 patients studied, passing both cranially and laterally from their internal opening through the sphincter on pre-operative MRI (Figure 4). These tracks would probably necessitate more extensive fistulotomy than is appreciable from clinical internal opening localisation, and are often difficult to probe. As such, this subset deserves careful attention.

Fistula assessment

Accurate assessment ensures all foci of infection are detected and eradicated to prevent recurrence. Even ostensibly simple primary fistula-in-ano may have extensions or internal openings that may be difficult to detect at initial surgery, but which may subsequently precipitate relapse [42]. Recurrent fistula-in-ano pose a

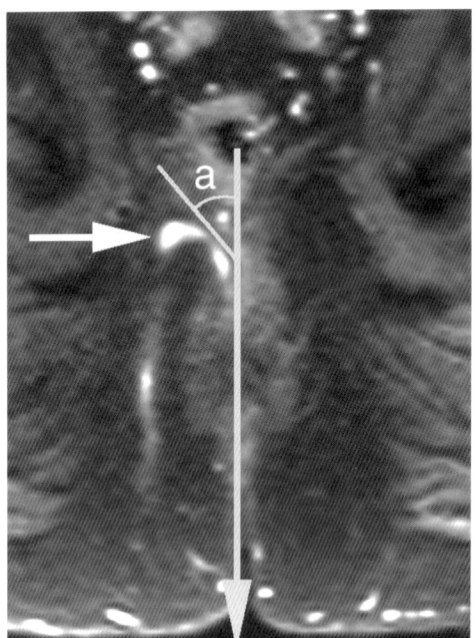

Figure 4. Acute-angle trans-sphincteric fistula. Coronal MRI of a trans-sphincteric fistula (arrowed) passing through the sphincter complex at an acute (a) angle from its internal opening.

external opening and appreciation of Goodsall's rule help determine internal opening location - this rule states that external openings situated behind the transverse anal line open into the anal canal in the midline posterior, whereas anteriorly placed external openings are usually associated with radial tracks [43]. Internal opening location may be confirmed by inspection, palpation or instillation of hydrogen peroxide [45] or methylene blue [46] via the external opening. Goodsall's rule is less accurate than hydrogen peroxide instillation [47] in predicting internal opening location.

The primary track may be palpable, or delineated using Lockhart-Mummery or lacrimal probes; however, forceful probing might precipitate iatrogenic tracks [34]. Supralevator induration suggests supralevator extension, suprasphincteric or extrasphincteric primary tracks, high intersphincteric extension or an apical ischiorectal extension (Figure 5) [34]. In difficult cases core-out fistulectomy [48] or circumferential exploratory incisions are useful as they do not divide the sphincter and facilitate evaluation of deep tracks.

difficult challenge, as scarring and distortion accompanying repeated surgery can further impair clinical assessment [2]. These patients become progressively harder to assess and treat. The key to breaking this loop is accurate initial pre-operative assessment.

Key points in delineating fistula-in-ano include [43] determining the location of the internal opening, external opening, primary track, any secondary track and presence of any underlying disease. Failure to identify and treat any one of these components can lead to recurrence [2].

Clinical assessment

Patients may present with acute anorectal sepsis or chronic peri-anal discharge. Surgeons have traditionally used EUA for assessment, though this can also be undertaken in the unanaesthetised patient.

Technique of clinical examination

Clinical evaluation of fistula-in-ano is well described [44]. The essential points include examination in either lithotomy or jack-knife positions. Visualisation of the

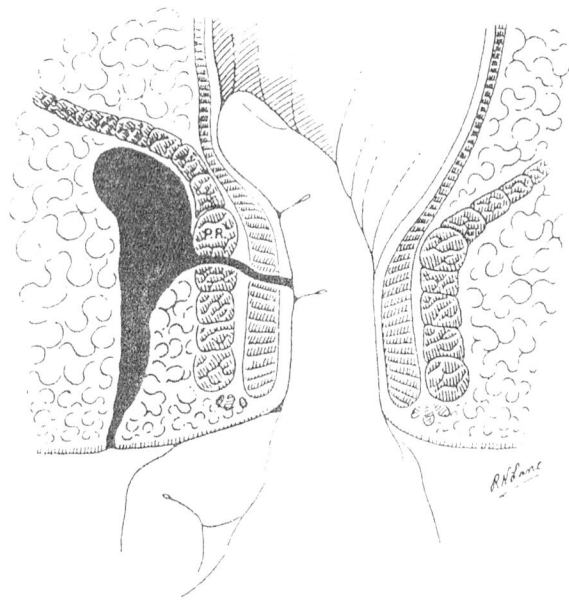

Figure 5. The classic St. Mark's anorectal fistula. Induration is felt above the anorectal ring, but the inflammation is restricted to the ischiorectal fossa. Reproduced with permission from John Wiley & Sons Ltd on behalf of the BJSS Ltd. © British Journal of Surgery Society Ltd. Parks AG, Gordon PH, Hardcastle JD. A classification of fistula-in-ano. Br J Surg 1976; 63: 1-12.

17 Frontiers in fistula

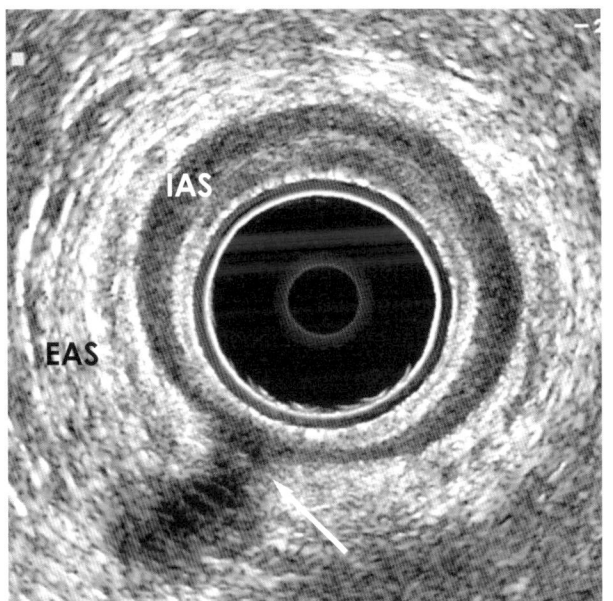

Figure 6. Fistula detected using AES: transsphincteric fistula, with internal opening (arrowed). IAS=internal, EAS=external sphincter.

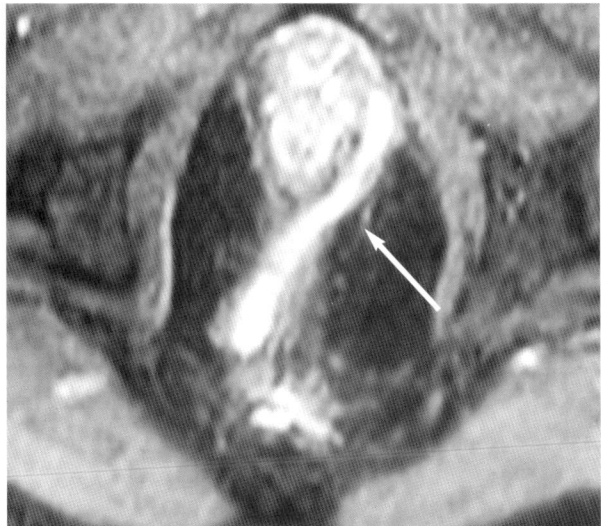

Figure 7. MRI of fistula-in-ano. Axial STIR sequence MRI: reveals a deep ishiorectal extension with a left-sided supralevator extension (arrow), unsuspected at EUA.

Accuracy of clinical assessment

Fistula is often easily treated by surgery alone [49]; however, simple fistulas can recur because of inadequate evaluation, often relating to missed internal openings, extensions [42] or skin bridging, a factor that can be diminished by Salmon's back cut [33].

While digital assessment by an experienced coloproctologist in one study was 85% accurate compared with surgery [50], surgical findings are not always correct, and others have failed to reproduce these results [51,52]. Subsequently, anal endosonography (AES) [53] and MRI [51] have been shown to be more accurate than surgical assessment, with MRI better predicting outcome [54] by depicting sepsis which surgery had failed to locate. While Schwartz et al [55] found EUA accurate in 90% of patients with Crohn's disease, 100% accuracy could be achieved if surgical findings were combined with findings obtained by either AES or MRI. Whilst in the majority of cases clinical assessment alone is adequate, assessment guided by imaging is essential in a proportion.

Fistula imaging

CT

CT can delineate pelvic collections, but it is inaccurate for fistula [56].

Fistulography

Fistulography is simple though only 20% accurate [57]. Contrast may only show part of the track, or reflux into the rectum leading to erroneous reporting of an extrasphincteric fistula [56]. As the sphincter is not visualised, accurate classification is not feasible, and fistulography is only useful where intra-abdominal disease is suspected, or if external openings lie distant from the anus.

Anal endosonography

Anal endosonography (AES) clearly delineates the sphincter, with fistulas appearing as hypoechoic tracks [58], occasionally containing focal bright echoes representing gas (Figure 6), and can be traced during probe withdrawal. Whilst initial reports suggested anal AES was no better than digital assessment [50], AES can alter management in 40% at surgery [59], also helping delineate sphincter damage and occult collections [60].

Magnetic resonance imaging

Short Tau Inversion Recovery (STIR) sequence MRI [61], which suppresses signals from fat and highlights fistulas (Figure 7), involves no contrast, internal coil or radiation, and demonstrates fistulas in axial and coronal images acquired relative to the longitudinal axis of the anal canal. Whilst STIR is simple, several other techniques are described [58].

Accuracy and utility of imaging

MRI-accuracy

Initial reports found pre-operative MRI correct in classifying all 16 patients with fistula-in-ano [61], with surgery incorrect in two cases. Subsequent reports of 94% accuracy [62], with sensitivity and specificity of 97% and 100% respectively for fistula classification in 42 subjects [51] are published.

MRI-impact

MRI-guided surgery probably provides the gold standard assessment for fistula-in-ano [63]. A recent prospective study of MRI-guided surgery in primary cryptoglandular fistula [64] used experienced radiologists and colorectal surgeons. MRI precipitated additional surgery in three of 30 patients (10%), of whom two would probably have recurred in the absence of imaging which revealed an internal opening where a sinus was initially diagnosed.

In contrast, a further prospective study from St. Mark's Hospital established that MRI is most beneficial in recurrent fistulas where occult sepsis missed at previous surgery predominates [65]. The therapeutic effect of MRI-guided surgery was 21.1%. Not only could MRI predict recurrence at the end of EUA, but surgeons acting on MRI had significantly fewer further recurrences versus those who ignored imaging; thus, MRI-guided surgery reduces further recurrence in this difficult group by 75%; surgeons ignore MRI findings at their peril.

MRI versus AES

While investigators have traditionally used surgical findings as their gold standard, it is clear that reference standards should incorporate findings at outcome [61,63,65]. With improvements in AES technology since the advent of the 10MHz probe [66] and refinements in fistula interpretation [67], a prospective study has reappraised the relative accuracies of digital examination, AES, and MRI for pre-operative fistula assessment in 104 patients [68], by comparison to an outcome-derived reference standard. AES using a 10MHz transducer was superior to digital examination, and while MRI remained superior to both, AES correctly identified the internal opening in 91% patients versus 97% patients with MRI, thus providing a viable alternative where MRI is unavailable or interpretation expertise is lacking. A list of current studies assessing fistula with AES is encompassed in Table 1. The majority of these studies relate accuracy of AES to surgical findings and do not include outcome to determine the "truth." Whilst in practical terms AES is a simple cheap examination, abnormality is altogether more definite on MRI and often more easily appreciated by the operating surgeon.

Contrast-enhanced AES

Improved efficacy of AES by levovist [69] or hydrogen peroxide enhancement (HPE) is reported [70,71], particularly in demonstrating the shape of the track [72] and extensions [53], although others have found HPE-AES inadequate at extension demonstration in complex tracks [73] (Figure 8). In direct comparison HPE-3D-AES provided an equivalent assessment to MRI [74]. Contrast enhancement is probably only useful in selected cases.

Treatment

Acute sepsis - relationship to fistula

The incidence of subsequent fistula-in-ano in patients presenting with peri-anal sepsis ranges from 26-66% [83,84]. Acute peri-anal sepsis should be drained. Whilst abscess cavities have traditionally been packed, a randomised trial has demonstrated that this confers no benefit [85].

In acute sepsis, patients undergoing fistulotomy report higher rates of flatus incontinence compared to those undergoing drainage alone [5]. While fistulectomy lowers recurrence, high incontinence rates may not be justifiable when this approach is used either routinely [5] or selectively [86]. In patients with proven internal openings [87], there is a trend towards recurrence in those treated with incision alone versus

Table 1. Endo-anal ultrasound in the evaluation of anal fistula. Concordance with surgical findings in primary track classification, identifying internal openings, abscesses, horseshoe or secondary extensions.

Authors	n	Recurrent	Probe MHz	Primary	Internal opening	Horse-shoe	Abscess
Law et al (1989) [75]	22	NS	7	92%	67%	100%	75%
Choen et al (1991) [50]	36	NS	7	80%	73%	NS	NS
Cheong et al (1993) [76]	2	100%	7	NS	NS	100%*	100%*
Cataldo et al (1993) [77]	19	NS	7	63%	28%	NS	NS
Lunniss et al (1994) [62]	20	57%	7	65%	50%	50%	62%
Deen et al (1994) [60]	18	100%	7	94%	11%	56%	NS
Hussain et al (1996) [78]	28	86%	7	61%	43%	100%	43%
Poen et al (1998) [52]	21	38%	7	62%	5%	50%	67%
				95%*	48%*	100%*	100%*
Orsoni et al (1999) [79]	22	23%	7	82%+	88%	NS	NS
Ratto et al (2000) [53]	26	0%	10	50%	54%	81%	65%
				77%*	54%*	92.3%*	89%*
Gustafsson et al (2001) [80]	23	87%	10	61%	74%	NS	65%
Schwartz et al (2001)** [55]	32	56%	7.5	91%	NS	NS	NS
Lindsey et al (2002) [59]	38	NS	10	84%	68%	NS	NS
Ortiz et al (2002)* [81]	143	10.5%	10	87%	62.5%	75%	85%
Lengyel et al (2002)* [82]	151	NS	10	82%	93%	NS	NS
Buchanan et al (2004) *** [68]	104	73%	10	81%	91%	56%	75%

NS=not stated in article; * patients who had hydrogen peroxide enhancement during endosonography; + includes both primary and secondary tracks; ** comparison made to standard defined by arbitration; *** comparison to outcome derived reference standard

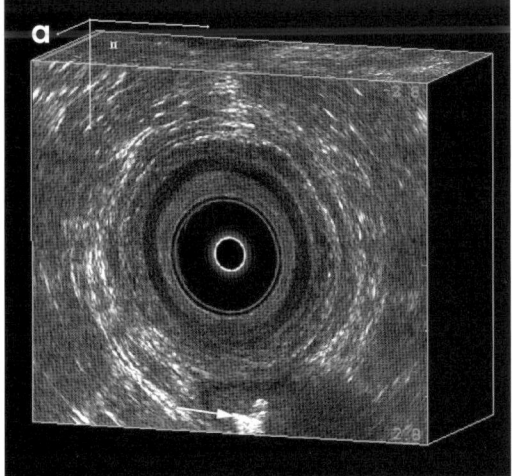
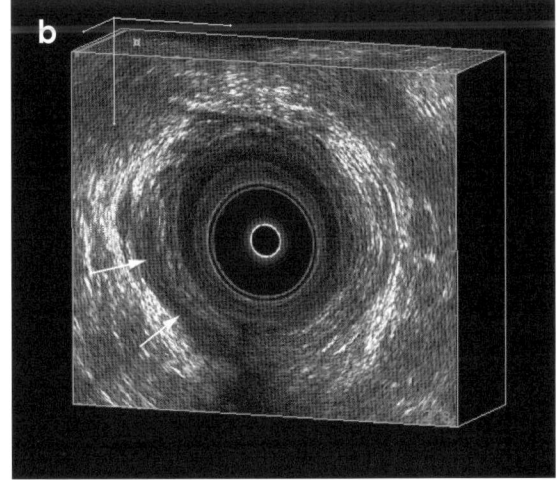

Figure 8. Gas failing to enter extension: a) 3-D anal ultrasound; axial images with gas (arrow) in a primary trans-sphincteric track at 6 o'clock, b) which failed to extend into the internal opening and secondary track (arrows) at a higher level.

fistulotomy. If patients presenting acutely have intersphincteric fistulas, the risk of incontinence on fistulotomy is small, with a significant decrease in recurrence [88]. A pragmatic approach, where low fistulas defined at acute presentation are laid open and high tracks are treated by staged setons, is justified by the reported functional outcome [89]. Such a protocol might be adopted where an experienced surgeon was available from the outset. Findings at surgery should be carefully documented on a fistula sheet (Figure 9).

Chronic fistula-in-ano

Fistulotomy

Fistulotomy, or lay open, is the surest method of cure, as tissue division overlying the track permits healing by secondary intention; extensions can be similarly treated [90]. By comparison, fistulectomy, or excision of the laid open track, delays healing [91]. Patients with HIV also display delayed healing [92]. Fistulotomy wounds heal faster after marsupialisation [93], and possibly also after radiofrequency fistulotomy [94].

Surgical strategy

Continuing problems after fistula surgery led to observations that a surgeon's reputation could be severely damaged by unsuccessful treatment [14]. Fistulotomy is usually undertaken where incontinence is unlikely to occur as a result, and this is where experience and judgement are required. Other factors considered when choosing surgical technique include the degree of pain, healing time, anal deformity [95] and the need for a seton or stoma. Although a small study found no relationship between fistula-in-ano and quality of life [96], a questionnaire assessment reported fistula recurrence, incontinence and its effects on lifestyle and social functioning predictive of patient dissatisfaction after surgery [97].

Outcome of treatment

Continence

Continence may be affected to a variable degree after fistula surgery, and anorectal physiology [98] provides quantitive measures of anorectal function, whilst continence scores enable patients to relay their degree of continence [99,100]. Diminished physiological parameters detected pre-operatively can prompt a surgeon to consider sphincter conservation instead of fistulotomy [101].

Whilst maintenance of the anorectal ring was previously considered the only necessity to maintain continence after fistulotomy [31], high EAS division which may occur with trans-sphincteric fistulas may lead to impaired continence, associated with lower distal anal canal pressure [102]. In a prospective study [103], 19 of 37 patients undergoing fistulotomy noted minor degrees of incontinence postoperatively. The severity of incontinence, the anal canal squeeze pressure and the anal canal length were similar when comparing those patients in whom the EAS was either preserved or divided; however, those patients with impaired continence had significantly lower resting pressure and higher sensory threshold than those remaining continent, suggesting that incontinence related primarily to IAS division and blunted mucosal sensation. Incidentally, the vast majority were satisfied with outcome.

In another study [104], factors predictive of diminished continence included a high internal opening and increasing fistula complexity (extra-sphincteric > suprasphincteric > trans-sphincteric > intersphincteric). Others have found female sex and a low pre-operative resting pressure [105] associated with incontinence in patients undergoing fistulotomy for intersphincteric fistulas.

A retrospective questionnaire-based study [106] reported that incontinence related to the amount of EAS divided at surgery; furthermore, quality of life in these patients related to the actual degree of incontinence. Interestingly, the ability to defer defecation has recently gained greater weight in modern scoring systems [100], which almost certainly reflects the importance attributed to maintaining EAS integrity. Fortunately, for those patients who become incontinent after fistulotomy, EAS repair achieves a satisfactory outcome for the majority [107].

Recurrence

Fistula may recur due to failure of technique such as an advancement flap, further sepsis caused by skin

Patient name: **Date of operation:**

Primary track
Sinus ☐
Superficial ☐
Intersphincteric ☐
Trans-sphincteric ☐
Suprasphincteric ☐
Extrasphincteric ☐

Internal opening
Site ____ o'clock
Level: Below dentate ☐
At dentate ☐
Above dentate ☐
Rectal ☐

External opening
Number
Sites ____ o'clock

Horse-shoeing
Intersphincteric ☐
Ischiorectal ☐
Supralevator ☐

Abscesses
Superficial ☐
Intersphincteric ☐
Ischiorectal ☐
Supralevator ☐

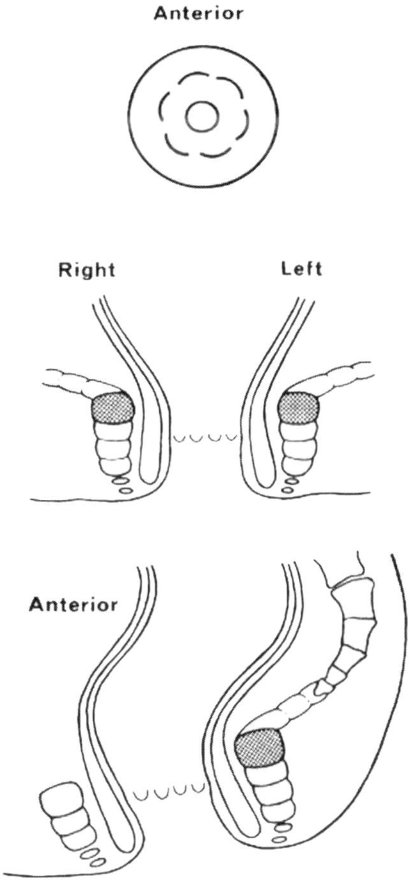

Figure 9. St. Mark's fistula sheet. This is beneficial for MRI reporting and accurately recording details of fistula surgery. (Designed by Mr. JPS Thomson).

bridging, or failure to detect and eradicate all tracks and openings at initial surgery. Recurrence after fistulotomy ranges from 0-26% [2, 108, 109], and increases with longer follow-up [110] and with proportionally higher fistula tracks [4].

Factors shown to precipitate recurrence include missed primary or secondary tracks [111], complex or horseshoe fistulas, previous fistula surgery, failure to identify internal openings, and even the individual surgeon performing the procedure [2,112]. It seems that missed tracks and openings remain a problem during fistula surgery; therefore, strategies to guide EUA seem worthwhile.

Sphincter-conserving surgery - traditional approaches

As fistulotomy may precipitate incontinence, sphincter-conservation is advocated in high fistula.

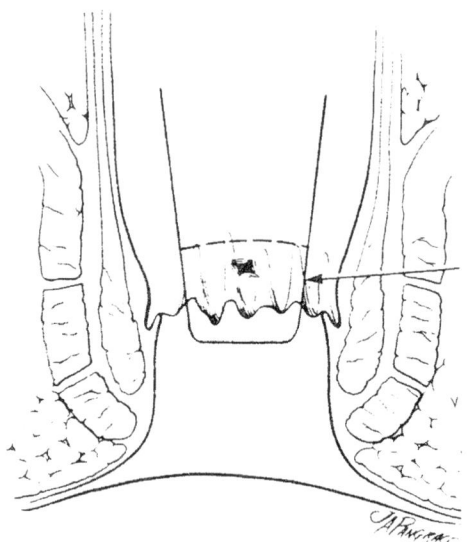

Figure 10. Rectal advancement flap raised. Apex of flap incorporating fistula orifice to be excised (arrow). Reproduced with permission from Springer and the authors. Springer © 1987. Jones IT, Fazio VW, Jagelman DG. The use of transanal rectal advancement flaps in the management of fistulas involving the anorectum. *Dis Colon Rectum* 1987; 30: 919-23.

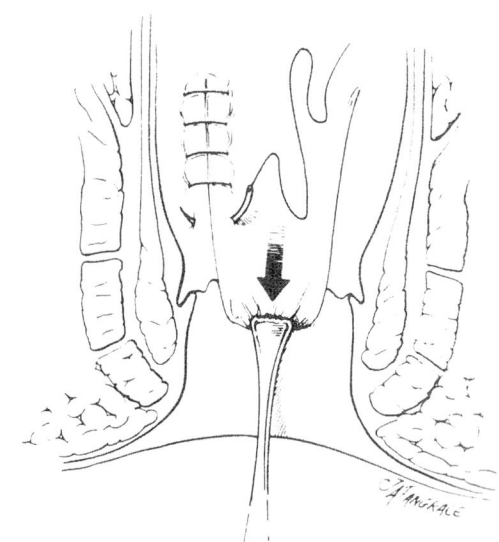

Figure 11. Flap advanced and sutured over anorectal defect. Reproduced with permission from Springer and the authors. Springer © 1987. Jones IT, Fazio VW, Jagelman DG. The use of transanal rectal advancement flaps in the management of fistulas involving the anorectum. *Dis Colon Rectum* 1987; 30: 919-23.

Core-out

The advantages of core-out fistulectomy, which involves fistula excision from the cutaneous perineal surface to the internal opening, include accurate visualisation of both primary and secondary tracks, avoidance of probing or developing false tracks, histological track assessment and depiction of the level of the track relative to the sphincter before dividing any muscle [48]. Core-out may be combined with seton placement [113] or a mucosal advancement flap [114]. Where the internal opening is closed [115] recurrence rates of 2% in low and 5% in high fistulas are reported, with others noting only minor functional disturbance [116] (although some experienced surgeons would consider these statistics very optimistic).

Advancement flap

Advancement flaps are usually employed where cure is sought but yet where fistulotomy might compromise function too much. Anocutaneous flaps do not involve sphincter division, and describe a mobilised flap of skin advanced cranially into the anal canal, whereas endorectal flaps usually consist of some internal sphincter, mucosa and submucosa [114,117] (Figures 10-11) advanced caudally over the defect. A double-flap using a combination of these two techniques is also described [118]. Furthermore, a labial fat pad (Martius flap) has proved a successful addition in complex rectovaginal and suprasphincteric fistulas in the medium term [119].

Whilst the size of the flap both circumferentially and longitudinally can vary [120], it is important that its base is wider than its apex [121]. Some report that long-term success is similar in those with cryptoglandular and Crohn's fistulas [122], whilst others have found Crohn's predictive of flap failure [123,124]. Smoking certainly has a deleterious effect on success [125]. Recurrence has been observed from 15 months to 5 years later [122,124]. An advancement flap is more likely to be successful if one or fewer previous procedures had been employed [126,127]. Where a flap fails, patients must be warned that the internal opening is often bigger and

Table 2. Success of advancement flap for treatment of fistula-in-ano.

Author and year	No.	Flap type	Success (%)	Incontinence (%)
Oh (1983) [130]	15	RMAF	87	Not stated
Aguilar et al (1985) [131]	21	RMAF	98.5	10
Wedell et al (1987) [132]	27	RMAF	100	0
Jones et al (1987) [117]	12	RMAF	66.7	Not stated
Reznick et al (1988) [133]	7	RMAF	86	0
Lewis et al (1990) [134]	8	RMAF	75	12.5
Kodner et al (1993) [135]	31	RMAF	87	Not stated
Athanasiadis et al (1994) [136]	224	RMAF	89	21
Lewis et al (1995) [137]	11	RMAF	100	0
Miller et al (1998) [138]	18	RMAF	83	0
Hyman (1999) [139]	5	RMAF	80	0
Schouten et al (1999) [126]	44	RMAF	75	35
Ortiz et al (2000) [140]	103	RMAF	93	8
Sonoda et al (2002) [124]	62	RMAF	76	Not stated
Gustafsson et al (2002) [141]	34	RMAF	59	Not stated
Lasheen (2004) [142]	50	RMAF	98	0
Del Pino et al (1996) [143]	8	AC	88	Not stated
Robertson et al (1998) [144]	14	AC	78	7
Jun et al (1999) [145]	40	AC	98	0
Zimmerman et al (2001) [127]	26	AC	46	30
Amin et al (2003) [146]	18	AC	83	0

RMAF=rectal mucosal advancement flap; AC=anocutaneous advancement flap

their symptoms may thus be worsened. The table above illustrates success and incontinence rates in reported series (Table 2). Again, some experienced surgeons would consider these success rates optimistic. As an alternative to a flap, careful direct internal opening closure in layers heals between 59-75% of fistulas [128,129].

Seton

Chemical seton

Chemical setons, which are strongly alkaline and have a caustic action, provide an ayurvedic method of treatment. In a randomised trial involving over 500 patients, healing times were longer than conventional surgery [147], although recurrence and incontinence rates were lower. A subsequent trial in low fistula [148] reported no difference in healing or function comparing fistulotomy and chemical seton; however, the latter technique was initially more painful. Chemical setons have not found worldwide usage due to licensing issues.

Tight seton

Tight (or cutting) setons are thought to act through slow transection of the enclosed sphincter [149], with fibrosis preventing sphincter disruption. A retrospective study of 20 patients with complex fistula-in-ano using a Penrose drain seton [150] reported median time to cut through of 14 days, with continence disturbance minimal (3 of 20 patients). While division of the overlying skin and anoderm enables painless tightening [113], some believe that internal sphincterotomy prior to use of a cutting seton is unnecessary and provokes incontinence [151]. Some employ a Rubber Band Ligator to tighten cutting setons [152], whilst others pass a new seton through a loop tied in the knotted suture [153] or even use a "hangman's tie" [154]. Some use a looped seton from the outset [155].

An alternative technique is two-stage seton fistulotomy (TSSF) [156], involving loose-seton placement to mark the track, which proponents believe stimulates fibrosis, and delayed secondary fistulotomy. Often, a proximal partial EAS sphincterotomy is performed, along with division of the peri-anal skin and underlying IAS, followed by delayed division of the caudal EAS. In one study, this was only necessary in 38%, although this latter group reported worse postoperative function [157]. Whilst direct comparison found cutting setons and TSSF equivalent for high fistula-in-ano in fistula eradication, both techniques rendered equally high numbers of patients incontinent (31/47 vs 8/12) [158].

Loose seton

A seton can drain fistula-in-ano [159], may stimulate fibrosis [157] and when marking the track [160] assists decision making regarding fistulotomy on subsequent palpation [161]. Long-term setons are useful in AIDS [156] and Crohn's fistulas [162]. The loose seton technique (LST) involves seton placement and subsequent removal after successfully eradicating secondary tracks and acute sepsis. Short-term success rates of 44-86% are reported [159,160,163,164]. In the long term the EAS is frequently preserved [165], although more patients relapsed than noted in the short term (16 versus seven of 20 respectively).

Other techniques

The Soave procedure, which involves rectal excision followed by colo-anal pull through and anastomosis, is applicable in pelvic sepsis associated with extrasphincteric fistulas without loss of anal sphincter musculature. As the anastomosis is constructed caudal to the infected field, healing inevitably takes place. The only report of five cases found satisfactory functional results, with all patients healing successfully [166].

A technique aimed at preserving the whole sphincter [167] involves intersphincteric dissection, internal opening suture and core-out with primary repair. Although successful in nine of 13 patients with complex trans-sphincteric and suprasphincteric fistulas, no long-term data are available.

A carbon dioxide laser with a focus-guide permitted core-out fistulectomy in three cases [168], with no recurrence or altered continence reported at 5 months; however, long-term data are not available. A technique involving core-out and re-routing of the fistula track medially with repair of sphincter defects is described, with excellent short-term results in five patients with complex tracks [169]; however, long-term data are unavailable.

Sphincter-conserving fistula surgery - novel approaches

Fibrin sealant

Fibrin sealants, which are derived from blood and accelerate the last steps of the coagulation cascade, offer an attractive treatment for fistula-in-ano. Two component solutions (component 1: fibrinogen, factor XIII; component 2: thrombin, calcium chloride) form a sealant when mixed during application. The sealant adheres to exposed collagen, remaining *in vivo* for several days, aided by the anti-fibrinolytic agent, aprotinin. The sealant acts as a plug, thus preventing contamination and also forms a fibrin mesh, providing the natural environment for unimpeded fibroblast proliferation, and hence, wound healing.

Fibrin sealant has been used with a wide variation in success (see Table 3); while some advocate sealant in all fistulas [170], others report failure in 100% [171], even after initial skin healing. Success is limited in Crohn's or HIV-related fistulas [172], those with high internal openings [173] or short tracks [174].

Most studies report track curettage as preparation [171,175-178]. In the only randomised controlled trial of fibrin sealant vs. conventional treatment (fistulotomy or loose seton insertion with or without a subsequent advancement flap), there was no advantage for sealant in simple fistulas; however,

Table 3. Success of fibrin sealant in fistula-in-ano.

Author	Year	Patients	Follow-up	Success
Hjortrup A et al [175]	1991	8	12-26 months	6
Abel ME et al [172]	1993	5	3-12 months	2
Aitola P et al [171]	1999	10	6 months	0
Venkatesh KS et al [176]	1999	30	Median 26 months	18
Cintron JR et al [177]	1999	26	Mean 3.5 months	22
Park JJ et al [178]	2000	25	Mean 6 months	17
Cintron JR et al [180]	2000	79	One year	38
Tocchi A et al [173]	2000	30	-	17
Patrlj L et al [174]	2000	69	Median 28 months	51
Sentovich SM [170]	2001	20	Mean 10 months	17
Lindsey I et al [179]	2002	19	-	12
Buchanan GN et al [181]	2003	22	Mean 16 months	3
Zmora O et al [182]	2003	37	Mean 12 months	15
Sentovich SM [183]	2003	48	Median 22 months	33

sealant healed more complex fistulas than conventional treatment, with higher satisfaction [179].

Longer follow-up [180] suggests that sealant effectiveness declines with time. A further prospective study used clinical assessment and MRI to determine healing after sealant instillation in patients with complex cryptoglandular fistula-in-ano without extension [181]. Despite skin healing in 77% at a median of 14 days after treatment, only 14% remained healed at 16 months, a result anticipated by MRI. However, sealant remains a simple treatment, and the addition of internal opening closure [183] or an advancement flap [182] has proved a useful adjunct.

Combination treatment

Whilst individual treatments are outlined, in practice combinations are often employed, particularly in complex fistula-in-ano. Initial surgery may involve lay open of secondary tracks and seton drainage, with delayed tight seton/advancement flap/fistulotomy of the main track.

Crohn's fistula

Two schools of thought predominate in the management of Crohn's fistula, which can affect up to 50% of patients. Conservative surgeons drain sepsis and use setons to preserve function, whereas bolder surgeons attempt to eradicate sepsis [184]. The key is treatment on an individual patient basis. A multidisciplinary approach with combined immunosuppressive and surgical therapy is the optimum strategy; however, despite best efforts, 20% of patients with severe peri-anal Crohn's currently require proctectomy [185].

Infliximab

Medical treatments for Crohn's fistula have previously not been curative [186], however, a randomised trial [187] reported a lower rate of "draining" fistulas in patients treated by infliximab, a mouse-human monoclonal antibody to TNF-alpha, versus placebo. Whilst pre-treatment with seton drainage may improve infliximab's efficacy [188], complete track resolution is only observed in a minority on both MRI [189] and AES [190]. This suggests that infliximab does not cure most fistulas, especially as tracks persisting on AES seem more likely to recur [191]. Infliximab, whilst useful in ameliorating symptoms, has so far proved disappointing in terms of cure, and its routine use does not currently seem cost-effective [192], particularly in light of the attendant risks of severe infection, hypersensitivity and unwanted malignancy [187].

Where are we going?

The parent abscess may be detectable at an earlier stage in the acute setting, allowing targeted aspiration or indeed image-guided surgery from the outset. With appropriate surgical expertise, immediate fistulotomy could reduce the incidence of simple fistula altogether. Although sex differences in fistula-in-ano are well documented, these are not explicable by circulating sex hormone levels [6], and further research is merited looking at end organ androgen sensitivity of anal glands.

Further recurrence in complex cases should be minimised by MRI-guided surgery [65]; increasing availability of AES or MRI may even prevent primary fistula recurring altogether - this hypothesis deserves further study. As recurrence is associated with dissatisfaction [97], the link between primary and recurrent fistula and quality of life needs to be established, so that surgeons can deliver appropriate treatments for this benign anorectal condition.

A high risk group of trans-sphincteric fistulas has been identified using MRI [41], and this risk may be quantifiable in terms of a structural and functional pressure-profile measurement using 3D-AES, manometry and modern continence scoring which takes greater account of external sphincter dysfunction [100]. This is an important area for further study, which could potentially help individualize ablative or conservative surgical treatments.

Excision of epithelialised tissue surrounding fistula tracks, not purely curettage, along with the development of more durable sealants may further improve the efficacy of fibrin sealant treatment. Whilst infliximab has shown some promise in Crohn's fistula, this treatment may at best assist preparation of inflamed tissues prior to definitive surgery; if, however, infliximab impacted on the proctectomy rate in severe peri-anal Crohn's disease, this would represent a major leap forward. In treatments using sealant and infliximab, MRI is essential to define cure beneath the skin [189] as the clinical term "closure" is unreliable.

References

1. Sainio P. Fistula-in-ano in a defined population. Incidence and epidemiological aspects. *Ann Chir Gynaecol* 1984; 73: 219-24.
2. Garcia-Aguilar J, Belmonte C, Wong WD, et al. Anal fistula surgery. Factors associated with recurrence and incontinence. *Dis Colon Rectum* 1996; 39: 723-9.
3. Ewerth S, Ahlberg J, Collste G, et al. Fistula-in-ano. A six year follow-up study of 143 operated patients. *Acta Chir Scand Suppl* 1978; 482: 53-5.
4. Sainio P, Husa A. Fistula-in-ano. Clinical features and long-term results of surgery in 199 adults. *Acta Chir Scand* 1985; 151: 169-76.
5. Schouten WR, van Vroonhoven TJ. Treatment of anorectal abscess with or without primary fistulectomy. Results of a prospective randomized trial. *Dis Colon Rectum* 1991; 34: 60-3.
6. Lunniss PJ, Jenkins PJ, Besser GM, et al. Gender differences in incidence of idiopathic fistula-in-ano are not explained by circulating sex hormones. *Int J Colorectal Dis* 1995; 10: 25-8.
7. McColl I. The comparative anatomy and pathology of anal glands. Arris and Gale lecture delivered at the Royal College of Surgeons of England on 25th February 1965. *Ann R Coll Surg Engl* 1967; 40: 36-67.
8. Marks CG, Ritchie JK, Lockhart-Mummery HE. Anal fistulas in Crohn's disease. *Br J Surg* 1981; 68: 525-7.
9. Shukla HS, Gupta SC, Singh G, et al. Tubercular fistula in ano. *Br J Surg* 1988; 75: 38-9.
10. Culp CE. Chronic hidradenitis suppurativa of the anal canal. A surgical skin disease. *Dis Colon Rectum* 1983; 26: 669-76.
11. Parks AG, Gordon PH. Fistula-in-ano: perineal fistula of intra-abdominal or intrapelvic origin simulating fistula-in-ano - report of seven cases. *Dis Colon Rectum* 1976; 19: 500-6.
12. Fry RD, Birnbaum EH, Lacey DL. Actinomyces as a cause of recurrent perianal fistula in the immunocompromised patient. *Surgery* 1992; 111: 591-4.
13. Seow C, Leong AF, Goh HS. Acute anal pain due to ingested bone. *Int J Colorectal Dis* 1991; 6: 212-3.
14. Lockhart-Mummery JP. Discussion on fistula-in-ano. *Proc R Soc Med* 1929; 22: 1331-41.
15. Jensen SL, Shokouh-Amiri MH, Hagen K, Harling H, Nielsen OV. Adenocarcinoma of the anal ducts. A series of 21 cases. *Dis Colon Rectum* 1988; 31: 268-72.
16. La Quaglia MP, Feins N, Eraklis A, et al. Rectal duplications. *J Pediatr Surg* 1990; 25: 980-4.

17. Eisenhammer S. A new approach to the anorectal fistulous abscess on the high intramuscular lesion. *Surg Gynecol Obstet* 1958; 106: 595-9.
18. Parks AG. Pathogenesis and treatment of fistula-in-ano. *BMJ* 1961; 1: 463-9.
19. Parks AG, Morson BC. The pathogenesis of fistula-in-ano. *Proc R Soc Med* 1962; 55: 751-4.
20. Herrmann G, Desfossess L. Sur la muqueuse de la region cloacale du rectum. *C R Acad Sci* [III] 1880; 90: 1301-2.
21. Seow-Choen F, Ho JM. Histoanatomy of anal glands. *Dis Colon Rectum* 1994; 37: 1215-8.
22. Fenger C. Histology of the anal canal. *Am J Surg Pathol* 1988; 12: 41-55.
23. Grace RH, Harper IA, Thompson RG. Anorectal sepsis: microbiology in relation to fistula-in-ano. *Br J Surg* 1982; 69: 401-3.
24. Eykyn SJ, Grace RH. The relevance of microbiology in the management of anorectal sepsis. *Ann R Coll Surg Engl* 1986; 68: 237-9.
25. Hamalainen KP, Sainio AP. Incidence of fistulas after drainage of acute anorectal abscesses. *Dis Colon Rectum* 1998; 41: 1357-61.
26. Lunniss PJ, Phillips RK. Surgical assessment of acute anorectal sepsis is a better predictor of fistula than microbiological analysis. *Br J Surg* 1994; 81: 368-9.
27. Seow-Choen F, Hay AJ, Heard S, et al. Bacteriology of anal fistulae. *Br J Surg* 1992; 79: 27-8.
28. Lunniss PJ, Faris B, Rees HC, et al. Histological and microbiological assessment of the role of microorganisms in chronic anal fistula. *Br J Surg* 1993; 80: 1072.
29. Lunniss PJ, Sheffield JP, Talbot IC, et al. Persistence of idiopathic anal fistula may be related to epithelialization. *Br J Surg* 1995; 82: 32-3.
30. Classic articles in colonic and rectal surgery. Diseases of the anus and rectum, DH Goodsall and W Ernest Miles. *Dis Colon Rectum* 1982; 25: 262-78.
31. Milligan ETC, Morgan CN. Surgical anatomy of the anal canal with special reference to anorectal fistulae. *Lancet* 1934; 2: 1150-6, 1213-7.
32. Goligher JC. Fistula-in-ano: management of perianal suppuration. *Dis Colon Rectum* 1976; 19: 516-7.
33. Thompson HR. The orthodox conception of fistula-in-ano and its treatment. *Proc R Soc Med* 1962; 55: 754-6.
34. Parks AG, Gordon PH, Hardcastle JD. A classification of fistula-in-ano. *Br J Surg* 1976; 63: 1-12.
35. Steltzner F. *Die anorectalen Fistein*. Springer-Verlag, Berlin, 1959.
36. Marks CG, Ritchie JK. Anal fistulas at St. Mark's Hospital. *Br J Surg* 1977; 64: 84-91.
37. Abcarian H, Dodi G, Girona J, et al. Fistula-in-ano. *Int J Colorectal Dis* 1987; 2: 51-71.
38. Eisenhammer S. The final evaluation and classification of the surgical treatment of the primary anorectal cryptoglandular intermuscular (intersphincteric) fistulous abscess and fistula. *Dis Colon Rectum* 1978; 21: 237-54.
39. Fucini C. One-stage treatment of anal abscesses and fistulas. A clinical appraisal on the basis of two different classifications. *Int J Colorectal Dis* 1991; 6: 12-6.
40. Malouf AJ, Buchanan GN, Carapeti EA, et al. A prospective audit of fistula-in-ano at St. Mark's Hospital. *Colorectal Dis* 2002; 4: 13-9.
41. Buchanan GN, Williams AB, Bartram CI, et al. Potential clinical implications of direction of a trans-sphincteric anal fistula track. *Br J Surg* 2003; 90: 1250-5.
42. Sangwan YP, Rosen L, Riether RD, et al. Is simple fistula-in-ano simple? *Dis Colon Rectum* 1994; 37: 885-9.
43. Goodsall DH, Miles WE. *Diseases of the anus and rectum*. Longmans, Green and Company, London, 1900.
44. Nicholls RJ. Clinical assessment. In: *Anal fistula: surgical evaluation and management*. Phillips RKS, Lunniss PJ, Eds. Chapman & Hall Medical, London, 1996: 47-51.
45. Glen DL. Anal fistula. *Br J Surg* 1993; 80: 1626-7.
46. Dunphy JE, Pikula J. Fact and fancy about fistula-in-ano. *Surg Clin North Am* 1955; 1469-77.
47. Gunawardhana PA, Deen KI. Comparison of hydrogen peroxide instillation with Goodsall's fule for fistula-in-ano. *ANZ J Surg* 2001; 71: 472-4.
48. Lewis AAM. Core out. In: *Anal fistula: surgical evaluation and management*. Phillips RKS, Lunniss PJ, Eds. Chapman & Hall, London, 1996: 81-6.
49. Shouler PJ, Grimley RP, Keighley MR, et al. Fistula-in-ano is usually simple to manage surgically. *Int J Colorectal Dis* 1986; 1: 113-5.
50. Choen S, Burnett S, Bartram CI, et al. Comparison between anal endosonography and digital examination in the evaluation of anal fistulae. *Br J Surg* 1991; 78: 445-7.
51. Beckingham IJ, Spencer JA, Ward J, et al. Prospective evaluation of dynamic contrast enhanced magnetic resonance imaging in the evaluation of fistula in ano. *Br J Surg* 1996; 83: 1396-8.
52. Poen AC, Felt-Bersma RJ, Eijsbouts QA, et al. Hydrogen peroxide-enhanced transanal ultrasound in the assessment of fistula-in-ano. *Dis Colon Rectum* 1998; 41: 1147-52.
53. Ratto C, Gentile E, Merico M, et al. How can the assessment of fistula-in-ano be improved? *Dis Colon Rectum* 2000; 43: 1375-82.
54. Chapple KS, Spencer JA, Windsor AC, et al. Prognostic value of magnetic resonance imaging in the management of fistula-in-ano. *Dis Colon Rectum* 2000; 43: 511-6.
55. Schwartz DA, Wiersema MJ, Dudiak KM, et al. A comparison of endoscopic ultrasound, magnetic resonance imaging, and exam under anesthesia for evaluation of Crohn's perianal fistulas. *Gastroenterology* 2001; 121: 1064-72.
56. Halligan S. Imaging fistula-in-ano. *Clin Radiol* 1998; 53: 85-95.
57. Kuijpers HC, Schulpen T. Fistulography for fistula-in-ano. Is it useful? *Dis Colon Rectum* 1985; 28: 103-4.
58. Bartram C, Buchanan G. Imaging anal fistula. *Radiol Clin North Am* 2003; 41: 443-57.
59. Lindsey I, Humphreys MM, George BD, et al. The role of anal ultrasound in the management of anal fistulas. *Colorectal Disease* 2002; 4: 118-22.
60. Deen KI, Williams JG, Hutchinson R, et al. Fistulas in ano: endoanal ultrasonographic assessment assists decision making for surgery. *Gut* 1994; 35: 391-4.

61. Lunniss PJ, Armstrong P, Barker PG, et al. Magnetic resonance imaging of anal fistulae. Lancet 1992; 340: 394-6.
62. Lunniss PJ, Barker PG, Sultan AH, et al. Magnetic resonance imaging of fistula-in-ano. Dis Colon Rectum 1994; 37: 708-18.
63. Beets-Tan RG, Beets GL, van der Hoop AG, et al. Preoperative MR imaging of anal fistulas: does it really help the surgeon? Radiology 2001; 218: 75-84.
64. Buchanan GN, Halligan S, Williams AB, et al. Magnetic resonance imaging for primary fistula in ano. Br J Surg 2003; 90: 877-81.
65. Buchanan G, Halligan S, Williams A, et al. Effect of MRI on clinical outcome of recurrent fistula-in-ano. Lancet 2002; 360: 1661-2.
66. Frudinger A, Halligan S, Bartram CI, et al. Female anal sphincter: age-related differences in asymptomatic volunteers with high-frequency endoanal US. Radiology 2002; 224: 417-23.
67. Cho DY. Endosonographic criteria for an internal opening of fistula-in-ano. Dis Colon Rectum 1999; 42: 515-8.
68. Buchanan GN, Halligan S, Bartram CI, et al. Clinical examination, endosonography, and MR imaging in preoperative assessment of fistula in ano: comparison with outcome-based reference standard. Radiology 2004; 233: 674-81.
69. Chew SS, Yang JL, Newstead GL, et al. Anal fistula: Levovist-enhanced endoanal ultrasound: a pilot study. Dis Colon Rectum 2003; 46: 377-84.
70. Kruskal JB, Kane RA, Morrin MM. Peroxide-enhanced anal endosonography: technique, image interpretation, and clinical applications. Radiographics 2001; 21: 173-89.
71. Sudol-Szopinska I, Jakubowski W, Szczepkowski M. Contrast-enhanced endosonography for the diagnosis of anal and anovaginal fistulas. J Clin Ultrasound 2002; 30: 145-150.
72. Navarro-Luna A, Garcia-Domingo MI, Rius-Macias J, et al. Ultrasound study of anal fistulas with hydrogen peroxide enhancement. Dis Colon Rectum 2004; 47: 108-14.
73. Buchanan GN, Bartram CI, Williams AB, et al. Value of hydrogen peroxide enhancement of three-dimensional endoanal ultrasound in fistula-in-ano. Dis Colon Rectum 2005; 48: 141-7.
74. West RL, Zimmerman DD, Dwarkasing S, et al. Prospective comparison of hydrogen peroxide-enhanced three-dimensional endoanal ultrasonography and endoanal magnetic resonance imaging of perianal fistulas. Dis Colon Rectum 2003; 46: 1407-15.
75. Law PJ, Talbot RW, Bartram CI, et al. Anal endosonography in the evaluation of perianal sepsis and fistula in ano. Br J Surg 1989; 76: 752-5.
76. Cheong DM, Nogueras JJ, Wexner SD, et al. Anal endosonography for recurrent anal fistulas: image enhancement with hydrogen peroxide. Dis Colon Rectum 1993; 36: 1158-60.
77. Cataldo PA, Senagore A, Luchtefeld MA. Intrarectal ultrasound in the evaluation of perirectal abscesses. Dis Colon Rectum 1993; 36: 554-8.
78. Hussain SM, Stoker J, Schouten WR, et al. Fistula in ano: endoanal sonography versus endoanal MR imaging in classification. Radiology 1996; 200: 475-81.
79. Orsoni P, Barthet M, Portier F, et al. Prospective comparison of endosonography, magnetic resonance imaging and surgical findings in anorectal fistula and abscess complicating Crohn's disease. Br J Surg 1999; 86: 360-4.
80. Gustafsson UM, Kahvecioglu B, Astrom G, et al. Endoanal ultrasound or magnetic resonance imaging for preoperative assessment of anal fistula: a comparative study. Colorectal Dis 2001; 3: 189-97.
81. Ortiz H, Marzo J, Jimenez G, et al. Accuracy of hydrogen peroxide-enhanced ultrasound in the identification of internal openings of anal fistulas. Colorectal Dis 2002; 4: 280-3.
82. Lengyel AJ, Hurst NG, Williams JG. Pre-operative assessment of anal fistulas using endoanal ultrasound. Colorectal Dis 2002; 4: 436-40.
83. Scoma JA, Salvati EP, Rubin RJ. Incidence of fistulas subsequent to anal abscesses. Dis Colon Rectum 1974; 17: 357-9.
84. Henrichsen S, Christiansen J. Incidence of fistula-in-ano complicating anorectal sepsis: a prospective study. Br J Surg 1986; 73: 371-2.
85. Tonkin DM, Murphy E, Brooke-Smith M, et al. Perianal abscess: a pilot study comparing packing with nonpacking of the abscess cavity. Dis Colon Rectum 2004; 47: 1510-4.
86. Seow-Choen F, Leong AF, Goh HS. Results of a policy of selective immediate fistulotomy for primary anal abscess. ANZ J Surg 1993; 63: 485-9.
87. Tang CL, Chew SP, Seow-Choen F. Prospective randomized trial of drainage alone vs. drainage and fistulotomy for acute perianal abscesses with proven internal opening. Dis Colon Rectum 1996; 39: 1415-7.
88. Ho YH, Tan M, Chui CH, et al. Randomized controlled trial of primary fistulotomy with drainage alone for perianal abscesses. Dis Colon Rectum 1997; 40: 1435-8.
89. Oliver I, Lacueva J, Perez VF, et al. Randomized clinical trial comparing simple drainage of anorectal abscess with and without fistula track treatment. Int J Colorectal Dis 2003; 18: 107-10.
90. Abcarian H. The "Lay open" technique. In: Anal fistula: surgical evaluation and management. Phillips RK, Lunniss PJ, Eds. Chapman & Hall, London, 1996: 73-80.
91. Kronborg O. To lay open or excise a fistula-in-ano: a randomized trial. Br J Surg 1985; 72: 970.
92. Nadal SR, Manzione CR, Galvao VM, et al. Healing after anal fistulotomy: comparative study between HIV+ and HIV- patients. Dis Colon Rectum 1998; 41: 177-9.
93. Ho YH, Tan M, Leong AF, et al. Marsupialization of fistulotomy wounds improves healing: a randomized controlled trial. Br J Surg 1998; 85: 105-7.
94. Filingeri V, Gravante G, Baldessari E, et al. Radiofrequency fistulectomy vs. diathermic fistulotomy for submucosal fistulas: a randomized trial. Eur Rev Med Pharmacol Sci 2004; 8: 111-6.
95. Mazier WP. Keyhole deformity. Fact and fiction. Dis Colon Rectum 1985; 28: 8-10.
96. Sailer M, Bussen D, Debus ES, et al. Quality of life in patients with benign anorectal disorders. Br J Surg 1998; 85: 1716-9.
97. Garcia-Aguilar J, Davey CS, Le CT, et al. Patient satisfaction after surgical treatment for fistula-in-ano. Dis Colon Rectum 2000; 43: 1206-12.

98. Jorge JM, Wexner SD. Anorectal manometry: techniques and clinical applications. *South Med J* 1993; 86: 924-31.
99. Rockwood TH, Church JM, Fleshman JW, et al. Patient and surgeon ranking of the severity of symptoms associated with fecal incontinence: the fecal incontinence severity index. *Dis Colon Rectum* 1999; 42: 1525-32.
100. Vaizey CJ, Carapeti E, Cahill JA, et al. Prospective comparison of faecal incontinence grading systems. *Gut* 1999; 44: 77-80.
101. Pescatori M, Maria G, Anastasio G, et al. Anal manometry improves the outcome of surgery for fistula-in-ano. *Dis Colon Rectum* 1989; 32: 588-92.
102. Belliveau P, Thomson JP, Parks AG. Fistula-in-ano. A manometric study. *Dis Colon Rectum* 1983; 26: 152-4.
103. Lunniss PJ, Kamm MA, Phillips RK. Factors affecting continence after surgery for anal fistula. *Br J Surg* 1994; 81: 1382-5.
104. Van Tets WF, Kuijpers HC. Continence disorders after anal fistulotomy. *Dis Colon Rectum* 1994; 37: 1194-7.
105. Chang SC, Lin JK. Change in anal continence after surgery for intersphincteral anal fistula: a functional and manometric study. *Int J Colorectal Dis* 2003; 18: 111-5.
106. Cavanaugh M, Hyman N, Osler T. Fecal incontinence severity index after fistulotomy: a predictor of quality of life. *Dis Colon Rectum* 2002; 45: 349-53.
107. Engel AF, Lunniss PJ, Kamm MA, et al. Sphincteroplasty for incontinence after surgery for idiopathic fistula in ano. *Int J Colorectal Dis* 1997; 12: 323-5.
108. Hanley PH, Ray JE, Pennington EE, et al. Fistula-in-ano: a ten-year follow-up study of horseshoe-abscess fistula-in-ano. *Dis Colon Rectum* 1976; 19: 507-15.
109. Lilius HG. Fistula-in-ano, an investigation of human foetal anal ducts and intramuscular glands and a clinical study of 150 patients. *Acta Chir Scand* Suppl 1968; 383: 7-88.
110. Grace R. Fistulotomy in the management of acute anorectal sepsis. *Dis Colon Rectum* 1997; 40: 1130-1.
111. Seow C, Phillips RK. Insights gained from the management of problematical anal fistulae at St. Mark's Hospital, 1984-88. *Br J Surg* 1991; 78: 539-41.
112. Barwood N, Clarke G, Levitt S, et al. Fistula-in-ano: a prospective study of 107 patients. *ANZ J Surg* 1997; 67: 98-102.
113. Ustynoski K, Rosen L, Stasik J, et al. Horseshoe abscess fistula. Seton treatment. *Dis Colon Rectum* 1990; 33: 602-5.
114. Stone JM, Goldberg SM. The endorectal advancement flap procedure. *Int J Colorectal Dis* 1990; 5: 232-5.
115. Lewis A. Excision of fistula in ano. *Int J Colorectal Dis* 1986; 1: 265-7.
116. Christiansen J, Ronholt C. Treatment of recurrent high anal fistula by total excision and primary sphincter reconstruction. *Int J Colorectal Dis* 1995; 10: 207-9.
117. Jones IT, Fazio VW, Jagelman DG. The use of transanal rectal advancement flaps in the management of fistulas involving the anorectum. *Dis Colon Rectum* 1987; 30: 919-23.
118. Pescatori M, Interisano A, Mascagni D, et al. Double flap technique to reconstruct the anal canal after concurrent surgery for fistulae, abscesses and haemorrhoids. *Int J Colorectal Dis* 1995; 10: 19-21.
119. Pinedo G, Phillips R. Labial fat pad grafts (modified Martius graft) in complex perianal fistulas. *Ann R Coll Surg Engl* 1998; 80: 410-2.
120. Berman IR. Sleeve advancement anorectoplasty for complicated anorectal/vaginal fistula. *Dis Colon Rectum* 1991; 34: 1032-7.
121. Zimmerman DD, Briel JW, Schouten WR. Endoanal advancement flap repair for complex anorectal fistulas. *Am J Surg* 2001; 181: 576-7.
122. Ozuner G, Hull TL, Cartmill J, et al. Long-term analysis of the use of transanal rectal advancement flaps for complicated anorectal/vaginal fistulas. *Dis Colon Rectum* 1996; 39: 10-4.
123. Mizrahi N, Wexner SD, Zmora O, et al. Endorectal advancement flap: are there predictors of failure? *Dis Colon Rectum* 2002; 45: 1616-21.
124. Sonoda T, Hull T, Piedmonte MR, et al. Outcomes of primary repair of anorectal and rectovaginal fistulas using the endorectal advancement flap. *Dis Colon Rectum* 2002; 45: 1622-8.
125. Zimmerman DD, Delemarre JB, Gosselink MP, et al. Smoking affects the outcome of transanal mucosal advancement flap repair of trans-sphincteric fistulas. *Br J Surg* 2003; 90: 351-4.
126. Schouten WR, Zimmerman DD, Briel JW. Transanal advancement flap repair of trans-sphincteric fistulas. *Dis Colon Rectum* 1999; 42: 1419-22.
127. Zimmerman DD, Briel JW, Gosselink MP, et al. Anocutaneous advancement flap repair of trans-sphincteric fistulas. *Dis Colon Rectum* 2001; 44: 1474-80.
128. Thomson WH, Fowler AL. Direct appositional (no flap) closure of deep anal fistula. *Colorectal Dis* 2004; 6: 32-6.
129. Athanasiadis S, Helmes C, Yazigi R, et al. The direct closure of the internal fistula opening without advancement flap for trans-sphincteric fistulas-in-ano. *Dis Colon Rectum* 2004; 47: 1174-80.
130. Oh C. Management of high recurrent anal fistula. *Surgery* 1983; 93: 330-2.
131. Aguilar PS, Plasencia G, Hardy TG, Jr., et al. Mucosal advancement in the treatment of anal fistula. *Dis Colon Rectum* 1985; 28: 496-8.
132. Wedell J, Meier zu EP, Banzhaf G, et al. Sliding flap advancement for the treatment of high level fistulae. *Br J Surg* 1987; 74: 390-1.
133. Reznick RK, Bailey HR. Closure of the internal opening for treatment of complex fistula-in-ano. *Dis Colon Rectum* 1988; 31: 116-8.
134. Lewis P, Bartolo DC. Treatment of trans-sphincteric fistulae by full thickness anorectal advancement flaps. *Br J Surg* 1990; 77: 1187-9.
135. Kodner IJ, Mazor A, Shemesh EI, et al. Endorectal advancement flap repair of rectovaginal and other complicated anorectal fistulas. *Surgery* 1993; 114: 682-9.
136. Athanasiadis S, Kohler A, Nafe M. Treatment of high anal fistulae by primary occlusion of the internal ostium, drainage of the intersphincteric space, and mucosal advancement flap. *Int J Colorectal Dis* 1994; 9: 153-7.
137. Lewis WG, Finan PJ, Holdsworth PJ, et al. Clinical results and manometric studies after rectal flap advancement for

infra-levator trans-sphincteric fistula-in-ano. *Int J Colorectal Dis* 1995; 10: 189-92.
138. Miller GV, Finan PJ. Flap advancement and core fistulectomy for complex rectal fistula. *Br J Surg* 1998; 85: 108-10.
139. Hyman N. Endoanal advancement flap repair for complex anorectal fistulas. *Am J Surg* 1999; 178: 337-40.
140. Ortiz H, Marzo J. Endorectal flap advancement repair and fistulectomy for high trans-sphincteric and suprasphincteric fistulas. *Br J Surg* 2000; 87: 1680-3.
141. Gustafsson UM, Graf W. Excision of anal fistula with closure of the internal opening: functional and manometric results. *Dis Colon Rectum* 2002; 45: 1672-8.
142. Lasheen AE. Partial fistulectomy and fistular wall flap for the treatment of high perianal fistulas. *Surg Today* 2004; 34: 977-80.
143. Del Pino A, Nelson RL, Pearl RK, et al. Island flap anoplasty for treatment of transsphincteric fistula-in-ano. *Dis Colon Rectum* 1996; 39: 224-6.
144. Robertson WG, Mangione JS. Cutaneous advancement flap closure: alternative method for treatment of complicated anal fistulas. *Dis Colon Rectum* 1998; 41: 884-6.
145. Jun SH, Choi GS. Anocutaneous advancement flap closure of high anal fistulas. *Br J Surg* 1999; 86: 490-2.
146. Amin SN, Tierney GM, Lund JN, et al. V-Y advancement flap for treatment of fistula-in-ano. *Dis Colon Rectum* 2003; 46: 540-3.
147. Shukla NK, et al. Multicentric randomized controlled clinical trial of Kshaarasootra (Ayurvedic medicated thread) in the management of fistula-in-ano. Indian Council of Medical Research. *Indian J Med Res* 1991; 94: 177-85.
148. Ho KS, Tsang C, Seow-Choen F, et al. Prospective randomised trial comparing ayurvedic cutting seton and fistulotomy for low fistula-in-ano. *Tech Coloproctol* 2001; 5: 137-41.
149. McCourtney JS, Finlay IG. Setons in the surgical management of fistula in ano. *Br J Surg* 1995; 82: 448-52.
150. Culp CE. Use of Penrose drains to treat certain anal fistulas: a primary operative seton. *Mayo Clin Proc* 1984; 59: 613-7.
151. McCourtney JS, Finlay IG. Cutting seton without preliminary internal sphincterotomy in management of complex high fistula-in-ano. *Dis Colon Rectum* 1996; 39: 55-8.
152. Cirocco WC, Rusin LC. Simplified seton management for complex anal fistulas: a novel use for the rubber band ligator. *Dis Colon Rectum* 1991; 34: 1135-7.
153. Seow-Choen F, Leong AF. Simple method of tightening cutting setons. *Br J Surg* 1994; 81: 1214.
154. Loberman Z, Har-Shai Y, Schein M, et al. Hangman's tie simplifies seton management of anal fistula. *Surg Gynecol Obstet* 1993; 177: 413-4.
155. Jain BK, Gupta A. Simple method of tightening cutting setons. *Br J Surg* 1995; 82: 1002.
156. Pearl RK, Andrews JR, Orsay CP, et al. Role of the seton in the management of anorectal fistulas. *Dis Colon Rectum* 1993; 36: 573-7.
157. Parks AG, Stitz RW. The treatment of high fistula-in-ano. *Dis Colon Rectum* 1976; 19: 487-99.
158. Garcia-Aguilar J, Belmonte C, Wong DW, et al. Cutting seton versus two-stage seton fistulotomy in the surgical management of high anal fistula. *Br J Surg* 1998; 85: 243-5.
159. Thomson JP, Ross AH. Can the external anal sphincter be preserved in the treatment of trans-sphincteric fistula-in-ano? *Int J Colorectal Dis* 1989; 4: 247-50.
160. Lunniss PJ, Thomson JPS. The loose seton. In: *Anal fistula: surgical evaluation and management.* Phillips RKS, Lunniss PJ, Eds. Chapman and Hall, London, 1996: 92-3.
161. Hawley PR. Anorectal fistula. *Clin Gastroenterol* 1975; 4: 635-49.
162. White RA, Eisenstat TE, Rubin RJ, et al. Seton management of complex anorectal fistulas in patients with Crohn's disease. *Dis Colon Rectum* 1990; 33: 587-9.
163. Kennedy HL, Zegarra JP. Fistulotomy without external sphincter division for high anal fistulae. *Br J Surg* 1990; 77: 898-901.
164. Williams JG, MacLeod CA, Rothenberger DA, et al. Seton treatment of high anal fistulae. *Br J Surg* 1991; 78: 1159-61.
165. Buchanan GN, Owen HA, Torkington J, et al. Long-term outcome following loose-seton technique for external sphincter preservation in complex anal fistula. *Br J Surg* 2004; 91: 476-80.
166. Maxwell-Armstrong CA, Phillips RK. Extrasphincteric rectal fistulas treated successfully by Soave's procedure despite marked local sepsis. *Br J Surg* 2003; 90: 237-8.
167. Matos D, Lunniss PJ, Phillips RK. Total sphincter conservation in high fistula in ano: results of a new approach. *Br J Surg* 1993; 80: 802-4.
168. Slutzki S, Abramsohn R, Bogokowsky H. Carbon dioxide laser in the treatment of high anal fistula. *Am J Surg* 1981; 141: 395-6.
169. Mann CV, Clifton MA. Re-routing of the track for the treatment of high anal and anorectal fistulae. *Br J Surg* 1985; 72: 134-7.
170. Sentovich SM. Fibrin glue for all anal fistulas. *J Gastrointest Surg* 2001; 5: 158-61.
171. Aitola P, Hiltunen KM, Matikainen M. Fibrin glue in perianal fistulas - a pilot study. *Ann Chir Gynaecol* 1999; 88: 136-8.
172. Abel ME, Chiu YS, Russell TR, et al. Autologous fibrin glue in the treatment of rectovaginal and complex fistulas. *Dis Colon Rectum* 1993; 36: 447-9.
173. Tocchi A, Mazzoni G, Miccini M. Fibrin sealant in the repair of anorectal fistulae. *Arch Surg* 2000; 135: 989.
174. Patrlj L, Kocman B, Martinac M, et al. Fibrin glue-antibiotic mixture in the treatment of anal fistulae: experience with 69 cases. *Dig Surg* 2000; 17: 77-80.
175. Hjortrup A, Moesgaard F, Kjaergard J. Fibrin adhesive in the treatment of perineal fistulas. *Dis Colon Rectum* 1991; 34: 752-4.
176. Venkatesh KS, Ramanujam P. Fibrin glue application in the treatment of recurrent anorectal fistulas. *Dis Colon Rectum* 1999; 42: 1136-9.
177. Cintron JR, Park JJ, Orsay CP, et al. Repair of fistulas-in-ano using autologous fibrin tissue adhesive. *Dis Colon Rectum* 1999; 42: 607-13.
178. Park JJ, Cintron JR, Orsay CP, et al. Repair of chronic anorectal fistulae using commercial fibrin sealant. *Arch Surg* 2000; 135: 166-9.
179. Lindsey I, Smilgin-Humphreys MM, Cunningham C, et al. A randomized, controlled trial of fibrin glue vs. conventional treatment for anal fistula. *Dis Colon Rectum* 2002; 45: 1608-15.

180. Cintron JR, Park JJ, Orsay CP, et al. Repair of fistulas-in-ano using fibrin adhesive: long-term follow-up. *Dis Colon Rectum* 2000; 43: 944-9.
181. Buchanan GN, Bartram CI, Phillips RK, et al. Efficacy of fibrin sealant in the management of complex anal fistula: a prospective trial. *Dis Colon Rectum* 2003; 46: 1167-74.
182. Zmora O, Mizrahi N, Rotholtz N, et al. Fibrin glue sealing in the treatment of perineal fistulas. *Dis Colon Rectum* 2003; 46: 584-9.
183. Sentovich SM. Fibrin glue for anal fistulas: long-term results. *Dis Colon Rectum* 2003; 46: 498-502.
184. Scott HJ, Northover JM. Evaluation of surgery for perianal Crohn's fistulas. *Dis Colon Rectum* 1996; 39: 1039-43.
185. Bell SJ, Williams AB, Wiesel P, et al. The clinical course of fistulating Crohn's disease. *Aliment Pharmacol Ther* 2003; 17: 1145-51.
186. Sandborn WJ, Present DH, Isaacs KL, et al. Tacrolimus for the treatment of fistulas in patients with Crohn's disease: a randomized, placebo-controlled trial. *Gastroenterology* 2003; 125: 380-8.
187. Sands BE, Anderson FH, Bernstein CN, et al. Infliximab maintenance therapy for fistulizing Crohn's disease. *N Engl J Med* 2004; 350: 876-85.
188. Regueiro M, Mardini H. Treatment of perianal fistulizing Crohn's disease with infliximab alone or as an adjunct to exam under anesthesia with seton placement. *Inflamm Bowel Dis* 2003; 9: 98-103.
189. Bell SJ, Halligan S, Windsor AC, et al. Response of fistulating Crohn's disease to infliximab treatment assessed by magnetic resonance imaging. *Aliment Pharmacol Ther* 2003; 17: 387-93.
190. Rasul I, Wilson SR, MacRae H, et al. Clinical and radiological responses after infliximab treatment for perianal fistulizing Crohn's disease. *Am J Gastroenterol* 2004; 99: 82-8.
191. Ardizzone S, Maconi G, Colombo E, et al. Perianal fistulae following infliximab treatment: clinical and endosonographic outcome. *Inflamm Bowel Dis* 2004; 10: 91-6.
192. Arseneau KO, Cohn SM, Cominelli F, et al. Cost-utility of initial medical management for Crohn's disease perianal fistulae. *Gastroenterology* 2001; 120: 1640-56.

Chapter 18

Haemorrhoid surgery

Per-Olof Nyström MD PhD, Consultant Colorectal Surgeon
Roger Gerjy MD, Registrar in Colorectal Surgery
University Hospital, Linköping, Sweden

What is the issue?

Two seminal text books on colorectal surgery, Goligher's and Corman's, both treat haemorrhoids extensively [1, 2]. Only the chapters on cancer of the colon and rectum are longer. One would think that the nature of haemorrhoids is so well understood that its treatment has matured beyond major improvement. Yet only the past few years have seen a revolution in our knowledge about this disease. As so often, it was presaged by the introduction of new concepts of treatment and the availability of several new devices. Although there is a tradition of conducting studies of haemorrhoids in the form of randomised controlled trials, many studies have been uncontrolled. This is unfortunate, because it is difficult to be sure that the patients who have been selected for treatment and the claimed difference of pre-treatment and post-treatment symptoms is genuinely a measure of success. No strict correlation exists between the surgeons' assessment of the anatomy and the degree of symptoms. Nor is it clear to what degree patients are given lasting cure, although the majority of patients are improved by any treatment, at least for a period.

The result of haemorrhoid treatment is worse than usually stated in textbooks and scientific reports, which all too frequently have observation periods that are simply too short. Not only can serious complications occur after all treatments, such as Fournier's gangrene, protracted anal pain or anal stenosis, but long-term follow-up demonstrates that the functional result is often inferior with many patients complaining of disturbed continence or continuing symptoms from their haemorrhoids [3-5]. Short-term improvement is common, even without treatment; such improvement is certainly seen in the large majority after any specific intervention, but is it a satisfactory state when so many recur years later?

An operation for haemorrhoids is associated with significant postoperative pain that may last for 2 or more weeks in many patients. Not every patient suffers extensive pain and it is not known why the pain experienced is so different among patients. Certainly, the wound to the anal canal contributes markedly to the pain. Treatments that avoid anal canal wounds can be expected to cause much less pain and such methods merit further exploration, so long as they are effective.

Haemorrhoid surgery is sufficiently minor even to be suitable for day surgery under local anaesthetic. But such local blocks need a skilled technique to avoid the discomfort and pain that injection of the anus may cause the patient. Acceptable methods that can be applied by the operating surgeon have been

Table 1. The pre-operative history of manual reduction of mucosal/haemorrhoidal prolapse according to a self-reported symptom questionnaire in 257 patients (for questionnaire details, see Table 3). All patients were operated for what the surgeon described as prolapsing haemorrhoids. But according to the patient, about a third of the patients were in fact grade II.

Age group	Number of patients	With prolapse n (%)	Prolapse score* (when present)	Total symptom score*
20-40 years	51	38 (74.5)	2.2	8.1
41-60 years	132	90 (68.2)	2.4	8.2
61-80 years	74	46 (62.2)	2.5	8.0

* Mean score. The maximum prolapse score is 3 points (a daily need manually to reduce prolapse) and the maximum total symptom score is 15 points.

described but need further exploration [6-8]. Traditions are very strong, however, and most patients in Europe have in-hospital treatment under general anaesthesia or axonal block, perhaps unnecessarily increasing expense [9, 10].

To make the transition to day surgery under local anaesthetic, both patients and surgeons must be confident that the operation can be done without undue pain in the majority of patients. In addition, are there perhaps surgical methods that are consistently associated with less pain? Can the operation be performed in a way that limits injury to the anal canal? Are we good at selecting those who will benefit most from surgery, permitting smaller interventions in the others? These issues are important for patient and community alike and should result in faster and better treatments.

Where are we now?

Classification of haemorrhoids

Symptomatic haemorrhoids are treated with one of several modalities depending on the stage of the disease. It is inadequate to apply the general terms "symptomatic haemorrhoids" or "prolapsing haemorrhoids" to describe the group of patients that have been treated. We need stage-specific results to understand the effectiveness of each treatment; but even the randomised controlled trials are surprisingly vague about the stage. One finds descriptions such as "irreducible prolapsing haemorrhoids" or "all patients were of third or fourth degree haemorrhoids", but closer examination raises doubt as to how many patients really did suffer from prolapse. In a recent randomised trial of 70 patients, 27 were rated as grade IV ("the prolapsed haemorrhoid could no longer be reduced"); so how could only three patients have complained of prolapse and only two describe mucus discharge? [11] The relative merits of different methods to treat haemorrhoids must depend on more accurate use of an agreed classification. Part of the current problem has been the excessive staging seen in many reports.

The presence of prolapse is probably the most important staging factor when selecting treatment. But we must distinguish between a patient who gives a history of manual reduction of prolapse and the surgeon's proctoscopic interpretation as surgeons tend to overstate the situation by comparison with the patient's history (Table 1) [12]. In the established grading, it is the patient's version (i.e. that the patient applies manual reduction of the prolapse) that is the discriminator of grade III from grade II haemorrhoids [1, 12]. Such a history of manual repositioning clearly indicates a sliding down of rectal mucosa with the haemorrhoid and lining of the anal canal. Grade II is by definition an intermittent prolapse, one that spontaneously reduces, but the demarcation of this stage from grade I is obviously subjective and depends on the surgeon's assessment

Table 2. Amended anatomical classification of haemorrhoids.

Grade I		Intact anal canal
Grade II		Patient denies manual reduction but examination reveals mucohaemorrhoidal prolapse
Grade III		Patient gives positive history of manual reduction of mucohaemorrhoidal prolapse
External component	A.	No external component
	B.	One or more soft skin folds
	C.	Circumferential tags and anodermal polyps

Traditional grade IV has been replaced by a grading of the external component that is its main feature. Patients are grade IIC or grade IIIC depending on their history of manual reduction.

and tradition. A practical definition could be those patients who themselves deny manual reduction but who actually have a prolapse in the opinion of the surgeon. This leaves grade I patients who must have an intact anal canal. We believe that the size of the haemorrhoid should be no part of the grading. It is a great help to ask the patient to strain while the proctoscope is withdrawn to guide any prolapsing mucosa outside the anal verge. Should it reduce spontaneously and should the patient deny manual reduction when passing a motion, then this is by definition a grade II haemorrhoid.

Grade IV haemorrhoids are defined as haemorrhoids that cannot be reduced by the patient. This entity is also difficult because it usually designates a large external component of deformed anoderm with tags and anal polyps. A mucosal/haemorrhoidal prolapse may or may not be present, and if it is, the patient not infrequently may be able to reduce this component. The dentate line has also often descended to lie near the lower margin of the internal sphincter. We believe a better grading is one that accounts for the external component separately but remains true to the grades II and III with respect to the patient's denial or affirmation of manual reduction (Table 2).

The anatomical grading is highly relevant for the patient as both the presence of a prolapse is a disturbing feature much as the presence of an external component. The patient reasonably expects that treatment will remove both components. By the same token, the classification aids assessment of efficacy of each treatment. For example, stapled anopexy effectively removes the prolapse but is frequently inadequate to deal with the external component. The best result therefore can be expected for grade IIIA, but grade IIIC requires a Milligan-Morgan operation or a hybrid operation where anopexy is combined with excision of the external component. Similarly, rubber banding may be adequate for grade IIA, but it is obviously less suitable when the external component is significant (grades IIB and C). This grading can also be applied postoperatively to describe the anatomical result of treatment.

Classification of the symptoms of haemorrhoids

Defaecatory bleeding is the second most important indication for treating haemorrhoids. However, there may be associated symptoms of pain, soiling and anal pruritus in many patients. These symptoms may well be directly related to the prolapse. Murie *et al* examined the prevalence of anal pain, pruritus ani and faecal soiling in 82 haemorrhoid patients before haemorrhoidectomy or rubber banding and again 1 year after treatment. The results were compared with 82 subjects without haemorrhoids. This was a randomised trial in which haemorrhoidectomy and rubber banding treated the associated symptoms equally well. One year after treatment, however, significantly more patients had residual associate symptoms than found among the control subjects [13].

Table 3. Sample of questions from self-reported symptoms questionnaire with regard to haemorrhoids. Statistical analysis is done on a nominal scale: never=0, less than once a week=1, etc., maximum score 15 points.

The following questions deal with haemorrhoids. Your answers should reflect the latest two-week period.

1. How often do you have pain from the anus?	☐ Never	☐ Less than once a week	☐ 1-6 times weekly	☐ Every day (always)
2. How often do you have itching or discomfort of the anus?	☐ Never	☐ Less than once a week	☐ 1-6 times weekly	☐ Every day (always)
3. How often do you have bleeding when passing a motion?	☐ Never	☐ Less than once a week	☐ 1-6 times weekly	☐ Every day (always)
4. How often do you soil your underclothes (soiling from the anus)?	☐ Never	☐ Less than once a week	☐ 1-6 times weekly	☐ Every day (always)
5. How often do you reduce a prolapsing haemorrhoid with your hand when passing a motion?	☐ Never	☐ Less than once a week	☐ 1-6 times weekly	☐ Every day (always)

The natural history of symptomatic haemorrhoids was investigated in a randomised study of grade II haemorrhoids [3]. The definition was very clear: "...during maintained straining and withdrawal of the proctoscope till it first emerged from the anal orifice, the anal mucosa projected out of the anal orifice and disappeared immediately as soon as the patient ceased to strain and the proctoscope was withdrawn completely." Ninety-eight such patients were randomised to rubber band ligation and 91 to observation. Patients in both groups were followed 6-monthly for a median of 48 months. After repeated sessions of rubber banding, 88% were initially considerably improved and then followed. Sixty-six percent of the patients with expectant management were also considerably improved without treatment and they too were followed. After a median of 48 months a third of those with rubber banding had recurred but 66% remained improved. Expectant management, after initial spontaneous improvement, resulted in 62% recurrence, but even so 38% remained well.

A questionnaire study of 418 patients with a haemorrhoidectomy 2-11 years previously, showed that as many as 33% claimed symptoms of faecal incontinence [5]. Another report on long-term follow-up of a randomised clinical trial which had compared haemorrhoidectomy with Lord´s dilatation showed that 52% of patients were symptom-free 17 years after haemorrhoidectomy, but 26% had recurrent haemorrhoids and 11% had had repeated treatment, Twenty percent had incontinence complaints after haemorrhoidectomy which was actually similar to the pre-operative status. Lord´s anal sphincter stretch produced incontinence in half the patients [4].

By rating the frequency of all five symptoms, a scale can be obtained which describes the symptom load before and after treatment in each patient (Table 3).

Table 4. Patient self-reported residual symptoms 6-12 months after a Milligan-Morgan operation or stapled anopexy. From the questionnaire of Table 3. Mean pre-operative symptoms score was 8 points, see Table 1. Unpublished data by the authors.

Operation	No of patients	Asymptomatic score 0	Symptom score 1-4	Symptom score 5-15
Milligan-Morgan patients (%)	69	25 (36.2)	30 (43.5)	14 (20.3)
Stapled anopexy patients (%)	184	60 (32.6)	92 (50.0)	32 (17.4)
All patients (%)	253	85 (33.6)	122 (48.2)	46 (18.2)

Table 5. Pre-operative classification of haemorrhoids with respect to patient denial of need for manual reduction of prolapse (grade II) or affirmation of reduction (grade III). The surgeon classified the presence of an external component: A none, B one or few tags, C circumferential tags and dermal polyps. The associated symptoms score for each group, based on self-reported pre-operative symptoms score and surgeons' assessment of the external anatomy at surgery, is given.

	No need for manual reduction			Needs manual reduction		
Grade of disease	IIA	IIB	IIC	IIIA	IIIB	IIIC
Number of patients	12	40	18	47	84	28
(%)	(5.2)	(17.5)	(7.9)	(20.5)	(36.7)	(12.2)
Symptom score	5.1	6.4	6.2	8.9	8.7	9.5
Mean (range)	(1-9)	(1-11)	(2-12)	(5-15)	(3-15)	(4-13)
Prolapse score excluded	5.1	6.4	6.2	6.3	6.4	7.2

Either some or all of these symptoms may be present but their intensity may vary over time. Using this self-reported scale we have found that residual symptoms are common among patients operated upon whether by Milligan-Morgan haemorrhoidectomy or stapled anopexy (Table 4). The mean pre-operative symptom score, however, is unrelated to the anatomical stage (Table 5); this may be a reason why surgical and non-operative methods of treatment apparently provide a similar result in the short run.

Treatments for haemorrhoids

The many methods to treat haemorrhoids call for some sort of taxonomy to understand their applicability relative to the haemorrhoidal stage. The following proposal attempts to group treatments that appear to work under a common principle.

- Group 1. Methods targeted at the origin of the cushion without excision: sclerosing injection, rubber band ligation, infrared coagulation, diathermy coagulation, cryotherapy, and Doppler-guided haemorrhoid artery ligation (HAL).
- Group 2. Methods of complete excision of the piles: Milligan-Morgan operation, Ferguson operation.
- Group 3. Methods that excise the haemorrhoid tissue with preservation and resuture of the mucosa and anoderm: Whitehead and Park's operations, radiofrequency ablation.
- Group 4. Method of excision of the mucosal prolapse and "pexy" of haemorrhoids: Longo stapled haemorrhoidopexy (anopexy).

Group 1: methods aimed at the origin of the pile without excision

All of these methods induce a discrete tissue necrosis or inflammation that results in fibrosis of the submucosa. The result is a restored fixation of the mucosa to the rectal wall. Because the prolapse is prevented its associated symptoms are relieved. These methods will be effective when the prolapse is minor or affects only a part of the circumference. They are more effective when the mucosa is thin than when it is thick. However, none of the trials have assessed these circumstances in detail.

The final result with these methods also depends on the number of haemorrhoidal sites treated in each session and the number of sessions. It is a matter of judgement how many sites can be treated at a time without causing ulceration of the mucosa and pain [14]. These treatments are applied without anaesthesia or with just local or topical anaesthetic.

Doppler-guided ligation of the haemorrhoid arteries (HAL) was proposed by Morinaga in Japan [15]. The haemorrhoids are obviously conceived as a vascular disease that can be treated by interrupting the arterial supply while retaining the distal venous return from the piles. Transmucosal suture ligation of the arteries is applied 1-2cm above the haemorrhoid by means of an anoscope fitted with a doppler probe and a window through which the suture is made. Two case series have been published and one randomised trial comparing HAL to Ferguson excision [11, 16, 17]. The randomised study showed similar symptom resolution after 1 year for both treatments. A mean of six sutures was applied, which would be very similar to an extensive transmucosal suture fixation of the muco-haemorrhoidal prolapse at the anorectal ring, an operation whose design disregards the role of the artery supply entirely [18, 19]. Further studies must therefore prove the necessity of the doppler identification of the arteries.

Several of these methods have been compared in randomised trials and two meta-analyses have been published [20, 21]. One such compared two studies of rubber band ligation versus infrared coagulation, two studies of banding versus injection sclerotherapy and one study that compared all three treatments. All the studies had a follow-up of 12 months. The proportion of "asymptomatic" patients at 12 months was assessed and the need for re-treatment. The pooled response rates showed that 42% and 43% were asymptomatic at 12 months after infrared coagulation and rubber band ligation respectively. However, 16% versus 5% of the patients required repeated therapy (p=0.0002). Pain was more common after rubber banding (20%) than after infrared coagulation (4%, p=0.02). The pooled response rates for injection sclerotherapy versus rubber band ligation showed that 25% versus 37% were asymptomatic at 12 months (p=0.07). Repeat treatment had been required in 23% and 9% respectively (p=0.009) and pain had been experienced by 53% after sclerotherapy and 48% after banding. It was concluded that rubber banding appears to be a more lasting treatment but can be associated with more pain [21]. A later study of combined rubber band ligation and sclerosing injections performed at the same session versus either treatment alone showed that the combination gave more lasting result with less need for additional treatment sessions but caused more discomfort and pain. Patients were followed for 4 years, by which time 46% of patients treated with the combination remained asymptomatic compared with only 8% of those with sclerosing injection [22].

As mentioned above, the treatment effect with these methods is related to the amount of tissue destruction and number of sites treated; but then the risk of pain increases. Three randomised trials have evaluated the use of local anaesthetic to prevent pain after multiple banding. Local anaesthetic was found to be effective in the first few hours after treatment, but it did not prevent later pain [23-25].

The low rate of asymptomatic patients after a year is a concern, but as shown earlier in Table 4, this is not improved by an operation when patients are asked. As might therefore be expected, rubber banding was found to be equally effective in controlling symptomatic prolapse but had a higher risk of recurrent symptoms when compared with stapled anopexy [26]. In an earlier randomised comparison of rubber band ligation and haemorrhoidectomy, equal symptom resolution was also demonstrated and this lasted for 3 years after treatment [27]. Another study of long-term follow-up (4.8 years) after rubber band ligation using patient questionnaires and clinical examination found that 44% of patients claimed to be symptom-free [28]. By contrast, a randomised study of stapled anopexy versus Milligan-Morgan with 42 patients in both groups, all with prolapse, claimed a much higher proportion of asymptomatic patients after 6-14 months with conventional surgery (78% anopexy and 85% conventional) [29]. It is obvious that only a minority is cured with any of the treatments available for haemorrhoids, a fact that surgeons should consider when counselling patients. The difference appears to be in the duration of the improvement, where sclerosing injections seem worse and rubber banding is better.

Group 2: excision of piles

Most surgeons excise the piles with conventional monopolar diathermy because it bleeds less. If the pile is put under tension diathermy excision can elegantly dissect out the pile with minimal damage and loss of tissue within the anal canal. The thin fascia covering the internal sphincter can often be preserved and the traditional ligature on the pedicle in the rectal mucosa can be omitted. The technique was described by Sharif in 1991 and has subsequently been used as the reference method in several trials [30]. By comparison with scissors excision, not one of three randomised trials found any advantage with respect to postoperative pain [31-33].

Excision by Ultracision shears or bipolar diathermy shears (Ligasure) offers less bleeding consequent upon the function of these devices. Ligasure in addition offers the choice of a completely closed excision if the piles are grasped within the shears, as this fuses the collagen and seals the wound. The internal sphincter is not exposed at all, so there is no need to suture the wound for those preferring a closed, Ferguson procedure. However, none of the studies mention whether the wounds remain fused throughout the healing process. Concerns that this "blind" excision might cause sphincter damage have been refuted by long-term follow-up compared with conventional haemorrhoidectomy [34]. The randomised studies show that operation time was halved compared with conventional operation, with operation times between 5 and 10 minutes [35-37].

The randomised trials show inconsistent results with regard to reduced postoperative pain with these new devices. The overall impression is one of little benefit, although two of five studies with Ligasure found less pain and one of three with Ultracision [35, 37-42].

Group 4: stapled haemorrhoidopexy

The Longo operation is a new concept. It is rooted in an understanding of symptomatic haemorrhoids as a disease of prolapse in which excessive mucosa of the lower rectum is the important component. The mucosal/haemorrhoidal prolapse is treated with "prolapsectomy" of the mucosa by means of the circular stapler. The haemorrhoids are not excised but should adhere to the staple line which is conventionally situated 2cm above the dentate line [43-46]. Cephalad elevation of the lining of the anal canal and the haemorrhoids is achieved - and hence the operation has been termed haemorrhoidopexy or anopexy.

More than 30 case series and randomised trials show that the principle seems valid to treat haemorrhoids [29, 47-58]. The prolapse is indeed effectively removed, but in cases with an external component of anodermal folds and polyps, these need complementary excision.

The finding that conventional excision and anopexy are equally effective suggests that the haemorrhoid itself may be immaterial (as it is retained in anopexy); it is the mucosa of the lower rectum that forms the prolapse and the associated symptoms. It seems that it is the scarring of the wounds that prevents further prolapse after both treatments, but in one the scar is longitudinal throughout the anal canal whereas the other is circular above the anal canal. In both methods the scar reaches equally high above the dentate line to excise part of (Milligan-Morgan) or the entire (anopexy) mucosal prolapse. The difference in the orientation and location of the wounds obviously is the reason for the lesser pain after anopexy consistently found in the randomised trials.

Pharmacologic methods to reduce pain

The immediate postoperative pain can be controlled with injection of a local anaesthetic agent at the time of surgery, either by infiltration anaesthesia or by regional block [59, 60]. The duration is only a few hours, but this is extremely useful for day surgery. Spasm of the internal sphincter, which is associated with and may indeed cause the severe pain in subsequent days, has been addressed in various ways. Anal sphincter stretch or internal sphincterotomy appears to provide no pain relief but adds to the risk of incontinence [1, 61, 62]. More recently, various pharmacological means known to relax the sphincters have been tried. These include trimebutine, nitroglycerine and Botulinum toxin [63-65]. Botox seems more interesting as its effect lasts for several weeks. In a recent double-blind randomised study, Botox provided lower pain scores for both daily average pain and the maximal pain, although statistical difference was only attained after the fifth day - compatible with the delayed effect seen when similarly treating anal fissure [65].

Metronidazole, an antibiotic active against anaerobic bacteria, in an oral dose of 400mg twice daily, was found to reduce postoperative pain on days 5-7 after Milligan-Morgan haemorrhoidectomy [66]. Another British randomised study with the same dose of metronidazole, but following Ferguson operation, failed to disclose a positive effect on pain [67]. Both of these studies evaluated the patients' expectation of pain and found that they rated pain as less than expected. A third study using excision with Ultracision and Ferguson closure with topical application of 2.5ml of a 10% metronidazole cream three times daily, again showed significantly less pain on days 7 and 14. (Interestingly, these authors had earlier shown a significantly lower pain score with Ultracision [VAS about 5, days 1-2] but excision with Ultracision in the metronidazole study showed a VAS about 7 for days 1 and 2 [38, 68]).

The ideal pharmacological means to treat postoperative pain after haemorrhoidectomy should have a duration of at least a week. What is available so far is either too short acting or has too delayed an effect. Furthermore, results are not consistent across the studies. A mix of agents is sometimes recommended, such as diclofenac, paracetamol, glyceryl-nitrate, metronidazole and lactulose, but the evidence supporting such poly-pharmacy remains to be established.

Pain after haemorrhoid surgery

After a haemorrhoid operation, patients display two components of pain. There is a steady, moderate pain during most of the day (daily average pain). Standard oral analgesics will treat this pain quite well. There is also a peak pain of short duration which is usually experienced at attempts to defecate and which may linger for a period after defecation, similar to the pain with an anal fissure. This pain is sharp and often beyond the therapeutic limit of oral non-morphine analgesics. The overall maximum pain is usually experienced on the third or fourth postoperative day. From then on both types of pain resolve gradually over the next couple of weeks. Using a ten-pointed visual analogue scale (VAS), the peak pain is about 2 points more severe than the daily average pain (Figure 1). The total pain experience can be calculated by adding up the VAS per day for each type of pain.

Pain medication will obviously modify the pain score. Thus, scores can be similar between two study groups because the amount of pain medication has been different [31].

The method to measure and report postoperative pain is not standardised, which makes it difficult to compare the VAS across studies in an attempt to extract general conclusions about surgical technique in this respect. We are more or less limited to the differences observed in individual randomised trials; the general conclusion about a better method of pain control rests with the availability of several similar studies showing the same direction of change. Whatever limitation is associated with measuring pain, the VAS targets the key dimension for any attempt to find a less painful treatment.

Operation under local anaesthetic

The anus is particularly sensitive and injection into the anoderm or sphincters usually requires conscious sedation or topical local anaesthetic (EMLA cream) [7, 9, 10]. Marti described a technique of blocking the posterior ischiorectal fossa combined with infiltration of the commisure anterior to the anus but avoiding infiltration of the anus itself [6]. A series of 400 haemorrhoidectomies with this posterior block

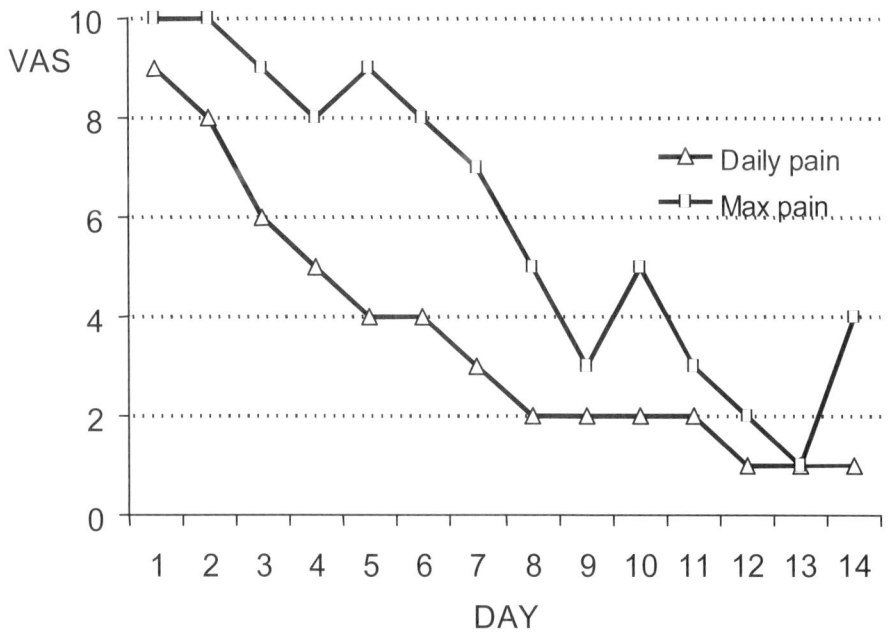

Figure 1. Example of self-reported postoperative pain using a 10-pointed visual analogue scale (VAS) in a patient operated for haemorrhoids, clearly showing the character of the two types of pain.

but supplemented with 360 degree subcutaneous infiltration and of the haemorrhoid pedicle, was reported. Only 6% of the patients needed supplementation with fentanyl intravenously. The duration of pain relief exceeded 5 hours in 68% [7]. Another report used this posterior block for stapled anopexy and supplemented the block with injection deep into the intersphincteric space under cover of intravenous fentanyl [69].

A simplification of the posterior block was described by the authors [8]. This peri-anal block targets the nerve endings to the anal sphincter by infiltration in the ischiorectal fat immediately peripheral to the sphincter. The anus itself is not injected at all, which avoids the necessity for conscious sedation. The peri-anal block renders the sphincters and the anal canal completely anaesthetised in its infralevator extension and is now our standard procedure for day cases. Inserting the mucosal suture in a case of a stapled anopexy is painless, but closure of the stapler can hurt because the staple line is at or above the levator. Infiltration of the submucosa under the purse string with a small amount of local anaesthetic prevents this pain.

Both the anaesthetic and surgical methods have developed to a point where the traditional infiltration of the anoderm, submucosa and intersphincteric space with adrenaline and local anaesthetic agent has become irrelevant. Apart from being painful we believe it also impairs precise diathermy dissection.

Day-case surgery

Ambulatory surgery is a strong incentive to modify operations and anaesthetic methods to become less painful, as the patient cannot be sent home with disturbing pain or if drowsy from opiate analgesics. The risk of postoperative bleeding must be made minimal. Because the operative field is dry there is no need for an anal pack or specific dressing. Such changes can be reflected in the postoperative care. The patients can be telephoned the next day and, if the situation is satisfactory, be seen in the outpatient

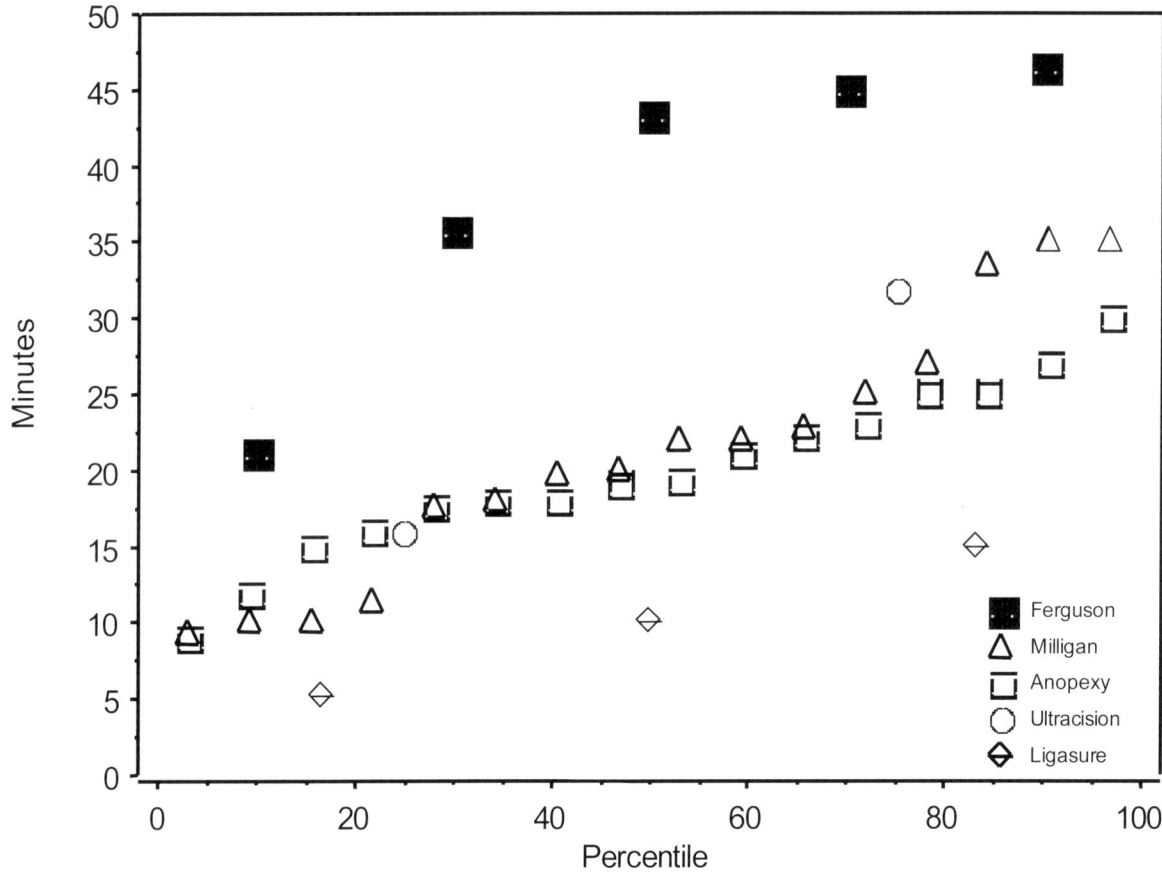

Figure 2. The distribution of operation time with regard to applied operation. Compiled from published randomised trials.

clinic only to record the final outcome after 2-4 months. A nurse in the outpatient clinic who patients can contact is desirable. Few patients (5%) will present as an emergency case because of urinary retention, excessive pain, or an unexpected bleed.

Day-case conventional haemorrhoidectomy has been described to work well, as has day-case stapled anopexy - which is easier because the pain is less [56, 69-74]. One randomised study of stapled anopexy versus diathermy haemorrhoidectomy showed that 80% and 97% respectively were managed as day cases. The failures were mainly due to anaesthetic adverse effects with dizziness and nausea or inability to void [57].

Where are we going?

The new surgical methods for treating prolapsed haemorrhoids have invited a large number of prospective randomised clinical trials. Indeed, symptomatic haemorrhoids are probably now the surgical disease that has the greatest evidence-based foundation. It has largely evolved through the application of new devices that have been the real subject of evaluation. Whether the choice is "ectomy", by whichever method, or "pexy", they both appear to provide similar results. In such circumstances, the ultimate preference might depend on what is cheaper, faster and easier. Traditional diathermy excision is certainly the cheapest, but it is neither easier nor faster than, for instance, Ultracision or Ligasure excision. The circular stapler needed for the anopexy operation costs more than the disposables needed for Ultracision and Ligasure, but it does not require the investment for the power generators of the latter.

The operation time is remarkably different, by at least a factor of two, across the randomised trials (Figure 2). It is unlikely that the difference is entirely explained by the variation between slow and fast surgeons. It probably reflects the fact that haemorrhoidectomy is not the same thing in the mind of all surgeons. Some surgeons painstakingly clean out as much as possible of the internal and external haemorrhoid plexa while others pay attention only to the prolapsing piles. Such a difference may in turn reflect how the surgeon understands the nature of the pathology involved in symptomatic haemorrhoids. In particular, do symptomatic haemorrhoids represent an enlargement of a vascular bed, making it a vascular disease as classified in ICD 10 and previous versions of the international classification of diseases?

We think it is likely that surgeons will increasingly view haemorrhoids as a disease of prolapse. One might speak of muco-anal prolapse, in which the haemorrhoid itself is a companion, or even an epiphenomenon, to the prolapsing excessive mucosa of the lower rectum. This would group muco-anal prolapse among intussusception and rectal prolapse as an entity by and in itself, although combined or intermediate forms of the three entities are occurring. The mucosal prolapse can be assessed by inserting a swab into the rectum of the anaesthetised patient, followed by retraction of the swab, to mimic the passage of a faecal bolus. The so visualised prolapse appears important to explain the symptoms. We find the evidence strongly in favour of Thompson, who examined three theories about the pathogenesis of haemorrhoids and concluded that prolapse was positively supported [75]. Thus, we expect that future versions of the ICD will re-classify haemorrhoids among anorectal diseases.

The evidence from the now many randomised clinical trials that have compared stapled anopexy with excison of the piles clearly shows that either operation effectively relieves the patient of a prolapse that required manual reduction. The associated symptoms, such as bleeding, pain, soiling and pruritus have also been greatly reduced. This leads to a conclusion that the collateral symptoms are a consequence of the prolapse. Extrapolated, it may be inferred that symptomatic haemorrhoids are always associated with muco-anal prolapse. Such an understanding may have implications for the choice of treatment, as any treatment must effectively remove, destroy or fix the prolapsing mucosa.

A meta-analysis has shown that surgery provides better symptom control of longer duration [20, 76]. Patients who present with frequent complaints of any of the haemorrhoid-associated symptoms and who have a thick rectal mucosa will stand a better chance of cure from an operation than from repetitive banding or injection. We believe the future management of muco-anal prolapse will be based on a single treatment session, more often an operation under local anaesthetic block, in day surgery.

It is time to disregard the former operations and their postoperative pain. The younger surgeon, unburdened with tradition and deficient training, might come to a fresh conclusion as to how haemorrhoids should be treated by a close examination of the recent literature. They might agree with us that the anatomy of the disease is excessive mucosa of the lower rectum and a sliding down of that mucosa together with the haemorrhoids into or outside the anal canal on moving the bowels. The symptoms then derive from trauma within the anal canal, especially the bleeding and pain. This means that the particular treatment must be capable of preventing the prolapse, by either its excision or its fixation. At hand are many choices, but the surgeon will chose three: rubber band ligation, diathermy excision and circular stapler anopexy. The selection is based upon published evidence of effectiveness; their mastery will allow the surgeon to manage all relevant situations. The surgeon will choose rubber banding for minor symptoms in patients who deny the need to reduce the prolapse manually. He or she will choose stapled anopexy whenever there is overt mucosal prolapse but an absence of a major external component of anodermal tags and polyps. Large external components are best treated by excision, either alone or combined with anopexy to remove the redundant mucosa first.

The operation will be performed in day surgery under local anaesthetic block. A small pre-operative enema to empty the rectum will suffice. Antibiotic prophylaxis is superfluous. The patient will be operated prone for the convenience of the patient and ergonometric concerns of the surgeon. The operation will target the prolapse but preserve as much as possible of the anoderm and lining of the anal canal. In particular, fascia covering the internal sphincter and under the anoderm will be preserved when excision is chosen. Intermediate haemorrhoids and the external plexus will be disregarded, as they are not part of the prolapse. The operation will take between 20 and 30 minutes. The operative field will be dry without need for a dressing. A non-steroidal anti-inflammatory drug, such as diclofenac, will control the pain in the majority. In cases of excision, a mild laxative such as Movicol (polyethylene glycol) postoperatively will be used, while anopexy patients do not need such help. About half the patients will return to work within a week. About 90% of patients selected for an operation will be treated in this way.

References

1. Goligher J. *Surgery of the Anus, Rectum and Colon*, 4th Ed. Balliere-Tindall, London, 1980.
2. Corman M. *Colon and Rectal Surgery*, 4th Ed. Lippincott-Raven, Philadelphia, 1998.
3. Jensen SL, Harling H, Arseth-hansen P, et al. The natural history of symptomatic haemorrhoids. *Int J Colorectal Dis* 1989; 4: 41-4.
4. Konsten J, Baeten CG. Hemorrhoidectomy vs. Lord's method: 17-year follow-up of a prospective, randomized trial. *Dis Colon Rectum* 2000; 43: 503-6.
5. Johannsson HO, Graf W, Pahlman L. Long-term results of haemorrhoidectomy. *Eur J Surg* 2002; 168: 485-9.
6. Marti M. Loco-regional anaesthesia in proctological surgery. *Ann Chir* 1993; 47: 250-5.
7. Gabrielli F, Cioffi U, Chiarelli M, et al. Hemorrhoidectomy with posterior perineal block: experience with 400 cases. *Dis Colon Rectum* 2000; 43: 809-12.
8. Nystrom PO, Derwinger K, Gerjy R. Local perianal block for anal surgery. *Tech Coloproctol* 2004; 8: 23-6.
9. Ho KS, Eu KW, Heah SM, et al. Randomized clinical trial of haemorrhoidectomy under a mixture of local anaesthesia versus general anaesthesia. *Br J Surg* 2000; 87: 410-3.
10. Read TE, Henry SE, Hovis RM, et al. Prospective evaluation of anesthetic technique for anorectal surgery. *Dis Colon Rectum* 2002; 45: 1553-8; discussion 1558-60.
11. Bursics A, Morvay K, Kupcsulik P, et al. Comparison of early and 1-year follow-up results of conventional hemorrhoid-ectomy and hemorrhoid artery ligation: a randomized study. *Int J Colorectal Dis* 2004; 19: 176-80.
12. Lunniss PJ, Mann CV. Classification of internal haemorrhoids: a discussion paper. *Colorectal Dis* 2004; 6: 226-32.
13. Murie JA, Sim AJ, Mackenzie I. The importance of pain, pruritus and soiling as symptoms of haemorrhoids and their response to haemorrhoidectomy or rubber band ligation. *Br J Surg* 1981; 68: 247-9.
14. Armstrong DN. Multiple hemorrhoidal ligation: a prospective, randomized trial evaluating a new technique. *Dis Colon Rectum* 2003; 46: 179-86.
15. Morinaga K, Hasuda K, Ikeda T. A novel therapy for internal hemorrhoids: ligation of the hemorrhoidal artery with a newly devised instrument (Moricorn) in conjunction with a Doppler flowmeter. *Am J Gastroenterol* 1995; 90: 610-3.
16. Arnold S, Antonietti E, Rollinger G, et al. [Doppler ultrasound-assisted hemorrhoid artery ligation. A new therapy in symptomatic hemorrhoids]. *Chirurg* 2002; 73: 269-73.
17. Narro JL. [Hemorrhoid therapy with Doppler-guided hemorrhoidal artery ligation via proctoscope KM-25. A new alternative to hemorrhoidectomy and rubber band ligation?]. *Zentralbl Chir* 2004; 129: 208-10.
18. Hussein AM. Ligation-anopexy for treatment of advanced hemorrhoidal disease. *Dis Colon Rectum* 2001; 44: 1887-90.
19. Aigner F, Bodner G, Conrad F, et al. The superior rectal artery and its branching pattern with regard to its clinical influence on ligation techniques for internal hemorrhoids. *Am J Surg* 2004; 187: 102-8.
20. MacRae HM, McLeod RS. Comparison of hemorrhoidal treatment modalities. A meta-analysis. *Dis Colon Rectum* 1995; 38: 687-94.
21. Johanson JF, Rimm A. Optimal nonsurgical treatment of hemorrhoids: a comparative analysis of infrared coagulation, rubber band ligation, and injection sclerotherapy. *Am J Gastroenterol* 1992; 87: 1600-6.
22. Kanellos I, Goulimaris I, Christoforidis E, et al. A comparison of the simultaneous application of sclerotherapy and rubber band ligation, with sclerotherapy and rubber band ligation applied separately, for the treatment of haemorrhoids: a prospective randomized trial. *Colorectal Dis* 2003; 5: 133-8.
23. Hooker GD, Plewes EA, Rajgopal C, et al. Local injection of bupivacaine after rubber band ligation of hemorrhoids: prospective, randomized study. *Dis Colon Rectum* 1999; 42: 174-9.
24. Law WL, Chu KW. Triple rubber band ligation for hemorrhoids: prospective, randomized trial of use of local anesthetic injection. *Dis Colon Rectum* 1999; 42: 363-6.
25. Gokalp A, Baskonus I, Maralcan G. A prospective randomised study of local anaesthetic injection after multiple rubber band ligation of haemorrhoids. *Chir Ital* 2003; 55: 213-7.

26. Peng BC, Jayne DG, Ho YH. Randomized trial of rubber band ligation vs. stapled hemorrhoidectomy for prolapsed piles. *Dis Colon Rectum* 2003; 46: 291-7; discussion 296-7.
27. Murie JA, Sim AJ, Mackenzie I. Rubber band ligation versus haemorrhoidectomy for prolapsing haemorrhoids: a long-term prospective clinical trial. *Br J Surg* 1982; 69: 536-8.
28. Steinberg DM, Liegois H, Alexander-Williams J. Long-term review of the results of rubber band ligation of haemorrhoids. *Br J Surg* 1975; 62: 144-6.
29. Correa-Rovelo J, Tellez O, Obregon L, et al. Stapled rectal mucosectomy vs. closed hemorrhoidectomy: a randomized, clinical trial. *Dis Colon Rectum* 2002; 45: 1374-5.
30. Sharif H, Lee L, Alexander-Williams J. Diathermy haemorrhoidectomy. *Int J Colorectal Dis* 1991; 6: 217-219.
31. Seow-Choen F, Ho YH, Ang HG, et al. Prospective, randomized trial comparing pain and clinical function after conventional scissors excision/ligation vs. diathermy excision without ligation for symptomatic prolapsed hemorrhoids. *Dis Colon Rectum* 1992; 35: 1165-9.
32. Andrews BT, Layer GT, Jackson BT, et al. Randomized trial comparing diathermy hemorrhoidectomy with the scissor dissection Milligan-Morgan operation. *Dis Colon Rectum* 1993; 36: 580-3.
33. Ibrahim S, Tsang C, Lee YL, et al. Prospective, randomized trial comparing pain and complications between diathermy and scissors for closed hemorrhoidectomy. *Dis Colon Rectum* 1998; 41: 1418-20.
34. Lawes DA, Palazzo FF, Francis DL, et al. One-year follow-up of a randomized trial comparing Ligasure with open haemorrhoidectomy. *Colorectal Dis* 2004; 6: 233-5.
35. Palazzo FF, Francis DL, Clifton MA. Randomized clinical trial of Ligasure versus open haemorrhoidectomy. *Br J Surg* 2002; 89: 154-7.
36. Jayne DG, Botterill I, Ambrose NS, et al. Randomized clinical trial of Ligasure versus conventional diathermy for day-case haemorrhoidectomy. *Br J Surg* 2002; 89: 428-32.
37. Franklin EJ, Seetharam S, Lowney J, et al. Randomized, clinical trial of Ligasure vs conventional diathermy in hemorrhoidectomy. *Dis Colon Rectum* 2003; 46: 1380-3.
38. Armstrong DN, Ambroze WL, Schertzer ME, et al. Harmonic scalpel vs. electrocautery hemorrhoidectomy: a prospective evaluation. *Dis Colon Rectum* 2001; 44: 558-64.
39. Khan S, Pawlak SE, Eggenberger JC, et al. Surgical treatment of hemorrhoids: prospective, randomized trial comparing closed excisional hemorrhoidectomy and the harmonic scalpel technique of excisional hemorrhoidectomy. *Dis Colon Rectum* 2001; 44: 845-9.
40. Chung CC, Ha JP, Tai YP, et al. Double-blind, randomized trial comparing harmonic scalpel hemorrhoidectomy, bipolar scissors hemorrhoidectomy, and scissors excision: ligation technique. *Dis Colon Rectum* 2002; 45: 789-94.
41. Jayne DG, Botterill I, Ambrose NS, et al. Randomized clinical trial of Ligasure™ versus conventional diathermy for day-case haemorrhoidectomy. *Br J Surg* 2002; 89: 428-32.
42. Chung YC, Wu HJ. Clinical experience of sutureless closed hemorrhoidectomy with LigaSure. *Dis Colon Rectum* 2003; 46: 87-92.
43. Longo A. Treatment of haemorrhoids disease by reduction of mucosa and hemorrhoidal prolapse with a circular suturing device: new procedure. In: 6th World Congress of Endoscopic Surgery. Rome, Italy, 3-6 June 1998; 777-90.
44. Longo A. Stapled anopexy and stapled hemorrhoidectomy: two opposite concepts and procedures. *Dis Colon Rectum* 2002; 45: 571-2; discussion 572.
45. Corman ML, Gravie JF, Hager T, et al. Stapled haemorrhoidopexy: a consensus position paper by an international working party - indications, contra-indications and technique. *Colorectal Dis* 2003; 5: 304-10.
46. Beattie G, Loudon M. Circumferential stapled anoplasty in the management of haemorrhoids and mucosal prolapse. *Colorectal Dis* 2000; 2: 170-5.
47. Shalaby R, Desoky A. Randomized clinical trial of stapled versus Milligan-Morgan haemorrhoidectomy. *Br J Surg* 2001; 88: 1049-53.
48. Rowsell M, Bello M, Hemingway DM. Circumferential mucosectomy (stapled haemorrhoidectomy) versus conventional haemorrhoidectomy: randomised controlled trial. *Lancet* 2000; 355: 779-81.
49. Mehigan BJ, Monson JR, Hartley JE. Stapling procedure for haemorrhoids versus Milligan-Morgan haemorrhoidectomy: randomised controlled trial. *Lancet* 2000; 355: 782-5.
50. Ganio E, Altomare DF, Gabrielli F, et al. Prospective randomized multicentre trial comparing stapled with open haemorrhoidectomy. *Br J Surg* 2001; 88: 669-74.
51. Au-Yong I, Rowsell M, Hemingway DM. Randomised controlled clinical trial of stapled haemorrhoidectomy vs conventional haemorrhoidectomy; a three and a half year follow-up. *Colorectal Dis* 2004; 6: 37-8.
52. Ho YH, Cheong WK, Tsang C, et al. Stapled hemorrhoidectomy - cost and effectiveness. Randomized, controlled trial including incontinence scoring, anorectal manometry, and endoanal ultrasound assessments at up to three months. *Dis Colon Rectum* 2000; 43: 1666-75.
53. Pavlidis T, Papaziogas B, Souparis A, et al. Modern stapled Longo procedure vs. conventional Milligan-Morgan hemorrhoidectomy: a randomized controlled trial. *Int J Colorectal Dis* 2002; 17: 50-3.
54. Ortiz H, Marzo J, Armendariz P. Randomized clinical trial of stapled haemorrhoidopexy versus conventional diathermy haemorrhoidectomy. *Br J Surg* 2002; 89: 1376-81.
55. Racalbuto A, Aliotta I, Corsaro G, et al. Hemorrhoidal stapler prolapsectomy vs. Milligan-Morgan hemorrhoidectomy: a long-term randomized trial. *Int J Colorectal Dis* 2004; 19: 239-44.
56. Guy RJ, Ng CE, Eu KW. Stapled anoplasty for haemorrhoids: a comparison of ambulatory vs. in-patient procedures. *Colorectal Dis* 2003; 5: 29-32.
57. Kairaluoma M, Nuorva K, Kellokumpu I. Day-case stapled (circular) vs. diathermy hemorrhoidectomy: a randomized, controlled trial evaluating surgical and functional outcome. *Dis Colon Rectum* 2003; 46: 93-9.
58. Boccasanta P, Capretti PG, Venturi M, et al. Randomised controlled trial between stapled circumferential mucosectomy and conventional circular hemorrhoidectomy in advanced

hemorrhoids with external mucosal prolapse. *Am J Surg* 2001; 182: 64-8.
59. Luck AJ, Hewett PJ. Ischiorectal fossa block decreases posthemorrhoidectomy pain: randomized, prospective, double-blind clinical trial. *Dis Colon Rectum* 2000; 43: 142-5.
60. Vinson-Bonnet B, Coltat JC, Fingerhut A, *et al*. Local infiltration with ropivacaine improves immediate postoperative pain control after hemorrhoidal surgery. *Dis Colon Rectum* 2002; 45: 104-8.
61. Asfar SK, Juma TH, Ala-Edeen T. Hemorrhoidectomy and sphincterotomy. A prospective study comparing the effectiveness of anal stretch and sphincterotomy in reducing pain after hemorrhoidectomy. *Dis Colon Rectum* 1988; 31: 181-5.
62. Mathai V, Ong BC, Ho YH. Randomized controlled trial of lateral internal sphincterotomy with haemorrhoidectomy. *Br J Surg* 1996; 83: 380-2.
63. Ho YH, Seow-Choen F, Low JY, *et al*. Randomized controlled trial of trimebutine (anal sphincter relaxant) for pain after haemorrhoidectomy. *Br J Surg* 1997; 84: 377-9.
64. Coskun A, Duzgun SA, Uzunkoy A, *et al*. Nitroderm TTS band application for pain after hemorrhoidectomy. *Dis Colon Rectum* 2001; 44: 680-5.
65. Davies J, Duffy D, Boyt N, *et al*. Botulinum toxin (botox) reduces pain after hemorrhoidectomy: results of a double-blind, randomized study. *Dis Colon Rectum* 2003; 46: 1097-102.
66. Carapeti EA, Kamm MA, McDonald PJ, *et al*. Double-blind randomised controlled trial of effect of metronidazole on pain after day-case haemorrhoidectomy. *Lancet* 1998; 351: 169-72.
67. Balfour L, Stojkovic SG, Botterill ID, *et al*. A randomized, double-blind trial of the effect of metronidazole on pain after closed hemorrhoidectomy. *Dis Colon Rectum* 2002; 45: 1186-90; discussion 1190-1.
68. Nicholson TJ, Armstrong D. Topical metronidazole (10 percent) decreases posthemorrhoidectomy pain and improves healing. *Dis Colon Rectum* 2004; 47: 711-6.
69. Gabrielli F, Chiarelli M, Cioffi U, *et al*. Day surgery for mucosal-hemorrhoidal prolapse using a circular stapler and modified regional anesthesia. *Dis Colon Rectum* 2001; 44: 842-4.
70. Carapeti EA, Kamm MA, McDonald PJ, *et al*. Randomized trial of open versus closed day-case haemorrhoidectomy. *Br J Surg* 1999; 86: 612-3.
71. Hunt L, Luck A, Rudkin G, *et al*. Day-case haemorrhoidectomy. *Br J Surg* 1999; 86: 255-8.
72. Singer MA, Cintron JR, Fleshman JW, *et al*. Early experience with stapled hemorrhoidectomy in the United States. *Dis Colon Rectum* 2002; 45: 360-7; discussion 367-9.
73. Cheetham MJ, Cohen CR, Kamm MA, *et al*. A randomized, controlled trial of diathermy hemorrhoidectomy vs. stapled hemorrhoidectomy in an intended day-care setting with longer-term follow-up. *Dis Colon Rectum* 2003; 46: 491-7.
74. Arroyo A, Perez F, Miranda E, *et al*. Open versus closed day-case haemorrhoidectomy: is there any difference? Results of a prospective randomised study. *Int J Colorectal Dis* 2004; 19: 370-3.
75. Thompson W. The nature of haemorrhoids. *Br J Surg* 1975; 62: 542-52.
76. MacRae HM, McLeod RS. Comparison of hemorrhoidal treatments: a meta-analysis. *Can J Surg* 1997; 40: 14-7.

Chapter 19

The treatment of anal fissures

Philip J Conaghan MA MRCS, Specialist Registrar, General Surgery
Ridzuan Farouk MCh FRCS (Glas) FRCS (Ed) FRCS, Consultant in Colorectal Surgery
Royal Berkshire Hospital, Reading, UK

What is the problem?

Anal fissures are tears in the skin of the distal anal canal usually presenting with severe anal pain and fresh rectal bleeding. The pain is often characterised as being worst at the time of a bowel action and lasting for several hours following this. Although they can occur at any age they are more common in young adults and those occurring in older patients need to be treated with a higher level of suspicion (see Table 1). Classical fissures-in-ano are single and in the midline, with 99% of these fissures in men and 90% in women in the posterior midline. Multiple or non-midline fissures should again raise the possibility of another anorectal process.

Fissures can be defined as acute or chronic based on the duration of symptoms and the morphology of the fissure and surrounding anal skin. The distinction, however, is arbitrary as far as treatment is concerned, although it does serve a purpose in defining entry criteria into trials of treatment since acute fissures are more likely to heal with conservative measures.

Treatment of anal fissures has evolved as the pathophysiology of the condition has been understood.

Pathophysiology of anal fissures

The traditional theory of the development of anal fissures involves a traumatic event in the anal canal in a susceptible patient with a hypertonic anal sphincter. The trauma is often caused by a hard stool. The subsequent failure to heal the wound is due to local ischaemia caused by the hypertonic sphincter. Studies have demonstrated a reduced perfusion of the anoderm [1] which improves following lateral sphincterotomy [2], and a reduced vessel density at the posterior midline [3]. In addition, clinical studies have demonstrated higher anal resting pressures in patients with fissures compared to normal controls [4] and this is associated with a reduction in the number of spontaneous relaxation events [5]. The hypertonia has been found to persist even after the fissure has healed [6].

However, there are problems with such a theory. The lack of a clear initiating event in the history of many patients with anal fissures raises the possibility that no overt traumatic event is necessary for the development of anal fissures. In addition, there is a subset of patients with normal or hypotonic sphincter pressures who develop fissures. This is most commonly seen in post-partum women [7]. We may simply have to regard these as a different pathology.

Table 1. Aetiology of anal fissures.

- Idiopathic
- Post-partum
- Secondary fissures
    Infection
        - Syphilis
        - TB
    Immunosuppression
    Crohn's disease
    Malignancy
- Trauma

Beyond conservative therapy, such as local anaesthesia, stool softeners and dietary modification, most treatments have been targeted at reducing the anal sphincter resting pressure, either pharmacologically or surgically.

Where are we now?

The move away from surgical to medical treatment as first-line therapy for chronic fissures has been largely due to the threat of incontinence that surgery carries. This review of current treatment will be subdivided into conservative, medical and surgical, although a combination of these categories is often what is employed.

Conservative treatment

Acute fissures are successfully healed by conservative measures in at least 50% of patients. These include dietary modifications, especially bran supplementation, stool softeners and local anaesthetic ointment. The reason that such measures are rarely successful in the surgical clinic is that few fissures persist by the time of a surgical consultation other than chronic. Acute fissures are seen by the primary care physician and if conservative therapy is successful, a surgical consultation is rarely requested. Most studies of conservative therapy are retrospective and, of course, contain patients who may have healed without any treatment. However, one randomised controlled trial (RCT) recruiting a useful number of patients with acute fissures noticed a significant reduction in relapse rates using 15g bran daily compared to placebo [8]. Studies comparing lignocaine, hydrocortisone or bran in a 3-way study showed healing rates of 60%, 82% and 88% respectively at 3 weeks, although there was no statistical difference between the groups [9].

Medical treatment

Pharmacological treatment for anal fissures has been aimed at reducing the resting tone of the anal sphincters. The internal anal sphincter is responsible for 70% of the resting tone of the sphincter complex and so most treatment has focused on this (Figure 1). The main advantage of such treatment over surgery is that it

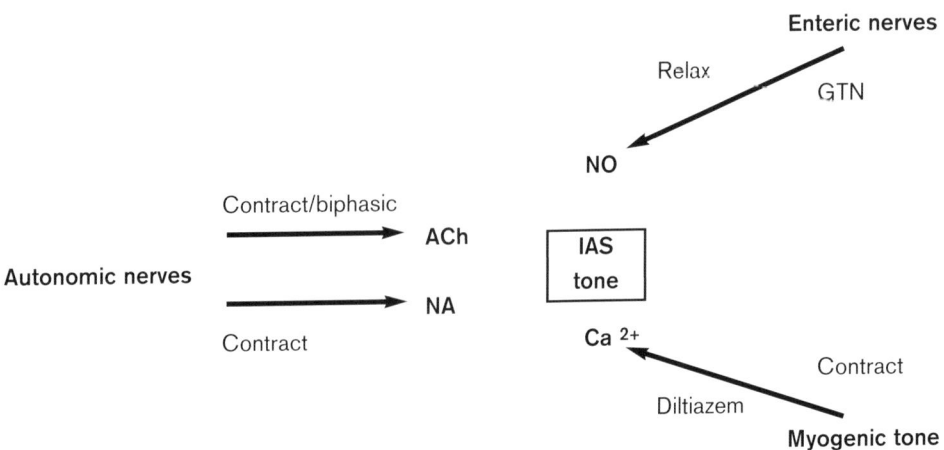

Figure 1. Internal anal sphincter neuropharmacology.

Table 2. Drugs used in clinical studies for anal fissures.

- Nitric oxide donors
    - GTN
    - ISDN
- Calcium-channel antagonists (oral and topical)
    - Nifedipine
    - Diltiazem
- Botulinum toxin A
- Cholinergic agonists
    - Bethanecol
- Alpha-1 adrenergic antagonists
    - Indoramin
- Hyperbaric O_2

produces a transient reduction in sphincter tone, which is reversed once the drug is stopped. Drugs that have been subject to study are listed in Table 2. Three main treatment groups have received most attention: nitrates, calcium-channel antagonists and botulinum toxin A.

Topical nitric oxide donors

Neurogenic relaxation of the internal anal sphincter is mediated by nitric oxide [10]; hence, the interest in topical preparations that will increase the local concentration of nitric oxide. The vast majority of studies have focused on GTN as the nitric oxide donor. Results have been varied. The first placebo-controlled double-blind RCT randomised 80 patients [11]. They found 68% healing in the treatment group compared with 8% treated with placebo at 8 weeks. This was associated with an increase in anodermal blood flow and a reduction in pain in the treatment group. Carapeti et al [12] also showed encouraging results with two different concentrations of GTN. They reported 67% healing in the GTN groups vs 32% receiving placebo at 8 weeks, but no advantage in using the higher GTN concentration. However, other studies show lower healing rates, especially those with longer follow-up. Libertiny et al [13] showed a 46% healing rate at 2 years after an initial 54% healed at 8 weeks in a study randomising patients to 0.2% GTN or lateral internal sphincterotomy (LIS). Richard et al [14], on behalf of the Canadian Colorectal Surgical Trials Group, published a multicentre trial, again randomising between GTN and LIS. Of the 44 patients taking GTN, only 29.5% had complete healing of the fissure. One large multicentre study in Italy [15] failed to show any benefit of GTN over placebo (49.2% healed with GTN vs 51.7% with placebo), although the large number of patients healed in the placebo group must give rise to questions about the number of acute fissures in this study. Randomised studies involving topical GTN are summarised in Table 3, where the results for the GTN itself are shown.

Table 3. Randomised trials involving topical 0.2% GTN for chronic anal fissures.

1st author	No. of patients in GTN group	Comparison	Duration of therapy	Duration of follow-up	Healing
Lund & Scholefield [11]	38	Placebo	8 weeks	4 months	68%
Carapeti [12]	46	Placebo	8 weeks	9 months	67%
Kennedy [16]	24	Placebo	4 weeks	29 months	46%
Brisinda [34]	25	BTA	6 weeks	16 months	60%
Altomare [15]	59	Placebo	4 weeks	29 months	49%
Richard [14]	44	LIS	6 weeks	6 months	27%
Evans [38]	33	LIS	8 weeks	5 months	61%
Libertiny [13]	39	LIS	8 weeks	2 years	46%
Ezri & Susmallian [27]	26	Nifedipine	11 weeks	8 months	58%

LIS=lateral internal sphincterotomy

An additional problem with GTN is the frequency of side effects, especially headaches, reported in the studies. This was as high as 84% in the Canadian multicentre study. In the placebo-controlled trials the frequency varied from 29-65%. This has led to the early cessation of treatment in some patients and may account for the high failure rates in some studies. Wearing gloves for cream application and pre-emptive analgesia have been suggested as ways of reducing side effects to help patients complete the course of treatment.

Recurrence rates with GTN have also caused concern in the literature. Five of 13 patients recurred in the Canadian Trials Group [14] with three responding to further GTN and one healing without further treatment. Carapeti reported a 33% relapse rate with GTN within 9 months [12]. In a retrospective study by Jonas et al [17], 49 of 72 patients were successfully treated initially with GTN but by 6 months 25 of these had recurrent symptoms, 16 of whom had further GTN with two failing this subsequent treatment. The high recurrence rate may be partly due to the definition of healing. Some studies use the absence of pain as a treatment success, although the fissure may persist despite the alleviation of symptoms. It may be that early recurrence is due to inadequately treated fissures in the first instance.

Isosorbide dinitrate has also been used as the nitric oxide donor in treatment regimens [18-19] and L-arginine has been used in physiological studies but not investigated for fissure healing [20].

Calcium-channel blockade

Calcium movement into cells and release from intracellular stores is known to be important in the maintenance of tone and contraction in the internal anal sphincter [21].

Both oral and topical calcium-channel blockers have been shown to reduce anal sphincter tone and to aid fissure healing. Most studies have looked at topical preparations. Jonas et al compared the two routes with 60mg diltiazem bd orally and 2% diltiazem gel bd topically [22]. They found that both preparations reduced the mean resting pressure of the anal sphincters but the topical preparation was more effective at healing fissures (15 of 26 patients) than the oral medication (9/24 patients) and with fewer side effects. One study did compare GTN (0.5%) with 2% diltiazem in 43 patients [23]. The healing in the GTN group was far higher than in other published series, which was unusual (86% for both treatments), but side effects were more prevalent in the GTN group (33% for GTN vs 0% for diltiazem). Conclusions from prospective studies using 2% diltiazem agree that it is as effective as GTN and has fewer side effects. Knight et al [24] treated 71 patients with 2% diltiazem with 51 (75%) healing after a median of 9 weeks' treatment and a further eight patients healing after a second 8-week treatment period. They noted recurrences in 17% of 41 patients that were available for long-term follow-up for as long as 67 weeks. A similar study by Griffin et al [25] showed fissure healing in 22/46 patients who had previously failed to heal with a course of GTN. A further ten patients in their study were improved symptomatically, requiring no further treatment.

Nifedipine cream has also been used with some success. A recent randomised study compared a nifedipine/local anaesthetic mixture to hydrocortisone/local anaesthetic in 110 patients. At 1 year they reported healing in 93% of fissures - two following a second course of diltiazem for recurrence of the fissure. This was compared with 16% in the hydrocortisone (control) group [26]. A further randomised trial [27] comparing the same ointment to GTN found that nifedipine was superior to GTN for healing (89 vs 58%; p<0.04) and with fewer side effects at 6 months (although both had high rates of recurrence within this time frame). In conclusion, the calcium-channel blockers applied as an ointment seem to be at least as effective as GTN, but with fewer side effects.

Botulinum toxin

Botulinum toxin A (BTA) has an expanding list of indications. There have been a number of studies since the first report in 1993 [28]. Studies have used a variety of doses and sites of injections. The mode of action in the treatment of anal fissures is still unclear. In striated muscle BTA reduces ACh-release (acetylcholine) from the pre-synaptic terminal of the neuromuscular junction, and the initial experience used injections into the striated external anal sphincter (EAS) as a way of reducing anal sphincter tone [29] with 82% healing reported at 3 months in a series of 100 patients, falling to 79% at 6 months. However, injection into the internal anal sphincter (IAS) has also been shown to reduce sphincter tone [30], despite the fact that cholinergic innervation to the IAS produces relaxation of the muscle. It has recently been suggested from *in vitro* studies that the action of BTA on the IAS may be through the blockade of sympathetic neural output, reducing NA release at the neuromuscular junction [31]. BTA may also act as an analgesic [32], thus reducing the additional pain-related sphincter spasm and so contribute to fissure healing.

Maria *et al* [33] reported a placebo-controlled randomised trial of 20 units of BTA injection into the IAS in 30 patients. In addition to showing a reduction in mean resting anal pressure in the BTA group, they found 73% healing at 2 months compared with 13% in the control group (p=0.003). In addition, 7/10 healed with BTA injection in the cross-over arm of the study. A double-blind randomised controlled trial [34] comparing 0.2% GTN and 20U BTA in 50 patients again found excellent healing in the BTA group (24/25 at 2 months) which was significantly better than GTN (15/25; p=0.005). The subsequent cross-over of 10 patients achieved healing for all of them. Certainly from studies available, BTA seems to be highly effective for first-line treatment of anal fissures with very few side effects, although cost and convenience remain issues.

Other medical treatments

Bethanecol, a cholinergic agonist [35], and hyperbaric oxygen [36] have both been used in small studies for the treatment of chronic anal fissures with some success. Indoramin, an alpha-1-adrenoreceptor antagonist, failed to heal fissures compared to placebo in a small randomised controlled trial, although it did reduce mean anal resting pressures [37].

Surgical treatment

Surgery remains the treatment most likely to heal an anal fissure. However, it carries with it not only the general risks of surgery and anaesthesia, but a risk of faecal or flatus incontinence. As far as the procedure of choice is concerned, the literature is consistent. Essentially for classical idiopathic anal fissures associated with raised sphincter tone, the lateral internal sphincterotomy is the treatment of choice. For those idiopathic fissures associated with normal or low pressure sphincters or in the presence of a previous sphincter injury, an anal advancement flap should be considered.

Lateral internal sphincterotomy (LIS)

The operative division of the internal sphincter has been subject to extensive investigation and is generally found to be efficacious compared to both medical treatment and other surgical techniques. Healing rates are generally high, but the incidence of incontinence has been variable. Early studies tended to lack standardisation of reporting of complications, but more recently, with some acceptance of incontinence scores, different studies are more amenable to comparison.

When compared with GTN ointment, which might have been considered the best available medical therapy, LIS tends to have a higher rate of healing. The Canadian Colorectal Surgical Trials Group [14] randomised 82 patients to LIS or GTN and assessed these at 6 weeks and 6 months. They found a better healing rate in the LIS group at 6 months (92% vs 27%) but interestingly, no disturbance in continence in the LIS group. Libertiny *et al* [13] randomised 70 patients to the same two groups with similar healing rates at a longer follow-up period of 2 years. LIS healed 34/35 patients (97%) compared to 46% with GTN. Very similar results were seen in an Australian study [38].

The complication profile of LIS remains a matter of debate, however. It is obviously important to identify factors which contribute to complications as a result of the procedure or impact on the rate of reporting of such complications. Four factors seem to predominate:

- Length and type of follow-up.
- Length of sphincterotomy.
- Operative injury to the external sphincter.
- Patient selection.

Nyam and Pemberton described a 13-year experience of 585 patients who underwent LIS [39]. They were followed-up by questionnaire after a mean of more than 5 years. Although transient incontinence was high (45%), this fell to 15% at the time of the questionnaire (14% flatus and minor soiling, 1% solid stool); 98% of patients reported being satisfied with the outcome of their surgery. However, much higher rates of incontinence have been reported. Garcia-Aguilar et al [40] had 549 (64%) respondents to a questionnaire in a retrospective review of patients who had undergone open or closed LIS an average of 3 years previously. They reported a 38% rate of incontinence (8% to solid stool) overall, with a higher rate in those undergoing open LIS compared with the closed procedure.

Although LIS has often been described as division of the sphincter up to the dentate line, the practice of this technique has been variable and the length of sphincterotomy is often not recorded. A study by Sultan et al [41] demonstrated that in women the extent of sphincterotomy is often more extensive than initially suspected. They used endo-anal ultrasound before and after LIS. In the 15 patients examined, one male had no defect visible and in 9/10 women the sphincterotomy involved the full length of the internal anal sphincter. They presumed that this was due to surgeons not accounting for the shorter length of the female anal canal. Evidence seems to support more conservative sphincterotomy reducing the risk of incontinence, with a move towards "tailored" sphincterotomy being recommended. This involves limiting the sphincterotomy to the length of the fissure.

Littlejohn and Newstead described their experience of this technique in a retrospective study at a single institution [42]. They report excellent results with only seven of 287 patients reporting incontinence or urgency and none of these with incontinence to stool. Five patients required repeat sphincterotomy.

Accidental damage to the external anal sphincter has also been reported during attempted LIS [43] and is a known factor in incontinence in the non-surgical population [44].

Persistence or recurrence of fissures after LIS is an uncommon problem. Garcia-Aguilar et al [40] reported 4% persistence of symptoms with 11% reporting recurrence of their fissures over a median of 3 years in their questionnaire review of 549 patients. However, Argov and Levandovsky quoted their recurrence rate at only 1% of over 2108 patients [45]. Although consideration must again be given to whether these fissures are secondary to another aetiology, the reason for persistence and recurrence after LIS is usually technical failure. Farouk et al performed endo-anal ultrasound scanning (USS) on 13 patients with a persistent fissure following LIS and found that 11 of these had no evidence of internal sphincterotomy but instead had an external sphincter defect [43]. There does not seem to be an advantage to carrying out the procedure in an open as opposed to a closed fashion [40]. A list of trials involving LIS is given in Table 4, quoting the incontinence rate after sphincterotomy.

Table 4. Randomised trials of lateral internal sphincterotomy (LIS) for treatment of chronic anal fissures.

1st author	No. of patients in LIS group	Comparison	Duration of follow-up	Healing	Incontinence
Kortbeek [46]	112	Open vs closed	6 weeks	96%	NS
Leong & Seow-Choen [54]	20	Anal advancement flap	26 weeks	100%	0%
Richard [14]	38	GTN	6 months	92%	0%
Evans [38]	27	GTN	5 months	97%	0%
Libertiny [13]	35	GTN	2 years	97%	3%
Mentes [47]	50	Botulinum toxin A	6 months	94%	16%
Parellada [48]	27	Isosorbide dinitrate	2 years	100%	15%
Wiley [49]	76	Open vs closed	1 year	96%	6.8%

LIS=lateral internal sphincterotomy

As mentioned earlier, patient selection is critical in fissure surgery. Patients with low to normal anal sphincter pressures are unlikely to benefit from techniques designed to reduce anal pressures, since sphincter hypertonia is not the aetiology of their fissure. The other group that needs consideration in this respect is those with secondary fissures (Table 1). Patients with Crohn's disease not uncommonly have anal fissures. In a French study, 101 consecutive patients referred with Crohn's were examined for peri-anal disease. They found 63% of patients with peri-anal ulcers of varying severity [50]. A study from St. Mark's in the UK [51] found 26% of patients with Crohn's disease had anal fissures and that Crohn's fissures will often heal with conservative therapy alone and Crohn's-specific therapy is often the best second-line treatment. Weakening the anal sphincters in patients already prone to diarrhoea can be disastrous. Patients on immunosuppression or those with HIV need special consideration also and LIS is rarely indicated in these circumstances, since the fissure is often a complication of these disease processes. However, a report from Brazil found no difference in the incidence of fissures in 1860 HIV-positive patients when compared with HIV-negative patients [52]. Other infections causing anal fissures, such as TB or syphilis, are now uncommon in Europe and the USA. Anal cancers can present as fissures or cause fissuring in proximity to the tumour, but these conditions are usually identifiable and rarely get confused with idiopathic fissures.

Anal advancement flaps

For patients with anal fissures in the presence of normal or low anal sphincter tone, LIS should clearly be avoided, given the risk of incontinence. Anal advancement flaps have proved successful in this group of patients. Nyam et al described success with this technique in all 21 patients in their observational study [53] without any disturbance of continence or serious complications. A randomised controlled trial [54] compared this technique with LIS in an unselected group of patients with anal fissures. Although the numbers were too small for adequate comparison, it allowed the technique of advancement flaps to be examined. Three of the 20 patients in the flap group failed to heal, but there was no reported incontinence.

The techniques of manual anal dilatation and posterior sphincterotomy will be briefly mentioned. The former in particular had such a poor complication profile [55], with ultrasound evidence of significant sphincter injury [56], that its use is no longer generally acceptable for the treatment of anal fissures. LIS also appears to have a lower complication rate than posterior sphincterotomy and as such takes precedence over its older relative [57]. Fissurectomy alone has been used with success in children who have failed conservative therapy [58], but it has not been tried alone in adults, perhaps because it does not treat the underlying problem causing the fissure. However, combinations which reduce sphincter tone and excise the fissure have been tried as a way of preserving the integrity of the anal sphincters. A Dutch study combined fissurectomy followed by isosorbide dinitrate in 17 patients with all fissures healing and no sphincter injuries [59]. In a similar way, Lindsey et al have reported patients treated with a combination of fissurectomy and botulinum toxin A injection, achieving healing in 28/30 patients [60].

A suggested plan of treatment is illustrated by the algorithm in Figure 2.

Where are we going?

The future of treatment for anal fissures must be directed in two areas. Firstly, it requires the continued investigation of medical treatment for those who fail to respond to the current selection of drugs on offer. This may involve both the development of new treatments and combinations of existing preparations. Secondly, the development of successful sphincter-sparing surgery or reducing the morbidity of sphincter division whilst maintaining the same healing rates.

As far as medical treatment is concerned, botulinum toxin seems to be the most successful in healing fissures and has very few side effects [34]. In addition, it is given as a single dose which lasts a number of months. This prevents the regular application of the topical ointments and, compared

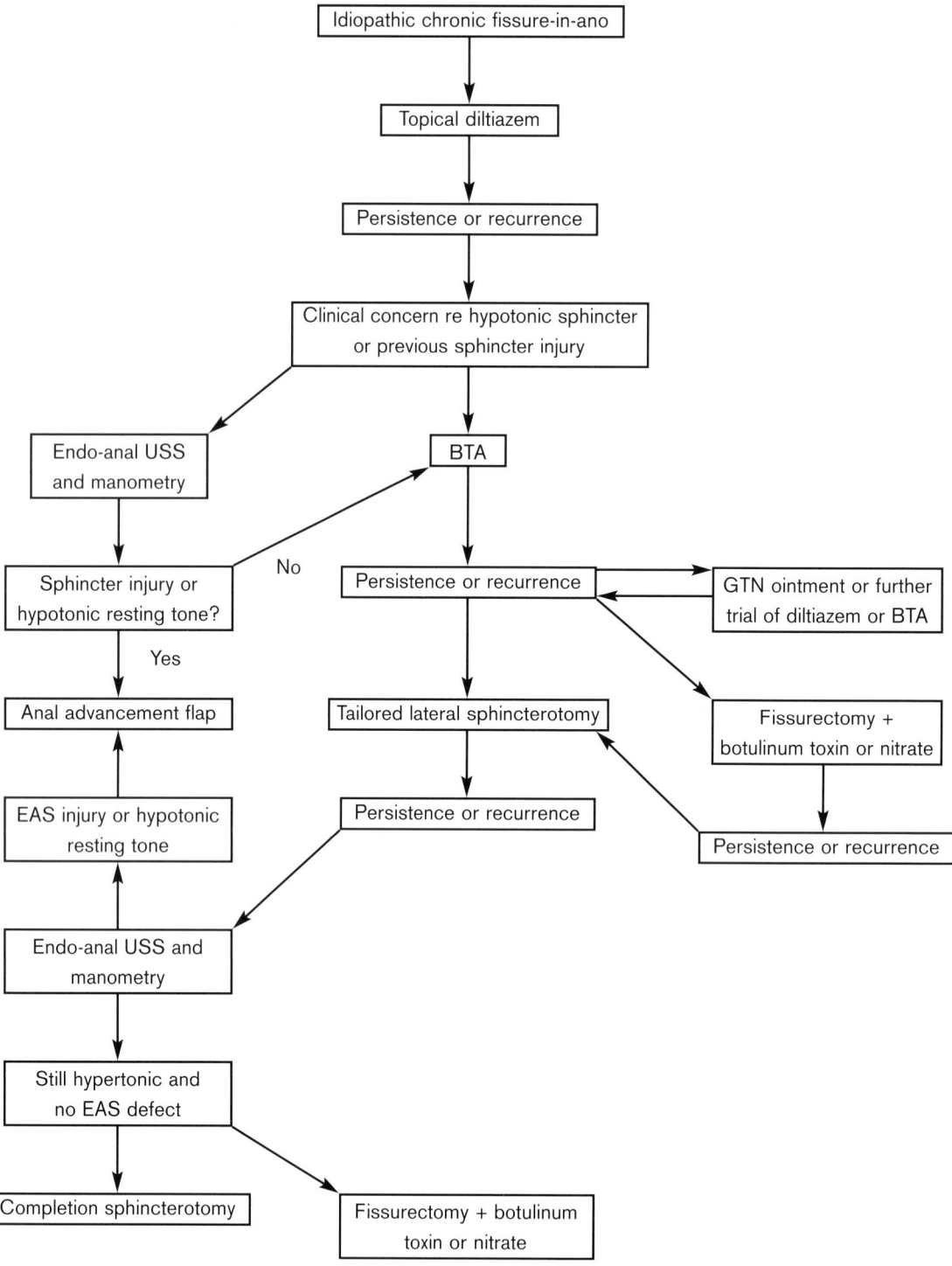

Figure 2. Algorithm for a suggested plan of treatment.

with GTN, it has fewer side effects. However, costing studies are becoming increasingly important in healthcare, and it may be this, rather than the evidence of efficacy, that will have a greater bearing on which treatment is used in the first line [61].

As for sphincter-sparing surgery, this has begun to receive consideration. The situation with anal advancement flaps in patients with known sphincter injuries or low sphincter tone has already been discussed. However, we need to become more proficient in detecting those at high risk, and we also need to offer an effective procedure but with less risk in those who do have high sphincter tone. On the subject of proficiency of clinical assessment, it may be necessary to advise endo-anal ultrasound and physiology on all women who have had children and present with fissures irrespective of what the subjective assessment of their anal tone is, since occult sphincter injuries are common. Sultan et al demonstrated that 35% of primiparous women and 44% of multiparous women demonstrated sphincter disruption after delivery but were asymptomatic [44].

For those with high-pressure sphincter tone, tailoring the sphincterotomy to the length of the fissure seems to be an important safety issue [42]. Further tailoring of the technique by ultrasound guidance during the operation has also been suggested, but no studies have been published. Another possibility for this group is avoiding dividing the sphincter altogether, and the small studies mentioned above combining fissurectomy with a temporary pharmacological lowering of anal sphincter tone may provide a better risk:benefit option. Obviously, further studies are required.

Conclusion

Chronic fissure-in-ano is a common problem which significantly impacts on a patient's quality of life [62]. The subject has received appropriate attention with well designed studies in evidence and further research in progress. It is clear from the evidence available that surgery is the most effective method of healing anal fissures, but its potential side effects, in particular incontinence, would caution its use as a first-line treatment when newer medical therapies with improving healing rates and side effect profiles are becoming available. Tailoring the length of the sphincterotomy to the length of the fissure seems to improve the incontinence risk without compromising significantly the chance of healing.

References

1. Schouten WR, Briel JW, Auwerda JJ. Relationship between anal pressure and anodermal blood flow. The vascular pathogenesis of anal fissures. *Dis Colon Rectum* 1994; 37: 664-9.
2. Schouten WR, Briel JW, Auwerda JJ, *et al*. Ischemic nature of anal fissure. *Br J Surg* 1996; 83: 63-5.
3. Lund JN, Binch C, McGrath J, *et al*. Topographical distribution of blood supply to the anal canal. *Br J Surg* 1999; 86: 496-8.
4. Gibbons CP, Read NW. Anal hypertonia in fissures: cause or effect? *Br J Surg* 1986; 73: 443-5.
5. Farouk R, Duthie GS, MacGregor AB, *et al*. Sustained internal sphincter hypertonia in patients with chronic anal fissure. *Dis Colon Rectum* 1994; 37: 424-9.
6. Lund JN, Parsons SL, Scholefield JH. Spasm of the internal sphincter in anal fissure - cause or effect? *Gastroenterology* 1996; 110: A711.
7. Corby H, Donnelly VS, O'Herlihy C, *et al*. Anal canal pressures are low in women with postpartum anal fissure. *Br J Surg* 1997; 84: 86-8.
8. Jensen SL. Maintenance therapy with unprocessed bran in the prevention of acute anal fissure recurrence. *J R Soc Med* 1987; 80: 296-8.
9. Jensen SL. Treatment of first episodes of acute anal fissure: prospective randomized study of lignocaine ointment versus hydrocortisone ointment or warm sitz baths plus bran. *Br Med J (Clin Res Ed)* 1986; 292: 1167-9.
10. O'Kelly T, Brading A, Mortensen N. Nerve mediated relaxation of the human internal anal sphincter: the role of nitric oxide. *Gut* 1993; 34: 689-93.
11. Lund JN, Scholefield JH. A randomized, prospective, double-blind, placebo-controlled trial of glyceryl trinitrate ointment in treatment of anal fissure [published erratum appears in *Lancet* 1997; 349: 656]. *Lancet* 1997; 349: 11-4.
12. Carapeti EA, Kamm MA, McDonald PJ, *et al*. Randomized controlled trial shows that glyceryl trinitrate heals anal fissures, higher doses are not more effective, and there is a high recurrence rate. *Gut* 1999; 44: 727-30.
13. Libertiny G, Knight JS, Farouk R. Randomized trial of topical 0·2% glyceryl trinitrate and lateral internal sphincterotomy for the treatment of patients with chronic anal fissure: long-term follow-up. *Eur J Surg* 2002; 168: 418-21.

14. Richard CS, Gregoire R, Plewes EA, et al. Internal sphincterotomy is superior to topical nitroglycerin in the treatment of chronic anal fissure: results of a randomized, controlled trial by the Canadian Colorectal Surgical Trials Group. Dis Colon Rectum 2000; 43: 1048-57.
15. Altomare DF, Rinaldi M, Milito G, et al. Glyceryl trinitrate for chronic anal fissure - healing or headache? Results of a multicenter, randomized, placebo-controlled, double-blind trial. Dis Colon Rectum 2000; 43: 174-9.
16. Kennedy ML, Sowter S, Nguyen H, et al. Glyceryl trinitrate ointment for the treatment of chronic anal fissure: results of a placebo-controlled trial and long-term follow-up. Dis Colon Rectum 1999; 42: 1000-6.
17. Jonas M, Lund JN, Scholefield JH. Topical 0·2% glyceryl trinitrate ointment for anal fissures: long-term efficacy in routine clinical practice. Colorectal Dis 2002; 4: 317-20.
18. Werre AJ, Palamba HW, Bilgen EJ, et al. Isosorbide dinitrate in the treatment of anal fissure: a randomized, prospective, double blind, placebo-controlled trial. Eur J Surg 2001; 167: 382-5.
19. Lysy J, Israelit-Yatzkan Y, Sestiere-Ittah M, et al. Treatment of chronic anal fissure with isosorbide dinitrate: long-term results and dose determination. Dis Colon Rectum 1998; 41: 1406-10.
20. Griffin N, Zimmerman DD, Briel JW, et al. Topical L-arginine gel lowers resting anal pressure: possible treatment for anal fissure. Dis Colon Rectum 2002; 45: 1332-6.
21. Cook TA, Brading AF, Mortensen NJ. Differences in contractile properties of anorectal smooth muscle and the effects of calcium channel blockade. Br J Surg 1999; 86: 70-5.
22. Jonas M, Neal KR, Abercrombie JF, et al. A randomized trial of oral vs. topical diltiazem for chronic anal fissures. Dis Colon Rectum 2001; 44: 1074-8.
23. Bielecki K, Kolodziejczak M. A prospective randomized trial of diltiazem and glyceryl trinitrate ointment in the treatment of chronic anal fissure. Colorectal Dis 2003; 5: 256-7.
24. Knight JS, Birks M, Farouk R. Topical diltiazem ointment in the treatment of chronic anal fissure. Br J Surg 2001; 88: 553-6.
25. Griffin N, Acheson AG, Jonas M, et al. The role of topical diltiazem in the treatment of chronic anal fissures that have failed glyceryl trinitrate therapy. Colorectal Dis 2002; 4: 430-5.
26. Perrotti P, Bove A, Antropoli C, et al. Topical nifedipine with lidocaine ointment vs. active control for treatment of chronic anal fissure: results of a prospective, randomized, double-blind study. Dis Colon Rectum 2002; 45: 1468-75.
27. Ezri T, Susmallian S. Topical nifedipine vs. topical glyceryl trinitrate for treatment of chronic anal fissure. Dis Colon Rectum 2003; 46: 805-8.
28. Jost WH, Schimrigk K. Use of botulinum toxin in anal fissure. Dis Colon Rectum 1993; 36: 974.
29. Jost WH. One hundred cases of anal fissure treated with botulin toxin: early and long-term results. Dis Colon Rectum 1997; 40: 1029-32.
30. Gui D, Cassetta E, Anastasio G, et al. Botulinum toxin for chronic anal fissure. Lancet 1994; 344: 1127-8.
31. Jones OM, Brading AF, Mortensen NJ. Mechanism of action of botulinum toxin on the internal anal sphincter. Br J Surg 2004; 91: 224-8.
32. Jost WH, Aoki KR. Botulinum toxin A in anal fissure: why does it work? Dis Colon Rectum 2004; 47: 257-8.
33. Maria G, Cassetta E, Gui D, et al. A comparison of botulinum toxin and saline for the treatment of chronic anal fissure. N Engl J Med 1998; 338: 217-20.
34. Brisinda G, Maria G, Bentivoglio AR, et al. A comparison of injections of botulinum toxin and topical nitroglycerin ointment for the treatment of chronic anal fissure. N Engl J Med 1999; 341: 65-9.
35. Carapeti EA, Kamm MA, Evans BK, et al. Topical diltiazem and bethanechol decrease anal sphincter pressure without side effects. Gut 1999; 45: 719-22.
36. Cundall JD, Gardiner A, Laden G, et al. Use of hyperbaric oxygen to treat chronic anal fissure. Br J Surg 2003; 90: 452-3.
37. Pitt J, Dawson PM, Hallan RI, et al. A double-blind randomized placebo-controlled trial of oral indoramin to treat chronic anal fissure. Colorectal Dis 2001; 3: 165-8.
38. Evans J, Luck A, Hewett P. Glyceryl trinitrate vs. lateral sphincterotomy for chronic anal fissure: prospective, randomized trial. Dis Colon Rectum 2001; 44: 93-7.
39. Nyam DC, Pemberton JH. Long-term results of lateral internal sphincterotomy for chronic anal fissure with particular reference to incidence of fecal incontinence. Dis Colon Rectum 1999; 42: 1306-10.
40. Garcia-Aguilar J, Belmonte C, Wong WD, et al. Open vs. closed sphincterotomy for chronic anal fissure: long-term results. Dis Colon Rectum 1996; 39: 440-3.
41. Sultan AH, Kamm MA, Nicholls RJ, et al. Prospective study of the extent of internal anal sphincter division during lateral sphincterotomy. Dis Colon Rectum 1994; 37: 1031-3.
42. Littlejohn DR, Newstead GL. Tailored lateral sphincterotomy for anal fissure. Dis Colon Rectum 1997; 40: 1439-42.
43. Farouk R, Monson JRT, Duthie GS. Technical failure of lateral sphincterotomy for the treatment of chronic anal fissure: a study using anal ultrasonography. Br J Surg 1997; 84: 84-5.
44. Sultan AH, Kamm MA, Hudson CN, et al. Anal-sphincter disruption during vaginal delivery. N Engl J Med 1993; 329: 1905-11.
45. Argov S, Levandovsky O. Open lateral sphincterotomy is still the best treatment for chronic anal fissure. Am J Surg 2000; 179: 201-2.
46. Kortbeek JB, Langevin JM, Khoo RE, et al. Chronic fissure-in-ano: a randomized study comparing open and subcutaneous lateral internal sphincterotomy. Dis Colon Rectum 1992; 35: 835-7.
47. Mentes BB, Irkorucu O, Akin M, et al. Comparison of botulinum toxin injection and lateral internal sphincterotomy for the treatment of chronic anal fissure. Dis Colon Rectum 2003; 46: 232-7.
48. Parellada C. Randomized, prospective trial comparing 0.2 percent isosorbide dinitrate ointment with sphincterotomy in treatment of chronic anal fissure: a two-year follow-up. Dis Colon Rectum 2004; 47: 437-3.
49. Wiley M, Day P, Rieger N, et al. Open vs. closed lateral internal sphincterotomy for idiopathic fissure-in-ano: a prospective, randomized, controlled trial. Dis Colon Rectum 2004; 47: 847-52.

50. Siproudhis L, Mortaji A, Mary JY, et al. Anal lesions: any significant prognosis in Crohn's disease? *Eur J Gastroenterol Hepatol* 1997; 9: 239-43.
51. Sweeney JL, Ritchie JK, Nicholls RJ. Anal fissure in Crohn's disease. *Br J Surg* 1988; 75: 56-7.
52. Nadal SR, Manzione CR, Galvao VM, et al. Perianal diseases in HIV-positive patients compared with a seronegative population. *Dis Colon Rectum* 1999; 42: 649-54.
53. Nyam DC, Wilson RG, Stewart KJ, et al. Island advancement flaps in the management of anal fissures. *Br J Surg* 1995; 82: 326-8.
54. Leong AF, Seow-Choen F. Lateral sphincterotomy compared with anal advancement flap for chronic anal fissure. *Dis Colon Rectum* 1995; 38: 69-71.
55. Collopy B, Ryan P. Comparison of lateral subcutaneous sphincterotomy with anal dilatation in the treatment of fissure in ano. *Med J Aust* 1979; 2: 461-462, 487.
56. Speakman CT, Burnett SJ, Kamm MA, et al. Sphincter injury after anal dilatation demonstrated by endosonography. *Br J Surg* 1991; 78: 1429-30.
57. Abcarian H. Surgical correction of chronic anal fissure: results of lateral internal sphincterotomy vs. fissurectomy - midline sphincterotomy. *Dis Colon Rectum* 1980; 23: 31-6.
58. Lambe GF, Driver CP, Morton S, et al. Fissurectomy as a treatment for anal fissures in children. *Ann R Coll Surg Engl* 2000; 82: 254-7.
59. Engel AF, Eijsbouts QA, Balk AG. Fissurectomy and isosorbide dinitrate for chronic fissure-in-ano not responding to conservative treatment. *Br J Surg* 2002; 89: 79-83.
60. Lindsey I, Francis C, Cunningham C, et al. Fissurectomy plus botulinum toxin: a novel sphincter-sparing procedure for medically-resistant chronic anal fissure. *Colorectal Dis* 2003; 5(Suppl 1): 1.
61. Christie A, Guest JF. Modelling the economic impact of managing a chronic anal fissure with a proprietary formulation of nitroglycerin (Rectogesic) compared to lateral internal sphincterotomy in the United Kingdom. *Int J Colorectal Dis* 2002; 17: 259-67.
62. Griffin N, Acheson AG, Tung P, et al. Quality of life in patients with chronic anal fissure. *Colorectal Dis* 2004; 6: 39-44.

Chapter 20

Incontinence

Carolynne J Vaizey MD FRCS (Gen) FCS (SA)
Consultant Colorectal Surgeon & Clinical Senior Lecturer
St. Mark's Hospital, Harrow, Middlesex, UK

What is the problem?

With increasing awareness of the magnitude of disability from faecal incontinence, this once taboo topic is now the subject of much focused research. With recent improvements in the assessment of treatment outcomes both in the long and the short term, many traditional therapies have now fallen from favour.

In the early 1990s, understanding of the aetiology of faecal incontinence was revolutionised following reports based on findings at endoanal sonography. Incomparable images of sphincter damage from obstetric trauma and surgical procedures, such as anal dilatation and sphincterotomy, radically altered thinking about vaginal deliveries and anal surgical procedures. The previously held view that pudendal nerve damage was the underlying cause of incontinence in most patients [1] was soon questioned and now even the accuracy of current methods of measurement of pudendal nerve terminal motor latencies is in doubt.

In the late 1990s, the concept of sphincter atrophy was formally introduced in an article in the *Lancet*, which described internal anal sphincter atrophy mainly defined on ultrasound criteria [2]. The external anal sphincter muscle is less distinct on ultrasound than the hypoechoic internal sphincter, so endocoil MRI was used to assess external sphincter atrophy [3-5]. The more recent introduction of three-dimensional endo-anal ultrasound further improves assessment of sphincter integrity.

The maintenance of faecal continence depends on stool consistency, colorectal activity and the harmonious functioning of the external and the internal anal sphincters [6]. As there are no reliable medications to counteract increased colonic activity or "irritable bowel syndrome", treatments classically focus on firming stools or on improving the sphincter mechanism. Results of surgery were poorly standardised prior to the introduction of validated continence scoring systems in the latter part of the 1990s. Before this, reports were generally of the operating surgeon's short-term subjective assessment of symptom improvement, with no regard to the need for anti-diarrhoeal medications and no assessment of quality of life. The St. Mark's Score correlates most closely with in-depth clinical symptom assessment [7]. This system, which is a modification of the Wexner continence score, together with a simple bowel diary and a disease-specific quality of life instrument, has revolutionised postoperative patient assessments and enabled more meaningful comparisons of treatment outcomes.

The post-anal repair is probably the best example of an operation which has not withstood current depths of analysis and duration of follow-up. Introduced by Parks in the 1970s, the post-anal repair was aimed at patients with idiopathic or "neurogenic incontinence" in the absence of a reparable defect. With long-term benefit maintained in only about a quarter of patients, this is now a redundant procedure.

Where are we now?

Loperamide or other stool-firming agents such as Lomotil or codeine phosphate should be used as first-line therapy for all incontinence patients who do not suffer from concomitant difficulty with defecation. Initially, these medications should be used in very small, carefully titrated doses, to avoid causing any discomfort or constipation. Loperamide can be obtained in syrup form to enable finer dose adjustments. A capsule contains 2mg of loperamide whereas a 5ml teaspoon contains only 1mg. A 2.5ml paediatric teaspoon contains only 0.5mg.

Biofeedback therapy, based around an exercise programme with visual computerised feedback to the patient, is now an established conservative therapy. It is particularly successful in patients who have intact but weakened sphincter muscles and, critically, it has no side effects [8].

The anal plug (Conveen; Coloplast Ltd, UK) is a tampon-like device worn inside the anus. It is coated with a dissolvable plastic-like cover and assumes a more mushroom-like shape when moist within the rectum, preventing anal leakage. However, only a minority find it sufficiently comfortable for long-term usage. In a recent study only six of 20 patients opted to continue with its usage [9].

Simple procedures and repairs

In the 1970s, Parks also developed overlapping sphincter repair for the defective external anal sphincter. The overlapping repair improves continence in 60-90% of patients in the short term, but this is said to drop to about 50% after an interval of 5 years [10]. However, this is a somewhat distorted figure as the groups examined so far in long-term studies all include a cohort of older women, continent post-sphincter trauma but incontinent with advancing age. These women must therefore have other factors contributing to their incontinence which cannot readily be reversed with a simple repair.

The new evidence on long-term results has led to a more cautious approach to the patient selection process and there is often an obligatory initial trial of conservative therapies.

Reparable defects of the anal sphincter muscles are most commonly due to obstetric trauma; surgical or traumatic injuries to the external sphincter or to both sphincters can usually be treated in the same manner. Isolated defects in the internal anal sphincter muscle usually follow surgical procedures. These are not amenable to simple surgical repair [11] as it is a smooth muscle, usually only about 2mm in thickness, which is in a state of constant contraction.

Repeat overlapping repair may be an attractive option for patients who fail an initial repair and are shown to have a persistent sphincter defect on endo-anal ultrasound [12]. In a study where patients were carefully selected on the basis of clinically good external anal sphincter muscle bulk and contractility, the short- and long-term results were good with about 60% acceptable function at both 20-month and 5-year follow-up.

Disruption of the anal sphincters not amenable to simple repair can range from a single defect in the internal sphincter to total disruption of the sphincter mechanism with little or no residual muscle. Internal sphincter defects are frequently due to common surgical procedures. Extensive external and internal anal sphincter damage can result from obstetric, surgical or other trauma, or follow previous unsuccessful surgery aimed at sphincter repair.

Following the demise of the post-anal repair, treatment options for patients without a reparable defect were limited. There was initial enthusiasm over topical treatment with the pharmacological agent, phenylephrine, applied peri-anally as a 10% cream. It was shown to enhance the function of the normal internal anal sphincter muscle [13] but its effects have been limited on the weak and atrophic sphincter [14].

The idea of bulking agents to promote closure of the lax anal canal followed decades of work by urologists using a similar concept to close down the urethra. The first report of the use of injectable bulking agents in the anal canal was in 1993 by Shafik [15]. Polytef (polytetrafluoroethylene paste, PTFE, Teflon; Dupont, Texas, USA) was injected into the "rectal neck submucosa" in 11 patients with improvement in all. In 1995, Shafik described the submucosal injection of autologous fat, harvested from the abdominal wall [16]. Fourteen patients with "partial" faecal incontinence were said to have had good short-term results. There was a further case report published in 1998 on a woman who required two injections of autologous fat to regain continence following a failed repair of an obstetric-related defect [17]. In 1998, Kumar *et al* used gluteraldehyde cross-linked collagen injections (Contigen; Bard, Covington, New Jersey, USA) in 17 patients, 11 of whom showed marked symptom improvement in the short term [18].

Bioplastique, similar to the silicone-based urological product Macroplastique, was used to inject ten patients with weak or disrupted internal anal sphincter muscles with mixed results. At 6 weeks three patients had a complete cessation of leakage and three a marked improvement; a further patient improved after a second injection. However, the effects were only maintained in two patients at a 6-month follow-up [19]. Five patients had pain and ulceration at the injection site with some having obvious back leakage of product. A repeat study using improved methodology showed that five of six patients had marked improvement and that this was sustained at 18 months [20].

This product is now known as PTQ Implants (Uroplasty Ltd; Reading, UK), and it is the only bulking agent currently licensed for use in faecal incontinence in the UK.

A further pilot study using carbon-coated zirconium oxide beads (Durasphere; Carbon Medical Technologies, Minnesota, USA) in 18 patients was reported to show significant improvement in continence grading and quality of life measurements [21]. Contigen and Durasphere are currently the only products with FDA approval in the USA.

The alternative therapy to use of a bulking agent is radio-frequency energy delivery to the anal canal, known as the Secca procedure. This can be performed under local anaesthesia, delivering thermal lesions deep to the mucosa at multiple sites and levels in the anal canal.

A study on ten female patients from Mexico showed a mean improvement in the Cleveland Clinic incontinence score from 13.8 out of 20 pre-procedure to 7.3 out of 20 at 2 years [22]. A further study from the USA on 43 females and seven males, showed a mean improvement in the Cleveland Clinic incontinence score from 14.5 to 11.1 and a mean improvement in the Short-Form-36 social function of 64.3 to 76 at 6 months [23].

Complex surgical options

Sacral nerve stimulation was first described as a treatment for faecal incontinence in 1995. It had been used in the treatment of patients with bladder dysfunction since 1981. Although classified as a complex surgical procedure, the complexity is more a function of our poor understanding of its mechanism of action than of the surgical procedure, which is actually quite straightforward. Initially, this therapy was reported as a treatment for faecal incontinence due to a weak but intact external sphincter [24], the implication being that its main action was to enhance sphincter function. Patients were instructed to turn off the stimulator prior to the passage of a stool just as with the dynamic graciloplasty.

A detailed physiological study published in 1999 failed to show a major effect on the external sphincter but did show an effect on rectal capacity and on rectal activity [25]. Additionally, there was a qualitative rather than a quantitative effect on the internal sphincter muscle with the induction of slow wave activity and a decrease in the number of spontaneous falls in pressure. Patients have now also been shown to pass stools without hindrance with the stimulator kept on at all times.

One of the unique features of this therapy is the possibility of a trial of stimulation prior to implantation of the permanent stimulator. A temporary electrode can be placed percutaneously, usually through the S3 foramen, and attached via a wire to an external stimulator, similar in size to a TENS machine. Symptomatic improvement over a 3-week test period then allows the patient to choose to proceed to a permanent implant of an electrode and stimulator. The permanent electrode can be implanted percutaneously with a tunnelled lead connecting it to an implanted stimulator in the buttock.

Larger studies have now confirmed the excellent results in earlier pilot studies. Forty-six permanent implants were reported from the UK [26]. At a median of 12 months, all but two had improved continence, with episodes of incontinence decreasing from a median of 7.5 to one episodes a week. There were no major complications and only one implant had to be removed.

A Danish study of 37 permanent implants reported difficulties with dislodgement of the test electrode and infection in the permanent implant, the latter relating to prolonged use of the temporary testing equipment. [27]. In a multicentre international trial, 37 patients had a median decrease in frequency of incontinence episodes from 16.4 per week pre-implantation to two a week at 2 years. Social function was also significantly improved [28].

The concept of a neosphincter embraces both the dynamic gracioplasty and the artificial bowel sphincter. As with sacral nerve stimulation these treatments are expensive; unlike sacral nerve stimulation they are associated with high morbidity and re-operation rates. However, there are patients with severe incontinence, unresponsive to other therapies, who may wish to avoid a stoma and who are prepared to accept the inherent risks of these procedures.

The use of a substitute skeletal muscle in place of the external anal sphincter has been described intermittently since 1952 when Pickrell first used the gracilis muscle as an "anal wrap". Poor results led to intermittent case reports on the use of other muscles, such as the gluteus maximus and obturator internus, but none has been accepted by the colorectal fraternity.

In 1991, Baeten in Maastricht and Williams in London both reported the use of an electrical stimulator to effect a chronic, sustained contraction of the gracilis muscle instead of relying on a tight wrap [29, 30]. Chronic stimulation of a skeletal muscle can convert fast twitch, fatiguable muscle into slow twitch muscle capable of continuous contraction [31].

The operative procedure is complex with two phases. The first involves mobilisation of the gracilis muscle, which is then wrapped scarf-like around the anal sphincters, with the distal end attached to one of the ischial tuberosities or to the skin. The fully implanted stimulator is the same as that used for sacral nerve stimulation; wires connect this to an electrode which either cuffs the nerve to gracilis or lies within its terminal branches at the proximal end of the muscle. A programme of incremental muscle stimulation usually spans a period of weeks before the muscle is fully trained to achieve a state of continuous contraction. For defecation the patient usually has to switch off the stimulator to allow the muscle to relax and this is achieved using a hand-held patient programmer which communicates with the stimulator by telemetry.

A temporary revival of the gracioplasty followed reports of good results from the Maastricht group [32,33], but these were rapidly followed by reports of high morbidity and re-operation rates from multicentre trials involving less experienced colorectal surgeons [34-36]. This complex surgery should really now be considered as a last resort in the treatment of incontinence, undertaken only in specialist centres with a high level of information and support supplied to the patients. It should not be performed in patients with pre-existing peri-anal sepsis, Crohn's disease or neurological disorders potentially resulting in weakness of the gracilis muscle.

The Acticon or artificial bowel sphincter (ABS) was first introduced in 1996. Modelled on the artificial urinary sphincter or AUS it was initially reported to provide near total continence in about 68% of cases.

Implantation of this device is simple compared to the creation of a dynamic graciloplasty. A hydraulic cuff encircles the anus, a balloon reservoir is placed in the pre-peritoneal plane in the lower abdomen and a valve pump in the labia or scrotum. The three components are connected by fully implanted silicone tubing and the device is filled with an isotonic, water-soluble, radio-opaque solution. The pump can be squeezed to achieve cuff deflation by temporary transfer of fluid into the balloon. Continence is restored passively over several minutes as the fluid drips back into the cuff with equilibration of pressures.

The results from a multicentre trial of 114 patients showed a success rate of 85% in patients with a functioning device, but only a 53% success rate calculated on an intention to treat basis. There were 73 revisional operations, 41 patients had the device completely removed and only seven of these were successfully re-implanted [37]. The incidence of infection has been higher than in the initial pilot studies, although mechanical failures have decreased [38,39]. Late postoperative complications are frequent [40].

Stomas and irrigations

Many patients with faecal incontinence fare extremely well with a colostomy with instant restoration of quality of life. Patients should be warned, however, that mucous leakage will still be expected in the presence of a retained rectum.

Stoma irrigations can provide further control and this strategy is also possible via the rectum in some patients without a stoma. There has been little written about this technique [41], but there is a specially designed tube called a Shandling tube which is available in the UK [CAMCARE Gels, UK]. The antegrade continence enema or ACE is still most commonly used in children with limited reported success in the adult population [42].

Where are we going?

As many of the complex treatments have not withstood the test of time, research has now focused on more simple treatments. The idea of a bulking agent has not been fully trialled with products currently licensed on the basis of pilot studies alone. No perfect filler material yet exists and many newer injectables are still undergoing investigation to determine their clinical efficacy and long-term safety. Newer products already tested in urinary incontinence include:

- Coaptite (Calcium hydroxylapatite; Bioform, Franksville, USA) which is made up of hydroxyapatite ceramic microspheres (CaHA) 75 to 125µm in size, suspended in a carrier gel of sodium carboxylmethylcellulose, glycerine and water. After injection they become enmeshed within a non-encapsulated stable soft collagen matrix which is said to result in maintenance of volume. It is easy to inject though a 21-gauge needle and is also radio-opaque [43].
- Deflux (Dextranomer/hyaluronic acid copolymer, Dx/HA, Zuidex; Q-Med, Uppsala, Sweden) consists of cross-linked molecules of dextran and a glucose-based polysaccharide used as a plasma expander. Dextranomer (Dx) microspheres are about 120µm in diameter which are suspended in a non-animal stabilised hyaluronic acid (NASHA). It is non-allergenic, non-immunogenic and non-migratory. It is subject to degradation but may retain its bulking effects through the formation and ingrowth of endogenous soft tissue fibrosis [44].
- Permacol (Tissue Science Laboratories, Aldershot, Hampshire, UK) is an acellular cross-linked porcine, dermal collagen which is, in effect, a fragmented version of the Permacol sheet used in abdominal wall reconstructions. It is non-allergenic and biocompatible. It is easy to inject through a 21-gauge needle and is said to be less biodegradable than Contigen. Once injected, revascularisation and cellular infiltration is said to occur [45].

The other current treatment which has yet to be fully investigated is nerve stimulation. Sacral nerve stimulation has recently been proposed as a treatment for faecal incontinence due to disruption of the external sphincter muscle. An initial pilot study has shown that all seven patients undergoing temporary nerve stimulation improved in terms of episodes of incontinence per week and urgency improved in three of the seven patients. Incontinence scores improved from 13.5/20 pre-procedure to 5/20 post-procedure. Five have already had a permanent implantation and two are planned for implantation [46].

Should larger studies confirm that this treatment is successful in patients with disrupted sphincter mechanisms, this should finally dispel the myth that it works by enhancing the function of the external anal sphincter muscle.

With so many treatments now known to be less successful than previously reported, the emphasis should be on prevention of sphincter damage in both the obstetric setting and during anal surgery. Unfortunately, many obstetric units continue to be manned by junior staff with little experience in assessment of sphincter disruption and a majority of obstetricians still do not feel sufficiently trained to deal with major tears [47].

References

1. Engel AF, Kamm MA, Bartram CI, Nicholls RJ. Relationship of symptoms in faecal incontinence to specific sphincter abnormalities. *Int J Colorectal Dis* 1995; 10: 152-5.
2. Parks AG, Swash M Urich H. Sphincter denervation in anorectal incontinence and rectal prolapse. *Gut* 1977; 19: 656-65.
3. Vaizey CJ, Bartram CI, Kamm MA. Primary degeneration of the internal anal sphincter as a cause of passive faecal incontinence. *Lancet* 1997; 349: 612-5.
4. Briel JW, Zimmerman DD, Stoker J, Rociu E, Lameris JS, Mooi WJ, Schouten WR. Relationship between sphincter morphology on endoanal MRI and histopathological aspects of the external anal sphincter. *Int J Colorectal Dis* 2000; 15: 87-90.
5. Briel JW, Stoker J, Rociu E, Lameris JS, Hop WC, Schouten WR. External anal sphincter atrophy on endoanal magnetic resonance imaging adversely affects continence after sphincteroplasty. *Br J Surg* 1999; 86: 1322-7.
6. Williams AB, Bartram CI, Modhwadia D, Nicholls T, Halligan S, Kamm MA, Nicholls RJ, Kmiot WA. Endocoil magnetic resonance imaging quantification of external anal sphincter atrophy. *Br J Surg* 2001; 88: 853-9.
7. Vaizey CJ, Carapeti E, Cahill J, Kamm MA. Prospective comparison of faecal incontinence grading systems. *Gut* 1999; 44: 77-80.
8. Norton C, Kamm MA. Outcome of biofeedback for faecal incontinence. *Br J Surg* 1999; 86: 1159-63.
9. Norton C, Kamm MA. Anal plug for faecal incontinence. *Colorectal Dis* 2001; 3: 323-7.
10. Malouf AJ, Norton CS, Engel AF, Nicholls RJ, Kamm MA. Long term results of overlapping anterior anal sphincter repair for obstetric trauma. *Lancet* 2000; 355: 260-5.
11. Leroi AM, Kamm MA, Weber J, Denis P, Hawley PR. Internal anal sphincter repair. *Int J Colorectal Dis* 1997; 12: 243-5.
12. Vaizey CJ, Norton C, Thornton MJ, Nicholls RJ, Kamm MA. Long-term results of repeat anterior anal sphincter repair. *Dis Colon Rectum* 2004; 47: 858-63.
13. Carapeti EA, Kamm MA, Evans BK, Phillips RKS. Topical phenylephrine increases anal sphincter resting pressure. *Br J Surg* 1999; 86: 267-70.
14. Carapeti EA, Kamm MA, Phillips RK. Randomized controlled trial of topical phenylephrine in the treatment of faecal incontinence. *Br J Surg* 2000; 87: 38-42.
15. Shafik A. Perianal injection of autologous fat for treatment of sphincteric incontinence. *Dis Colon Rectum* 1995; 38: 583-7.
16. Shafik A. Polytetrafluoroethylene injection for the treatment of partial faecal incontinence. *Int Surg* 1993; 78: 159-61.
17. Bernardi C, Favetta U, Pescatori M. Autologous fat injection for treatment of fecal incontinence: manometric and echographic assessment. *Plast Reconstr Surg* 1998; 102: 1626-8.
18. Kumar D, Benson M, Bland J. Gluteraldehyde cross-linked collagen in the treatment of faecal incontinence. *Br J Surg* 1998; 85: 978-9.
19. Malouf AJ, Vaizey CJ, Norton CS, Kamm MA. Internal anal sphincter augmentation for fecal incontinence using injectable silicone biomaterial. *Dis Colon Rectum* 2001; 44: 595-600.
20. Kenefick NJ, Vaizey CJ, Malouf AJ, Norton CS, Marshall M, Kamm MA. Injectable silicone biomaterial for faecal incontinence due to internal anal sphincter dysfunction. *Gut* 2002; 51: 225-8.
21. Davis K, Kumar D, Poloniecki J. Preliminary evaluation of an injectable anal sphincter bulking agent (Durasphere) in the management of faecal incontinence. *Aliment Pharmacol Ther* 2003; 18: 237-43.
22. Takahashi T, Garcia-Osogobio S, Valdovinos MA, Belmonte C, Barreto C, Velasco L. Extended two-year results of radio-frequency energy delivery for the treatment of fecal incontinence (the Secca procedure). *Dis Colon Rectum* 2003; 46: 711-5.
23. Efron JE, Corman ML, Fleshman J, Barnett J, Nagle D, Birnbaum E, Weiss EG, Nogueras JJ, Sligh S, Rabine J, Wexner SD. Safety and effectiveness of temperature-controlled radio-frequency energy delivery to the anal canal (Secca procedure) for the treatment of fecal incontinence. *Dis Colon Rectum* 2003; 46: 1606-18.
24. Matzel KE, Stadelmaier U, Hohenfeller M, Gall FP. Electrical stimulation of spinal nerves for treatment of faecal incontinence. *Lancet* 1995; 346: 1124-27.
25. Vaizey CJ, Kamm MA, Turner I, Nicholls RJ, Woloszko J. The results of short-term sacral nerve stimulation in the treatment of faecal incontinence. *Gut* 1999; 44: 407-12.

26. Jarrett ME, Varma JS, Duthie GS, Nicholls RJ, Kamm MA. Sacral nerve stimulation for faecal incontinence in the UK. *Br J Surg* 2004; 91: 755-61.
27. Rasmussen OO, Buntzen S, Sorensen M, Laurberg S, Christiansen J. Sacral nerve stimulation in fecal incontinence. *Dis Colon Rectum* 2004; 47: 1158-62; discussion 1162-3.
28. Matzel KE, Kamm MA, Stosser M, Baeten CG, Christiansen J, Madoff R, Mellgren A, Nicholls RJ, Rius J, Rosen H. Sacral spinal nerve stimulation for faecal incontinence: multicentre study. *Lancet* 2004; 363: 1270-6.
29. Baeten CG, Konsten J, Spaans F, Visser R, Habets AM, Bourgeois IM, Wagenmakers AJ, Soeters PB. Dynamic graciloplasty for treatment of faecal incontinence. *Lancet* 1991; 338: 1163-5.
30. Williams NS, Patel J, George BD, Hallan RI, Watkins ES. Development of an electrically stimulated neoanal sphincter. *Lancet* 1991; 338: 1166-9.
31. Salmons S, Henriksson J. The adaptive response of skeletal muscle to increased use. *Muscle and Nerve* 1981; 4: 94-105.
32. Baeten C, Geerdes BP, Adang EMM, *et al.* Anal dynamic graciloplasty in the treatment of intractable fecal incontinence. *N Engl J Med* 1995; 332: 1600-5.
33. Rongen MJ, Uludag O, El Naggar K, Geerdes BP, Konsten J, Baeten CG. Long-term follow-up of dynamic graciloplasty for fecal incontinence. *Dis Colon Rectum* 2003; 46: 716-21.
34. Wexner S, Gonzalez-Padron A, Rius J, Teoh T-A, Cheong DM, Nogueras JJ, Billotti VL, Weiss EG, Moon HK. Stimulated gracilis neosphincter operation: initial experience, pitfalls and complications. *Dis Colon Rectum* 1996; 39: 957-64.
35. Penninckx F; Belgian Section of Colorectal Surgery. Belgian experience with dynamic graciloplasty for faecal incontinence. *Br J Surg* 2004; 91: 872-8.
36. Madoff RD. Surgical treatment options for fecal incontinence. *Gastroenterology* 2004; 126(1 Suppl 1): S48-54.
37. Wong WD, Congliosi SM, Spencer MP, Corman ML, Tan P, Opelka FG, *et al.* The safety and efficacy of the artificial bowel sphincter for fecal incontinence. *Dis Colon Rectum* 2002; 45: 1139-53.
38. Malouf AJ, Vaizey CJ, Kamm MA, Nicholls RJ. Reassessing artificial bowel sphincters. *Lancet* 2000; 355: 2219-20.
39. Mundy L, Merlin TL, Maddern GJ, Hiller JE. Systematic review of safety and effectiveness of an artificial bowel sphincter for faecal incontinence. *Br J Surg* 2004; 91: 665-72.
40. Ortiz H, Armendariz P, DeMiguel M, Ruiz MD, Alos R, Roig JV. Complications and functional outcome following artificial anal sphincter implantation. *Br J Surg* 2002; 89: 877-81.
41. Christensen P, Olsen N, Krogh K, Bacher T, Laurberg S. Scintigraphic assessment of retrograde colonic washout in fecal incontinence and constipation. *Dis Colon Rectum.* 2003; 46: 68-76.
42. Krogh K, Laurberg S. Malone antegrade continence enema for faecal incontinence and constipation in adults. *Br J Surg* 1998; 85: 974-7.
43. van Kerrebroeck P, ter Meulen F, Farrelly E, Larsson G, Edwall L, Fianu-Jonasson A. Treatment of stress urinary incontinence: recent developments in the role of urethral injection. *Urol Res* 2003; 30: 356-62.
44. Puri P, Chertin B, Velayudham M, Dass L, Colhoun E. Treatment of vesicoureteral reflux by endoscopic injection of dextranomer/hyaluronic acid copolymer: preliminary results. *J Urol* 2003; 170: 1541-4.
45. Bano F, Barrington J and Dyer R. Comparison between porcine dermal implant (Permacol) and silicone injection (Macroplastique) for urodynamic stress incontinence. *International Urogynecology Journal and Pelvic Floor Dysfunction* 2005; in press.
46. Jarrett MED, Vaizey C, Cohen R, Nicholls RJ, Kamm MA. Sacral nerve stimulation for faecal incontinence secondary to obstetric damage: superior to sphincter repair. *Colorectal Dis* (Suppl) 2004; 6: 676-8.
47. Fernando RJ, Sultan AH, Radley S, Jones PW, Johanson RB. Management of obstetric anal sphincter injury: a systematic review and national practice survey. *BMC Health Serv Res* 2002; 2: 9.

# Chapter 21

Multimodal strategies for peri-operative optimisation

Sarah C Mills MRCS, Colorectal Fellow
Alastair C Windsor MD FRCS FRCS (Ed), Consultant Colorectal Surgeon
St. Mark's Hospital, Harrow, Middlesex, UK

What are the issues?

Patient morbidity and mortality associated with surgical procedures is determined by multiple factors. Although single interventions, such as antibiotic use and thrombo-embolic prophylaxis, have reduced morbidity and mortality, significant further reductions are only likely to result if the whole spectrum of modalities determining surgical outcome is addressed in an integrated, multidisciplinary fashion.

Organ dysfunction resulting from a surgical insult is the result of both endocrine and catabolic changes. The endocrine response is complex and manifests as elevated serum concentrations of the classic "stress" hormones, adrenaline and cortisol. Together with the accompanying elevations in corticotrophin, growth hormone and glucagons, this results in the hyperglycaemia and hypercatabolism that characterise the stress response. If volume depletion is present, vasopressin, renin and aldosterone secretion are stimulated which results in fluid retention and hyponatraemia. The catabolic response is mediated through the neuroendocrine axis. It is characterised by enhanced proteolysis and nitrogen excretion, gluconeogenesis and resistance of peripheral tissues to insulin. Its purpose is the release of energy from substrates, which is used for defence and tissue regeneration. The surgical stress response also encompasses changes in inflammatory responses and immunity. Although these stress responses have evolved to confer a survival advantage, they may, if amplified and prolonged, also contribute to reduction of body cell mass and physiological reserve capacity and ultimately result in multi-organ failure.

Multimodal intervention relies on a sound knowledge of the pathophysiology of the peri-operative period and a willingness to reassess and revise traditional, peri-operative surgical care principles. Its aim is to reduce surgical stress-induced organ dysfunction and the accompanying morbidity that results in a need for prolonged hospitalisation. It is a pre-requisite of such interventions that they are of proven efficacy, standardisation, safety and cost-effectiveness.

Where are we now?

Pre-operative fasting

Traditional guidelines recommend a 6-8 hour period of pre-operative fasting to reduce the risk of aspiration on induction of anaesthesia. This time period relates to gastric emptying of solid food. Gastric emptying of fluids, however, occurs within 2-3 hours. Long-term prospective studies and retrospective reviews of trials allowing consumption of up to a litre of clear fluids up until 2 hours pre-operatively, showed a subjective improvement in postoperative recovery and improved patient comfort with no increase in morbidity [1-3].

Pre-operative intake of a carbohydrate drink has been shown by meta-analysis to shorten length of hospital stay by reducing postoperative endocrine catabolic responses and improving insulin resistance [4,5].

Hydration status

Optimisation of intravascular volume status pre-operatively is essential for resuscitation of acutely ill patients and has been shown to decrease the risks of acute peri-operative renal failure, thrombo-embolism and fat embolus syndrome [6,7]. In elective patients, compensatory fluid administration for dehydration subjectively improves recovery and reduces discomfort [8]. Invasively-monitored fluid status optimisation in a high dependency unit for major elective cases has been shown to improve morbidity and mortality by optimising oxygen delivery to the tissues, but is rarely practised due to resource constraints [9].

Nutritional status

Malnutrition has long been recognised as having an adverse effect on surgical outcome. Despite this the rates of malnutrition in hospital in-patients are consistently reported to range from 30-50% [10]. Pre-operative nutritional supplementation of 5-7 days' duration has been shown to be of benefit in both well- and malnourished surgical patients in terms of reducing complication rates and length of stay [11,12]. Pre-operative supplementation is as effective as postoperative or peri-operative dietary supplementation. A meta-analysis of eight studies comparing modes of delivery of feeding showed that feeding via an enteral route had a infectious complication rate of 18% compared to a rate of 35% for parenteral feeding [13]. The benefits of enteral feeding have been attributed to the concept of gut origin sepsis. Experimental models have shown that avoidance of enteral feeding leads to a failure of gut barrier function, loss of gut mucosal immunity and mucosal atrophy, all of which contribute to translocation of bacteria across the gut mucosa [14].

Three meta-analyses have shown that compared to standard nutritional formulas the addition of immuno-active ingredients to the supplement results in shorter hospital stays and postoperative infectious complications in high risk patients [15-17]. Such nutritional interventions are cost-effective [10]. Further studies are needed to assess the benefits in moderate risk patients. There are inconsistencies in feeding trials for which there are several possible explanations. Firstly, there has been no standardisation of the combination of immuno-active agents used in nutritional formulations and, secondly, recent evidence has identified genetic polymorphisms which predict individual variation in response to immunomodulation [18].

Patients with diseases such as Crohn's disease must be assessed for specific micronutrients and vitamin deficiencies resulting from poor diet, malabsorption or the disease process itself, and these deficiencies corrected pre-operatively.

Medical comorbidity

Full evaluation of pre-existing medical comorbidities such as diabetes mellitus, chronic obstructive airways disease and cardiac disease should take place pre-operatively, allowing time for optimisation of the relevant organ function. Care should be taken to ensure that pre-operative fasting does not interfere with administration of regular medications, such as beta-blockers, antihypertensives and ACE inhibitors, as this has been linked to an increased incidence of cerebrovascular complications in the postoperative period [19].

Pharmacological means used to enforce alcohol abstinence for 4 weeks have resulted in lower morbidity and enhanced recovery in alcohol misusers [20]. One to two months of abstinence are required to improve pulmonary function in smokers and this should be encouraged [21].

Bowel preparation

Mechanical preparation of the bowel before elective colorectal surgery has long been believed to reduce the clinical effects of anastomotic leakage. Bowel preparation has significant adverse physiological effects [22]. These may not be detrimental in otherwise healthy patients who follow oral rehydration instructions, but the wisdom of subjecting high ASA grade patients to the fluid and electrolyte derangements that result from iatrogenic diarrhoea has been questioned. Evidence-based data in the surgical literature now suggest that mechanical bowel preparation may be unnecessary and possibly harmful [23]. Meta-analyses have revealed, however, that many of the trials were underpowered, and large, multicentre randomised controlled trials are required to clarify this issue.

Consent and patient education

No surgical procedure should be undertaken without the full consent of the patient. Patient education about the peri-operative care plan plays a significant role in reducing peri-operative anxiety and enhancing recovery [24,25]. Studies have indicated that the well-informed patient requires less analgesia and feels significantly less pain than the under-informed patient [26].

Operative factors

Maintenance of normothermia
Operating theatres are generally maintained at temperatures between 20-25°C, which is just below the zone of thermal neutrality for semi-clad patients. In addition, general anaesthesia alters the thermoregulatory set point for defence against cold exposure [27]. Spinal and epidural anaesthetics also alter central and peripheral thermoregulatory responses [27]. Hypothermia, with a fall in core temperature of 2-4°C, is often observed, especially with procedures lasting more than 2 hours. Falling core temperature is associated with the release of cortisol and catecholamines, which augments the surgical stress response [28]. Hypothermia has been associated with a two-fold to three-fold increase in surgical wound infections, significant increases in intra-operative blood loss, an increased incidence of peri-operative cardiac events and a 40% increase in nitrogen excretion [29-32]. Recent studies suggest that forced air heaters are the most effective way of maintaining intra-operative normothermia and their use is recommended in all major surgical procedures [33].

Thrombo-embolic prophylaxis
Surgery changes the coagulation/fibrinolytic balance in favour of coagulation hence increasing the risk of deep venous thrombosis (DVT) and pulmonary thrombo-embolism. Guidelines for thrombo-embolic prophylaxis have been established based on randomised controlled trials and meta-analyses [34]. Recent trials suggest that due to its sympatholytic actions, epidural anaesthesia increases venous flow in the leg thus aiding prevention of peri-operative venous stasis. This suggests a role for preferential selection of combined epidural and general anaesthetic in subjects at high risk for venous thrombo-embolism, particularly when optimal DVT prophylaxis is not possible due to limitations pertaining to the nature of surgery [35]. Other modalities of proven efficacy in thrombo-embolic prophylaxis are intra-operative, intermittent pneumatic compression, pre-operative autologous blood donation, expeditious surgery, minimising femoral vein occlusion and blood loss, patient mobilisation with foot exercises immediately after surgery, and early ambulation [36].

Antibiotic prophylaxis
Up to 2-5% of patients undergoing clean extra-abdominal operations and up to 20% undergoing intra-abdominal operations will develop a surgical site infection (SSI) [37]. Intravenous infusion of an appropriate antibiotic in the 60 minutes preceding the initial skin incision, to ensure peak tissue concentrations at the time of surgery, is recommended for almost all operations. The drug should be provided in an adequate dose on the basis of patient body weight, adjusted dosing weight, or body mass index, and administration should be repeated intra-operatively if the operation is still in progress two half-lives after the first dose to ensure adequate antimicrobial levels until wound closure [38]. The antimicrobial chosen should be active against bacteria that are likely to be encountered during the

particular type of operation being performed and should be safe for the patient and economical for the hospital.

Although a recent study suggests that in colorectal surgery the combination of oral prophylaxis with parenteral antimicrobial prophylaxis may result in lower SSI rates, this is not specified in any published guideline [39].

The majority of published evidence demonstrates that antimicrobial prophylaxis after wound closure is unnecessary, and most studies comparing single-dose prophylaxis with multiple-dose prophylaxis have not shown benefit of additional doses [40]. Prolonged use of prophylactic antimicrobials is associated with emergence of resistant bacterial strains, hence for the majority of operations the guidelines recommend that prophylaxis should end within 24 hours after the operation [38].

Minimal access surgery

The use of minimally invasive surgical techniques has not resulted in a significant reduction of the endocrine metabolic stress response to surgery but it has been associated with reductions in various inflammatory responses and immune dysfunctions [41]. Pulmonary function and postoperative hypoxemia does seem to be improved with laparoscopic surgery and postoperative ileus is reduced in clinical and experimental studies [8,42]. Subsequent studies have shown a shortened length of hospital stay, less pain and reduction of morbidity after minimal access surgery, but it is not clear whether this is due to altered pathophysiological responses to surgery or to concomitant changes in postoperative care pathways aimed at accelerated recovery. In studies where peri-operative care pathways were standardised, the same results were achieved with open and laparoscopic procedures.

In cases where minimal access surgery is inappropriate or impossible, thought should be given to the choice of wound. Horizontal abdominal incisions cause less pain and pulmonary dysfunction compared with longitudinal incisions [43].

Postoperative factors

Nasogastric tubes, urinary catheters and drains

Many of the guidelines for postoperative care are based on tradition and have not been validated by scientific studies. In the light of recent studies such approaches may hinder recovery or even contribute to morbidity. Meta-analysis has shown that the routine use of nasogastric tubes after elective abdominal surgery is unnecessary, and may contribute to pulmonary complications [44]. Furthermore, the presence of nasogastric tubes delays re-commencement of feeding and thereby hinders recovery. The routine use of drains in colonic surgery does not improve outcome as determined by randomised clinical trials [45,46].

Thus, in most cases, routine drainage can be avoided, or limited to a short period, allowing for earlier postoperative feeding and mobilisation. In operations where drainage has been proved efficacious, such as mastectomy, consideration should be given to home discharge with the drain in place and provision of appropriate support post-discharge.

The few controlled studies aimed at establishing optimal duration of urinary drainage suggest that after major, low rectal operations urinary drainage should be limited to 3 days and to 1 day after all other types of colonic surgery [47,48]. The use of low-dose thoracic bupivicaine-opioid epidurals should not be an indication for urinary drainage beyond 24 hours, despite continuous infusion as the risk of urinary retention is only 9% [48].

Postoperative hypoxaemia

Early postoperative hypoxaemia is closely related to the impairment of pulmonary function resulting from anaesthesia and a supine position. Late postoperative hypoxaemia may be persistent or take the form of episodic, nocturnal desaturations and is an important contributing factor to postoperative cardiac dysfunction and possibly myocardial infarction [49]. Modalities to improve postoperative pulmonary function include providing sufficient analgesia, positioning the patient optimally and early mobilisation. Postoperative pulmonary function is best improved by continuous epidural anaesthesia and reduced opioid use. The supine position is best avoided as this impairs pulmonary function and reduces oxygen saturation. Regular physiotherapy can also aid pulmonary function in the postoperative period.

Provision of early, supplemental oxygen has been shown to reduce nausea and vomiting, decrease the incidence of wound infection, reduce tachycardia, and improve cerebral dysfunction [49-52]. Although there are no controlled data available for the advantage or preventing late postoperative hypoxaemia, supplemental oxygen is recommended for high risk patients in the first 2-4 days if the patients are supine at night or their oxygen saturation is less than 93%.

Analgesia

Pain in the postoperative period results from several nociceptive mechanisms including nociceptive stimuli at the surgical wound site, injury-induced inflammation, sensitisation of peripheral somatic and visceral nociceptive nerve terminals and central neurons and loss of the local and descending inhibition of neurons in the brainstem and spinal cord [53]. It seems rational, therefore, to manage pain by combining treatment modalities that work on different mechanisms, hence harnessing their additive or synergistic effects whilst reducing side-effects. Combinations of local anaesthetic epidurals, opioids with NSAIDs, and NSAIDs with paracetamol have shown improved analgesia in several trials [54-58]. By blunting autonomic and somatic reflex responses, effective analgesia restores organ function and enables early mobilisation and food intake.

Epidural local anaesthetics result in effective pain relief and improved gastrointestinal function compared with opioid-based analgesia after abdominal surgery [59,60]. Addition of opioids relieves pain more effectively, but the effect on gastrointestinal motility of even small doses of opioid has not been quantified. Epidurals are safe and effective, easily managed on the ward and a prerequisite for accelerated recovery. If opioids are used, patient-controlled analgesic methods reduce the required dose but do not reduce morbidity or length of hospital stay [61]. The advent of cyclo-oxygenase-2 (COX-2) inhibitors, which have the analgesic potential to replace NSAIDs and their inherent side effects, might have had considerable benefit to the success of enhanced care pathways but for the recent concerns regarding cardiovascular safety.

New techniques and drugs also hold promise. Local anaesthetic administration into the surgical wound is of benefit in minor operations and continuous wound infusion with local anaesthetic has shown early promising results in larger wounds [62,63]. Gabapentin has shown an effective analgesic and opioid-sparing effect in acute pain in recent studies [64,65]. Pre-emptive analgesia has not been shown to be effective in meta-analysis [66].

Early enteral feeding

Traditional postoperative regimens restrict oral intake. The reasons cited for this approach include the presence of postoperative ileus (PI), the risk of anastomotic dehiscence, nausea and vomiting and loss of appetite. However, restricting intake results in catabolism with weight and skeletal muscle loss, increasing fatigue and duration of convalescence. Lack of an enteral diet also results in increased bowel mucosal permeability with possible bacterial translocation and an increase in infectious complications [67].

Scintigraphic measurement of entire gastrointestinal motility shows normalisation within 48 hours in patients undergoing open colonic resection with multimodal rehabilitation [68]. This observation underlies the numerous studies that have shown early enteral feeding after colonic surgery (open or laparoscopic) to be well tolerated and not associated with an increased incidence of complications, such as anastomotic leakage and intra-abdominal abscess formation. Men and patients undergoing total colectomy are more likely to be intolerant of early feeding [69-72].

Prolonged nutritional therapy post-surgery only appears to be of benefit in malnourished patients [73,74].

Postoperative nausea and vomiting

Postoperative nausea and vomiting (PONV) are two of the commonest problems preventing resumption of enteral feeding and slowing recovery. There are no controlled trials on multimodal approaches to reducing nausea and vomiting but there are results from good single modality trials. Propofol anaesthesia [75], ondansetron [76], pre-operative single-dose dexamethasone [77], early postoperative supplemental oxygen [78] and omission of nitrous oxide during anaesthesia have all been shown to be effective anti-emetics [79]. The use of NSAIDs, local anaesthesia and epidural infusions all have opioid-sparing effects, hence reducing their emetic effects. Metoclopramide is ineffective at reducing nausea and vomiting [80].

Postoperative ileus

Postoperative ileus (PI) is defined as an impairment of gastrointestinal motility after abdominal or other surgery. Its pathophysiology involves inhibitory neural reflexes and inflammatory mediators released from the site of injury. It is an inevitable response to surgery but has never been proven to have a purpose. Function normally returns to the bowel within 48-72 hours, but delayed return of function can increase patient discomfort, delay feeding, increase pulmonary morbidity and lengthen hospital stays.

The only modalities proven to decrease the incidence of PI are thoracic epidural with local anaesthetic [81-83], minimal access surgery [84,85], and opioid-sparing analgesic regimens [86]. The only beneficial pharmacological intervention is oral or intravenous cisapride [87-89]. Only one study has assessed the pro-kinetic effects of laxatives on PI. This showed a duration of ileus of 3 days with a 50% decrease in length of stay [90]. Early enteral feeding elicits a propulsive reflex response and releases hormones that have a stimulatory effect on gastrointestinal motility. Trials controlled for other multimodal factors, such as type of analgesia, have not been conducted, but some trials do show reduction in PI with early feeding [91-93]. Experimental studies suggest that kappa opioid agonists and peripheral μ-opioid antagonists may reduce ileus [94].

As with other post-surgical pathophysiology, the greatest reduction in duration of ileus is likely to be the result of a multimodal approach. In a study of 60 patients in an accelerated rehabilitation programme consisting of thoracic epidural with ketorolac or paracetamol, immediate removal of nasogastric tube post-surgery, mobilisation within 8 hours and enteral feeding from the day of surgery after open colorectal surgery, ileus was significantly reduced with 95% of patients tolerating normal food and defecating within 48 hours [95].

Fatigue, convalescence and return to activities of daily living

Early postoperative fatigue may be related to distorted sleep patterns as a result of noise, drugs (opioids, benzodiazepines) and the inflammatory response. Late postoperative fatigue is related to the magnitude of surgical injury, postoperative impairment of nutritional status with loss of weight and muscle mass, and postoperative impairment in cardiovascular adaptation to exercise. Single modality treatments have not significantly reduced postoperative fatigue, but a combined approach of minimal access surgery, effective pain control, early resumption of enteral feeding and early mobilisation is effective at reducing postoperative fatigue and length of convalescence after colonic surgery [96,97].

There appears to be no scientific basis for restrictions on activities of daily living. Studies in animals show resumption of strenuous activity within 2 weeks of an abdominal procedure without any detrimental effects [98]. Large, single centre studies of hernia surgery have shown that recommendations to commence immediate activity may shorten convalescence to a week without ill effect, instead of the traditional 2-4 weeks [99].

Early home discharge, which reduces costs and decreases the incidence of hospital-acquired infection, is only possible with the co-ordinated input of a multidisciplinary team comprised of anaesthetists, physiotherapists, occupational therapists, dieticians, stoma care and the primary healthcare practitioner.

Where are we going?

An understanding of the pathogenesis of postoperative morbidity is the key to modifying the surgical stress response with the aim of reducing morbidity and mortality. The multiple pathways constituting the stress response make it rational to address the numerous factors that hinder recovery after surgery by adopting a multimodal approach. Many controlled studies have already shown the benefits of accelerated care regimens in colorectal surgery [100-103].

However, if one were to be critical, most of the data have been generated by units with enthusiasm for this approach. Quite what constitutes the "ultimate package of care" has yet to be ascertained. In addition, the different peri-operative demands of the various surgical sub-specialities have yet to be accurately developed. There is little doubt that much of what we do as surgeons is controlled by conventional wisdom, not scientific fact, and further examination of a multimodal approach to surgical patients must constitute an advancement of the surgical craft.

References

1. Goodwin AP, Rowe WL, Ogg TW, Samaan A. Oral fluids prior to day surgery. The effect of shortening the pre-operative fluid fast on postoperative morbidity. *Anaesthesia* 1991; 46(12): 1066-8.
2. Gilbert SS, Easy WR, Fitch WW. The effect of pre-operative oral fluids on morbidity following anaesthesia for minor surgery. *Anaesthesia* 1995; 50(1): 79-81.
3. Scarlett M, Crawford-Sykes A, Nelson M. Preoperative starvation and pulmonary aspiration. New perspectives and guidelines. *West Indian Med J* 2002; 51(4): 241-5.
4. Ljungqvist O, Nygren J, Thorell A. Modulation of postoperative insulin resistance by pre-operative carbohydrate loading. *Proc Nutr Soc* 2002; 61(3): 329-36.
5. Nygren J, Soop M, Thorell A, Sree NK, Ljungqvist O. Preoperative oral carbohydrates and postoperative insulin resistance. *Clin Nutr* 1999; 18(2): 117-20.
6. Tang IY, Murray PT. Prevention of perioperative acute renal failure: what works? *Best Pract Res Clin Anaesthesiol* 2004; 18(1): 91-111.
7. McDermott ID, Culpan P, Clancy M, Dooley JF. The role of rehydration in the prevention of fat embolism syndrome. *Injury* 2002; 33(9): 757-9.
8. Holte K, Kehlet H. Compensatory fluid administration for preoperative dehydration - does it improve outcome? *Acta Anaesthesiol Scand* 2002; 46(9): 1089-93.
9. Wilson J, Woods I, Fawcett J, et al. Reducing the risk of major elective surgery: randomised controlled trial of preoperative optimisation of oxygen delivery. *BMJ* 1999; 318(7191): 1099-103.
10. Green C. Existence, causes and consequences of disease-related malnutrition in the hospital and community, and clinical and financial benefits of nutritional intervention. *Clinical Nutrition* 1999; 18 (Supplement 2): 3-28.
11. Gianotti L, Braga M, Nespoli L, et al. A randomized controlled trial of preoperative oral supplementation with a specialized diet in patients with gastrointestinal cancer. *Gastroenterology* 2002; 122(7): 1763-70.
12. Braga M, Gianotti L, Nespoli L, Radaelli G, Di C, V. Nutritional approach in malnourished surgical patients: a prospective randomized study. *Arch Surg* 2002; 137(2): 174-80.
13. Moore FA, Feliciano DV, Andrassy RJ, et al. Early enteral feeding, compared with parenteral, reduces postoperative septic complications. The results of a meta-analysis. *Ann Surg* 1992; 216(2): 172-83.
14. Mohr AJ, Leisewitz AL, Jacobson LS, et al. Effect of early enteral nutrition on intestinal permeability, intestinal protein loss, and outcome in dogs with severe parvoviral enteritis. *J Vet Intern Med* 2003; 17(6): 791-8.
15. Heyland DK, MacDonald S, Keefe L, Drover JW. Total parenteral nutrition in the critically ill patient: a meta-analysis. *JAMA* 1998; 280(23): 2013-9.
16. Beale RJ, Bryg DJ, Bihari DJ. Immunonutrition in the critically ill: a systematic review of clinical outcome. *Crit Care Med* 1999; 27(12): 2799-805.
17. Heys SD, Walker LG, Smith I, Eremin O. Enteral nutritional supplementation with key nutrients in patients with critical illness and cancer: a meta-analysis of randomized controlled clinical trials. *Ann Surg* 1999; 229(4): 467-77.
18. Grimble RF, Howell WM, O'Reilly G, et al. The ability of fish oil to suppress tumor necrosis factor alpha production by peripheral blood mononuclear cells in healthy men is associated with polymorphisms in genes that influence tumor necrosis factor alpha production. *Am J Clin Nutr* 2002; 76(2): 454-9.
19. Noble DW, Kehlet H. Risks of interrupting drug treatment before surgery. *BMJ* 2000; 321(7263): 719-20.
20. Tonnesen H, Rosenberg J, Nielsen HJ, et al. Effect of preoperative abstinence on poor postoperative outcome in alcohol misusers: randomised controlled trial. *BMJ* 1999; 318(7194): 1311-6.
21. Jackson CV. Preoperative pulmonary evaluation. *Arch Intern Med* 1988; 148(10): 2120-7.
22. Holte K, Nielsen KG, Madsen JL, Kehlet H. Physiologic effects of bowel preparation. *Dis Colon Rectum* 2004; 47(8): 1397-402.
23. Slim K, Vicaut E, Panis Y, Chipponi J. Meta-analysis of randomized clinical trials of colorectal surgery with or without mechanical bowel preparation. *Br J Surg* 2004; 91(9): 1125-30.
24. Daltroy LH, Morlino CI, Eaton HM, Poss R, Liang MH. Preoperative education for total hip and knee replacement patients. *Arthritis Care Res* 1998; 11(6): 469-78.

25. Klafta JM, Roizen MF. Current understanding of patients' attitudes toward and preparation for anesthesia: a review. *Anesth Analg* 1996; 83(6): 1314-21.
26. Egbert LD, Bant GE, Welch CE. Reduction of post-operative pain by encouragement and instruction of patients. *N Engl J Med* 1964; 207: 824-7.
27. Sessler DI. Mild perioperative hypothermia. *N Engl J Med* 1997; 336(24): 1730-7.
28. Frank SM, Higgins MS, Breslow MJ, et al. The catecholamine, cortisol, and hemodynamic responses to mild perioperative hypothermia. A randomized clinical trial. *Anesthesiology* 1995; 82(1): 83-93.
29. Kurz A, Sessler DI, Lenhardt R. Perioperative normothermia to reduce the incidence of surgical-wound infection and shorten hospitalization. Study of Wound Infection and Temperature Group. *N Engl J Med* 1996; 334(19): 1209-15.
30. Bock M, Muller J, Bach A, et al. Effects of preinduction and intraoperative warming during major laparotomy. *Br J Anaesth* 1998; 80(2): 159-63.
31. Kurz A, Sessler DI, Narzt E, et al. Postoperative hemodynamic and thermoregulatory consequences of intraoperative core hypothermia. *J Clin Anesth* 1995; 7(5): 359-66.
32. Carli F, Emery PW, Freemantle CA. Effect of peroperative normothermia on postoperative protein metabolism in elderly patients undergoing hip arthroplasty. *Br J Anaesth* 1989; 63(3): 276-82.
33. Ng SF, Oo CS, Loh KH, et al. A comparative study of three warming interventions to determine the most effective in maintaining perioperative normothermia. *Anesth Analg* 2003; 96(1): 171-6.
34. Clagett GP, Anderson FA, Jr., Geerts W, et al. Prevention of venous thromboembolism. *Chest* 1998; 114(5 Suppl): 531S-60S.
35. Delis KT, Knaggs AL, Mason P, Macleod KG. Effects of epidural-and-general anesthesia combined versus general anesthesia alone on the venous hemodynamics of the lower limb. A randomized study. *Thromb Haemost* 2004; 92(5): 1003-11.
36. Salvati EA. Multimodal prophylaxis of venous thrombosis. *Am J Orthop* 2002; 31(9 Suppl): 4-11.
37. National Nosocomial Infections Surveillance (NNIS) report, data summary from October 1986-April 1996, issued May 1996. A report from the National Nosocomial Infections Surveillance (NNIS) System. *Am J Infect Control* 1996; 24(5): 380-8.
38. Bratzler DW, Houck PM. Antimicrobial prophylaxis for surgery: an advisory statement from the National Surgical Infection Prevention Project. *Clin Infect Dis* 2004; 38(12): 1706-15.
39. Lewis RT. Oral versus systemic antibiotic prophylaxis in elective colon surgery: a randomized study and meta-analysis send a message from the 1990s. *Can J Surg* 2002; 45(3): 173-80.
40. McDonald M, Grabsch E, Marshall C, Forbes A. Single-versus multiple-dose antimicrobial prophylaxis for major surgery: a systematic review. *ANZ J Surg* 1998; 68(6): 388-96.
41. Kehlet H. Surgical stress response: does endoscopic surgery confer an advantage? *World J Surg* 1999; 23(8): 801-7.
42. Holte K, Kehlet H. Postoperative ileus: a preventable event. *Br J Surg* 2000; 87(11): 1480-93.
43. Grantcharov TP, Rosenberg J. Vertical compared with transverse incisions in abdominal surgery. *Eur J Surg* 2001; 167(4): 260-7.
44. Cheatham ML, Chapman WC, Key SP, Sawyers JL. A meta-analysis of selective versus routine nasogastric decompression after elective laparotomy. *Ann Surg* 1995; 221(5): 469-76.
45. Merad F, Yahchouchi E, Hay JM, et al. Prophylactic abdominal drainage after elective colonic resection and suprapromontory anastomosis: a multicenter study controlled by randomization. French Associations for Surgical Research. *Arch Surg* 1998; 133(3): 309-14.
46. Urbach DR, Kennedy ED, Cohen MM. Colon and rectal anastomoses do not require routine drainage: a systematic review and meta-analysis. *Ann Surg* 1999; 229(2): 174-80.
47. Benoist S, Panis Y, Denet C, et al. Optimal duration of urinary drainage after rectal resection: a randomized controlled trial. *Surgery* 1999; 125(2): 135-41.
48. Basse L, Werner M, Kehlet H. Is urinary drainage necessary during continuous epidural analgesia after colonic resection? *Reg Anesth Pain Med* 2000; 25(5): 498-501.
49. Rosenberg J, Kehlet H. Late post-operative hypoxemia. Kinney JM, Tucker HN, Eds. Lippincott-Raven, Philadelphia, 1997: 183-206.
50. Greif R, Laciny S, Rapf B, Hickle RS, Sessler DI. Supplemental oxygen reduces the incidence of postoperative nausea and vomiting. *Anesthesiology* 1999; 91(5): 1246-52.
51. Rosenberg-Adamsen S, Kehlet H, Dodds C, Rosenberg J. Postoperative sleep disturbances: mechanisms and clinical implications. *Br J Anaesth* 1996; 76(4): 552-9.
52. Greif R, Akca O, Horn EP, Kurz A, Sessler DI. Supplemental perioperative oxygen to reduce the incidence of surgical-wound infection. Outcomes Research Group. *N Engl J Med* 2000; 342(3): 161-7.
53. Carr DB, Goudas LC. Acute pain. *Lancet* 1999; 353(9169): 2051-8.
54. Romsing J, Moiniche S, Dahl JB. Rectal and parenteral paracetamol, and paracetamol in combination with NSAIDs, for postoperative analgesia. *Br J Anaesth* 2002; 88(2): 215-26.
55. Hyllested M, Jones S, Pedersen JL, Kehlet H. Comparative effect of paracetamol, NSAIDs or their combination in postoperative pain management: a qualitative review. *Br J Anaesth* 2002; 88(2): 199-214.
56. Kehlet H, Werner M, Perkins F. Balanced analgesia: what is it and what are its advantages in postoperative pain? *Drugs* 1999; 58(5): 793-7.
57. Jin F, Chung F. Multimodal analgesia for postoperative pain control. *J Clin Anesth* 2001; 13(7): 524-39.
58. Walker SM, Goudas LC, Cousins MJ, Carr DB. Combination spinal analgesic chemotherapy: a systematic review. *Anesth Analg* 2002; 95(3): 674-715.
59. Holte K, Kehlet H. Postoperative ileus: progress towards effective management. *Drugs* 2002; 62(18): 2603-15.

60. Jorgensen H, Wetterslev J, Moiniche S, Dahl JB. Epidural local anaesthetics versus opioid-based analgesic regimes on post-operative gastrointestinal paralysis, PONV and pain after abdominal surgery. *Cochrane Review*. Oxford, 2001: Issue 2.
61. Walder B, Schafer M, Henzi I, Tramer MR. Efficacy and safety of patient-controlled opioid analgesia for acute postoperative pain. A quantitative systematic review. *Acta Anaesthesiol Scand* 2001; 45(7): 795-804.
62. Moiniche S, Jorgensen H, Wetterslev J, Dahl JB. Local anesthetic infiltration for postoperative pain relief after laparoscopy: a qualitative and quantitative systematic review of intraperitoneal, port-site infiltration and mesosalpinx block. *Anesth Analg* 2000; 90(4): 899-912.
63. Rowlingson JC. How can local anesthetic in the wound not help? *Anesth Analg* 2001; 92(1): 3-4.
64. Dirks J, Fredensborg BB, Christensen D, et al. A randomized study of the effects of single-dose gabapentin versus placebo on postoperative pain and morphine consumption after mastectomy. *Anesthesiology* 2002; 97(3): 560-4.
65. Fassoulaki A, Patris K, Sarantopoulos C, Hogan Q. The analgesic effect of gabapentin and mexiletine after breast surgery for cancer. *Anesth Analg* 2002; 95(4): 985-91.
66. Moiniche S, Kehlet H, Dahl JB. A qualitative and quantitative systematic review of pre-emptive analgesia for postoperative pain relief: the role of timing of analgesia. *Anesthesiology* 2002; 96(3): 725-41.
67. Kudsk KA. Gut mucosal nutritional support - enteral nutrition as primary therapy after multiple system trauma. *Gut* 1994; 35(1 Suppl): S52-S54.
68. Basse L, Madsen JL, Kehlet H. Normal gastrointestinal transit after colonic resection using epidural analgesia, enforced oral nutrition and laxative. *Br J Surg* 2001; 88(11): 1498-500.
69. Reissman P, Teoh TA, Cohen SM, et al. Is early oral feeding safe after elective colorectal surgery? A prospective randomized trial. *Ann Surg* 1995; 222(1): 73-7.
70. Di Fronzo LA, Cymerman J, O'Connell TX. Factors affecting early postoperative feeding following elective open colon resection. *Arch Surg* 1999; 134(9): 941-5.
71. Khalili TM, Fleshner PR, Hiatt JR, et al. Colorectal cancer: comparison of laparoscopic with open approaches. *Dis Colon Rectum* 1998; 41(7): 832-8.
72. Milsom JW, Bohm B, Hammerhofer KA, et al. A prospective, randomized trial comparing laparoscopic versus conventional techniques in colorectal cancer surgery: a preliminary report. *J Am Coll Surg* 1998; 187(1): 46-54.
73. Jensen MB, Hessov I. Randomization to nutritional intervention at home did not improve postoperative function, fatigue or well-being. *Br J Surg* 1997; 84(1): 113-8.
74. Beattie AH, Prach AT, Baxter JP, Pennington CR. A randomised controlled trial evaluating the use of enteral nutritional supplements postoperatively in malnourished surgical patients. *Gut* 2000; 46(6): 813-8.
75. Tramer M, Moore A, McQuay H. Propofol anaesthesia and postoperative nausea and vomiting: quantitative systematic review of randomized controlled studies. *Br J Anaesth* 1997; 78(3): 247-55.
76. Tramer MR, Moore RA, Reynolds DJ, McQuay HJ. A quantitative systematic review of ondansetron in treatment of established postoperative nausea and vomiting. *BMJ* 1997; 314(7087): 1088-92.
77. Henzi I, Walder B, Tramer MR. Dexamethasone for the prevention of postoperative nausea and vomiting: a quantitative systematic review. *Anesth Analg* 2000; 90(1): 186-94.
78. Greif R, Laciny S, Rapf B, Hickle RS, Sessler DI. Supplemental oxygen reduces the incidence of postoperative nausea and vomiting. *Anesthesiology* 1999; 91(5): 1246-52.
79. Tramer M, Moore A, McQuay H. Omitting nitrous oxide in general anaesthesia: meta-analysis of intraoperative awareness and postoperative emesis in randomized controlled trials. *Br J Anaesth* 1996; 76(2): 186-93.
80. Henzi I, Walder B, Tramer MR. Metoclopramide in the prevention of postoperative nausea and vomiting: a quantitative systematic review of randomized, placebo-controlled studies. *Br J Anaesth* 1999; 83(5): 761-71.
81. Scheinin B, Asantila R, Orko R. The effect of bupivacaine and morphine on pain and bowel function after colonic surgery. *Acta Anaesthesiol Scand* 1987; 31(2): 161-4.
82. Bredtmann RD, Herden HN, Teichmann W, et al. Epidural analgesia in colonic surgery: results of a randomized prospective study. *Br J Surg* 1990; 77(6): 638-42.
83. Liu SS, Carpenter RL, Mackey DC, et al. Effects of perioperative analgesic technique on rate of recovery after colon surgery. *Anesthesiology* 1995; 83(4): 757-65.
84. Bohm B, Milsom JW, Fazio VW. Postoperative intestinal motility following conventional and laparoscopic intestinal surgery. *Arch Surg* 1995; 130(4): 415-9.
85. Davies W, Kollmorgen CF, Tu QM, et al. Laparoscopic colectomy shortens postoperative ileus in a canine model. *Surgery* 1997; 121(5): 550-5.
86. Ferraz AA, Cowles VE, Condon RE, et al. Nonopioid analgesics shorten the duration of postoperative ileus. *Am Surg* 1995; 61(12): 1079-83.
87. Brown TA, McDonald J, Williard W. A prospective, randomized, double-blinded, placebo-controlled trial of cisapride after colorectal surgery. *Am J Surg* 1999; 177(5): 399-401.
88. Boghaert A, Haesaert G, Mourisse P, Verlinden M. Placebo-controlled trial of cisapride in postoperative ileus. *Acta Anaesthesiol Belg* 1987; 38(3): 195-9.
89. Verlinden M, Michiels G, Boghaert A, de Coster M, Dehertog P. Treatment of postoperative gastrointestinal atony. *Br J Surg* 1987; 74(7): 614-7.
90. Fanning J, Yu-Brekke S. Prospective trial of aggressive postoperative bowel stimulation following radical hysterectomy. *Gynecol Oncol* 1999; 73(3): 412-4.
91. Schilder JM, Hurteau JA, Look KY, et al. A prospective controlled trial of early postoperative oral intake following major abdominal gynecologic surgery. *Gynecol Oncol* 1997; 67(3): 235-40.
92. Stewart BT, Woods RJ, Collopy BT, et al. Early feeding after elective open colorectal resections: a prospective randomized trial. *ANZ J Surg* 1998; 68(2): 125-8.
93. Cutillo G, Maneschi F, Franchi M, et al. Early feeding compared with nasogastric decompression after major oncologic gynecologic surgery: a randomized study. *Obstet Gynecol* 1999; 93(1): 41-5.

94. De Winter BY, Boeckxstaens GE, De Man JG, et al. Effects of mu- and kappa-opioid receptors on postoperative ileus in rats. *Eur J Pharmacol* 1997; 339(1): 63-7.
95. Basse L, Hjort JD, Billesbolle P, Werner M, Kehlet H. A clinical pathway to accelerate recovery after colonic resection. *Ann Surg* 2000; 232(1): 51-7.
96. Bardram L, Funch-Jensen P, Jensen P, Crawford ME, Kehlet H. Recovery after laparoscopic colonic surgery with epidural analgesia, and early oral nutrition and mobilisation. *Lancet* 1995; 345(8952): 763-4.
97. Moiniche S, Bulow S, Hesselfeldt P, Hestbaek A, Kehlet H. Convalescence and hospital stay after colonic surgery with balanced analgesia, early oral feeding, and enforced mobilisation. *Eur J Surg* 1995; 161(4): 283-8.
98. Alam MW, Martin JE. A survey of some physiological responses of domestic animals during the immediate post-surgical period. *Annals NY Acad Sci* 1958;(73): 438-43.
99. Callesen T, Klarskov B, Bech K, Kehlet H. Short convalescence after inguinal herniorrhaphy with standardised recommendations: duration and reasons for delayed return to work. *Eur J Surg* 1999; 165(3): 236-41.
100. Anderson AD, McNaught CE, MacFie J, et al. Randomized clinical trial of multimodal optimization and standard perioperative surgical care. *Br J Surg* 2003; 90(12): 1497-504.
101. Basse L, Thorbol JE, Lossl K, Kehlet H. Colonic surgery with accelerated rehabilitation or conventional care. *Dis Colon Rectum* 2004; 47(3): 271-7.
102. Basse L, Raskov HH, Hjort JD, et al. Accelerated postoperative recovery programme after colonic resection improves physical performance, pulmonary function and body composition. *Br J Surg* 2002; 89(4): 446-53.
103. Basse L, Jacobsen DH, Billesbolle P, Kehlet H. Colostomy closure after Hartmann's procedure with fast-track rehabilitation. *Dis Colon Rectum* 2002; 45(12): 1661-4.

Chapter 22

Anti-adhesion strategies

Michael C Parker BSc MS FRCS FRCS (Ed), Consultant Surgeon
Darent Valley Hospital, Dartford, Kent, UK

What is the problem?

Pathogenesis of adhesions

Adhesions can be defined as abnormal attachments that form between tissues and organs and may be either congenital or acquired [1]. Acquired adhesions develop in response to trauma to the peritoneum, which has an extremely delicate surface. Triggers for adhesion formation include: infection (e.g. appendicitis), chemical irritation (e.g. spillage of the contents of dermoid cysts) and endometriosis [2,3]. In addition, adhesions may be formed following surgical trauma, prompted by events such as exposure to infection/intestinal contents, ischaemia, irritation from foreign materials (e.g. sutures, gauze, glove dusting powder), abrasion, desiccation and overheating [4].

Adhesion formation is associated with peritoneal wound healing and re-epithelialisation of the peritoneal lining. Fibrin is deposited at the damaged peritoneal surface, which enlarges and forms a bridge to adjacent tissues if injured surfaces remain in apposition (Figure 1) [5]. The process of adhesion formation begins during surgery, and re-epithelialisation is achieved within 5-7 days. Whether or not an adhesion will develop is determined during the first 5 days following peritoneal trauma. Thus the time period immediately following surgery is crucial.

The impact of adhesions

The problem of adhesions is widespread; approximately 93% of patients develop adhesions following abdominopelvic surgery [6] and while many of these patients will remain asymptomatic, a significant proportion will develop adhesion-related problems. Some of the major clinical problems associated with adhesions include small bowel obstruction (of which up to 75% of cases are adhesion-related) [7], chronic and recurrent pelvic pain (of which approximately 40% of cases are adhesion-related) [8], secondary infertility in women (of which 20-40% of cases are adhesion-related) [9,10] and re-operative complications (of which approximately 56% of cases are adhesion-related) [11].

Not only do adhesions create problems for the patient in terms of hospitalisations and reduced quality of life but they also have a significant impact on surgeons. The high numbers of re-operations associated with adhesions considerably increase the workloads of surgeons. Surgical procedures are also prolonged and complicated by the presence of adhesions [12], with a 19% risk of inadvertent enterotomy [13], 10-25% risk of bowel injury [14], risks of injury to the bladder and blood vessels and increased risks of postoperative complications.

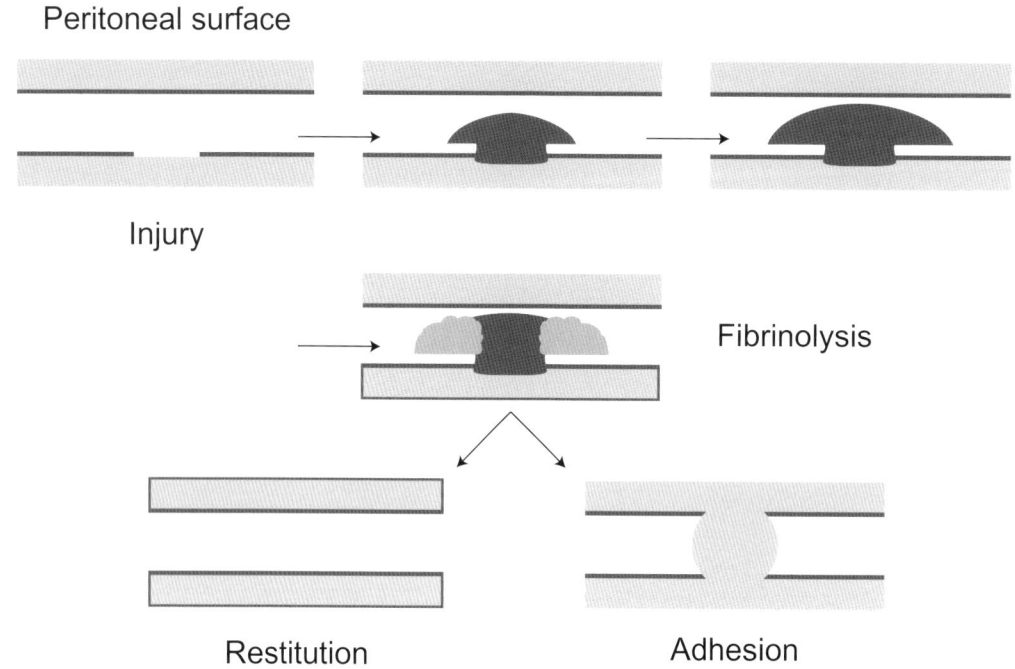

Figure 1. Pathogenesis of adhesions. Reproduced with permission from Elsevier. Holmdahl et al (1999) [5].

The burden of adhesions

Results from the SCAR study

Until recently, the scale of the problem of adhesions was unclear, since the unpredictable nature and time course of adhesion-related complications has made epidemiological assessments of adhesive disease difficult to perform. In 1992, the SCAR (Surgical and Clinical Adhesions Research) study was initiated with the purpose of determining the extent and burden of post-surgical adhesions [11,15,16]. The study involved a 10-year follow-up of nearly 30,000 patients who underwent open abdominal or pelvic surgery in Scotland in 1986 (including 12,584 patients who underwent lower abdominal surgery).

The study found that 32.6% of patients who underwent initial lower abdominal surgery in 1986 were readmitted an average of 2.2 times within the subsequent 10 years for procedures directly or possibly related to adhesions or for procedures that were complicated by adhesions. Most readmissions occurred within the first year of surgery, although readmissions continued to occur at a steady rate over the 10-year study period (Figure 2)[16]. Of the 8861 readmissions, 7.3% were considered to be directly related to adhesions. This risk varied according to the site of surgery; procedures on the colon and rectum were associated with the greatest risk of adhesion-related readmissions.

In summary, the SCAR study confirmed the extent and burden of adhesive disease and showed that adhesions occur most frequently following colorectal surgery, are associated with a high rate of patient readmissions, substantially increase workloads and exert a major impact on healthcare resources. Furthermore, they continue to be a problem even after 10 years.

Where are we now?

Have advances in surgery affected the burden of adhesions?

The SCAR study gave us a better understanding of the overall burden of adhesions in terms of patient readmissions and surgical workloads. However, surgical practices have changed since the completion

22 Anti-adhesion strategies

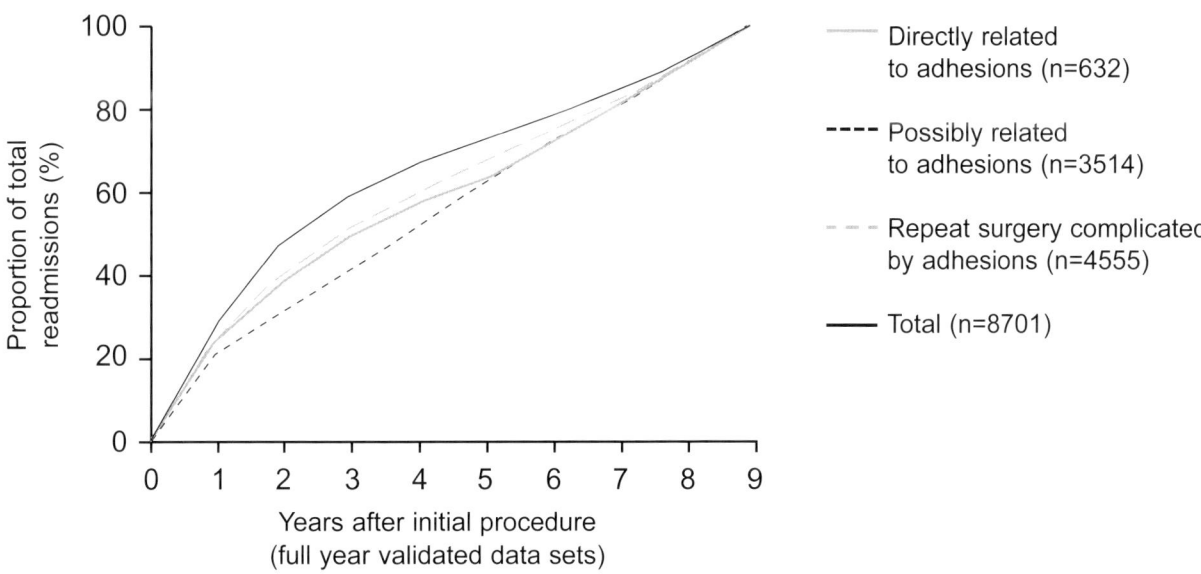

Figure 2. Timing of adhesion-related readmissions following initial open lower abdominal surgery in patients in the SCAR study. Reproduced with permission from Springer, © 2001. Parker *et al* (2001) [16].

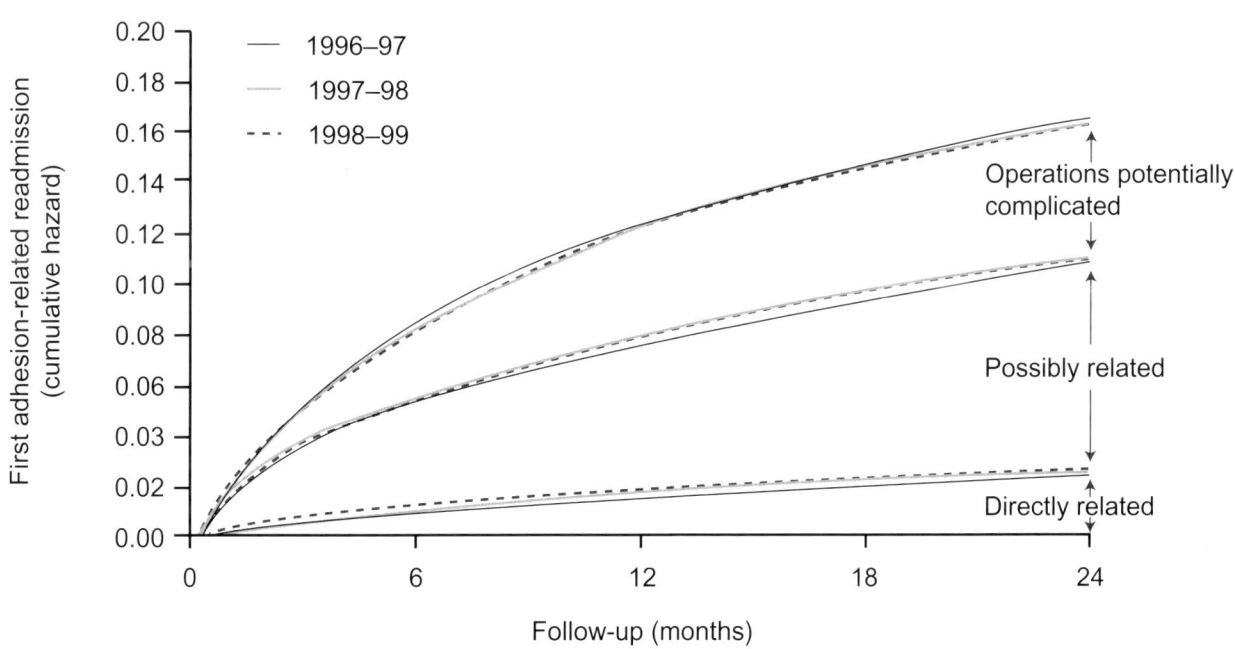

Figure 3. Cumulative risk of adhesion-related readmissions over 2 years following initial lower abdominal surgery in the 1996-97, 1997-98 and 1998-99 cohorts of the SCAR-2 study. Reproduced with permission from Blackwell Publishing Ltd. Sunderland (2003) [17].

Table 1. Summary of admission costs for surgical versus non-surgical management of adhesive small bowel obstruction in two UK hospitals over 2 years. Reproduced with permission from The Royal College of Surgeons of England, © 2001. Menzies et al (2001) [21].

Cost component	Mean cost of component per admission	
	Surgical	Non-surgical
Referral	£70.97	£77.79
Ward stay	£3,327.48	£1,267.92
Theatre	£832.32	N/A
Diagnostics	£282.73	£207.33
Drugs and fluids	£133.90	£28.29
Follow-up	£30.01	£24.82
Total	£4,677.41	£1,606.15

of the study (for example, laparoscopic surgery was in its infancy at that time) and the study did not evaluate the risk factors associated with patient readmission due to adhesions. Thus, a second study - SCAR-2 - was initiated to reassess the real-time burden of adhesion-related readmissions following lower abdominal surgery and assess the impact of previous surgery on adhesion-related outcomes [17,18]. Patients undergoing abdominopelvic surgery in the years 1996-97, 1997-98 and 1998-99 were compared and followed-up for at least 2 years.

Results for the 1996-97 incident cohort showed that 2.8% of readmission episodes occurring within the first year after surgery were directly related to adhesions, while a further 9.6% were possibly related to adhesions. The relative risk of a directly or possibly adhesion-related readmission episode following initial colorectal surgery rose from 12.4% in Year 1 (1996) to 29.7% in Year 4 (1999). Readmission rates were lower when patients who had undergone previous surgery were excluded, demonstrating the substantial impact of previous surgery on the risk of an adhesion-related readmission. The number of readmission episodes was greater than the number of patient readmissions, suggesting that many patients were readmitted more than once.

The cumulative risk of an adhesion-related readmission over 2 years was similar for each of the three incident cohorts (1996-97, 1997-98 and 1998-99; Figure 3). Thus, a key finding from this study was that, despite recent surgical advances, adhesions continue to present a significant burden to patients, surgeons and healthcare systems. Furthermore, the problem of adhesion-related events is expected to increase as greater numbers of patients undergo (often increasingly complex) surgical procedures. There is, therefore, an urgent need for the implementation of effective adhesion-prevention strategies.

Healthcare system expenditure

A number of studies have investigated the financial implications of postoperative adhesions and have shown that adhesions present a considerable financial burden to healthcare systems. A survey conducted in Sweden in 1993 found that the total costs relating to adhesive small bowel obstruction amounted to approximately US$13 million per year. Furthermore, the study did not include indirect costs, such as those for sick leave [19]. In the UK, where an estimated 158,000 lower abdominal surgery operations are conducted each year, the cumulative costs of adhesion-related readmissions over 10 years are estimated at £569 million [20]. A study analysing admissions for adhesive small bowel obstruction in two UK hospitals over 2 years found that 37% of the 110 adhesion-related admissions were treated surgically with a mean length of hospital stay of 16 days versus 7 days for non-surgical treatment, and a mean cost per surgical admission of £4677 (€7016) compared with £1606 (€2409) for non-surgical treatment (Table 1) [21].

Postoperative adhesion prevention

Surgical practice

A number of precautions can be taken during surgery to minimise the risk of adhesion formation, and it is recommended that the following techniques should be adopted by all surgeons:

- Careful surgical technique to minimise the risk of infection.
- Meticulous haemostasis.
- Minimal tissue handling.
- Avoidance of gastrointestinal contamination.
- Regular irrigation of the surgical field to minimise tissue drying.
- Minimal use of cautery and sutures.
- Avoidance of contamination by foreign bodies.
- The use of starch-free gloves [4].

Anti-adhesion adjuvants

Whilst adoption of the precautions outlined above will reduce the risks of post-surgical adhesive disease, they may not be sufficient to prevent adhesion formation, as evidenced by the SCAR study data. A number of anti-adhesion agents have become available in recent years, including pharmacological agents, physical barrier agents (solid mechanical barriers, bioabsorbable film/gel barriers) and solutions (Table 2). These anti-adhesion agents represent effective strategies to complement good surgical technique and reduce the risk of post-surgical adhesion formation; the principal agents currently in use are described in more detail below.

Interceed® (oxidised regenerated cellulose)

Interceed® is a bioabsorbable film that was introduced in 1990. The agent has been shown to reduce adhesion formation without affecting wound healing [22] and can be used at most intraperitoneal locations and during both laparoscopic and open surgical procedures. A meta-analysis of six studies assessing the efficacy of Interceed® following gynaecological laparotomies demonstrated that the agent was generally twice as effective as surgery alone in preventing postoperative adhesion formation [23]. However, Interceed® is relatively difficult to handle and turns black in the presence of blood, rendering it ineffective. It is therefore rarely used in general surgery, as meticulous haemostasis must be achieved before it can be applied.

Seprafilm® (Hyaluronic acid - carboxymethylcellulose)

Seprafilm® is the only agent that has been evaluated specifically for its adhesion-reducing potential during colorectal surgery. The film is placed under the suture line of the abdominal wound, where it persists during re-epithelialisation and is then spontaneously absorbed. In patients undergoing two-staged surgery, including colectomy with ileo pouch anal anastomosis and temporary diverting-loop ileostomy, Seprafilm® significantly reduced the incidence, extent, density and vascularisation of adhesions [24].

Data from a major multicentre colorectal study have recently been published, confirming the general safety of this agent. However, data from the same study also indicate that the use of Seprafilm® at the sites of anastomoses is to be avoided due to an increased risk of anastomotic leakage [25]. Additionally, the use of Seprafilm® in laparoscopy is extremely challenging and the agent is rarely used in these procedures.

SprayGel™ (synthetic polyethylene glycol solution)

SprayGel™ was approved for use in open and laparoscopic surgery in Europe in 2001. It consists of two water-based synthetic polyethylene glycol (PEG) solutions that mix to form a hydrogel film when sprayed onto target tissues. One solution is clear, while the other is coloured with methylene blue, so that it is easy to see where it has been used. The barrier remains in place for up to 7 days before it is absorbed and excreted renally.

SprayGel™ has shown efficacy in reducing the incidence, severity and extent of adhesions in preliminary clinical trials [26,27]. However, its use is limited by the skill, time and complex set-up of equipment required to spray and coat tissues evenly with this agent. In addition, SprayGel™ is relatively expensive to use and is site-specific, limiting its action to the sites where it is administered.

Adept® (icodextrin 4% solution)

Adept® is a solution of 4% icodextrin, which was approved in Europe in 1999 for the reduction of

Frontiers in Colorectal Surgery

Table 2. The key anti-adhesion agents in use or in development.

Agent	Current status	Mode of action/type of agent	Limitations
Pharmacological agents			
Anti-inflammatory drugs	Experimental	Reduce inflammation, preventing formation of adhesions [42]	• Doubtful clinical efficacy • Inadequate drug delivery [47]
Fibrinolytics	Experimental	Reduce fibrinogenesis, preventing formation of adhesions	• Required doses are associated with risk of impaired wound healing and haemorrhage [47]
Solid mechanical barrier			
Preclude®	Approved in Europe, withdrawn in the USA	Site-specific solid mechanical barrier	• Must be sutured in place and removed at second-look laparoscopy
Bioabsorbable films			
Interceed®	Approved in Europe and the USA	Site-specific bioabsorbable film	• Difficult to handle - rarely used in laparoscopy • Incompatible with blood; difficult to use during general surgery [48,49]
Seprafilm®	Approved in Europe and the USA	Site-specific bioabsorbable film	• Handling limitations - rarely used in laparoscopy • Associated with increased rates of anastomotic leakage [25]
SurgiWrap™	Approved in Europe	Site-specific bioabsorbable film	• Must be sutured in place (dissolves after 1 year)
Bioabsorbable gels			
Hyalobarrier® gel	Approved in Europe	Site-specific bioabsorbable gel	• Not widely available or widely used
SprayGel™	Approved in Europe	Site-specific bioabsorbable gel (consists of two water-based synthetic polyethylene glycol solutions)	• Complex equipment necessary • Use of the agent requires time • Expensive
Intergel®	Withdrawn	Broad-coverage bioabsorbable gel	• Withdrawn due to late-onset postoperative pain [50]
Solutions			
Hyskon®	Never approved as an anti-adhesion agent	Dextran solution (broad coverage) Hysteroscopy fluid	• Not found to be effective in clinical trials [51] • Associated with anaphylaxis [52]
Crystalloids - saline, lactated Ringer's solution and Hartmann's solution	Widely used, but not approved specifically for adhesion reduction	Fluid barrier - hydroflotation	• Rapidly absorbed from the peritoneal cavity [53,54]
Adept®	Approved in Europe	Fluid barrier - hydroflotation	• Efficacy demonstrated following major US study [31,32] • Full publication awaited, along with results from a major European study

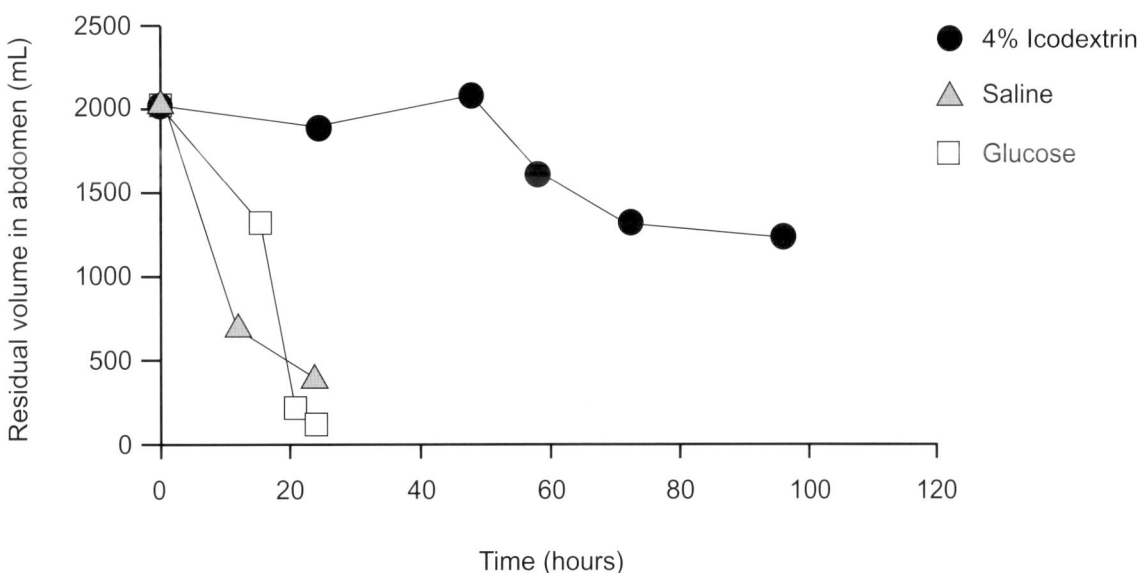

Figure 4. Intraperitoneal residence duration of Adept®. Reproduced with permission from Taylor & Francis, Inc., © 2001, http://www.taylorandfrancis.com. Hosie et al (2001) [28].

adhesions following surgery. Icodextrin 7.5% solution has been used safely and successfully as a peritoneal dialysate for a number of years. Adept® has a long intraperitoneal residence time and works by a process of "hydroflotation", remaining within the peritoneal cavity and keeping the abdominal organs apart during the critical post-surgical period when adhesion formation occurs (Figure 4) [28].

Pre-clinical studies have confirmed the efficacy of Adept® in reducing the incidence, severity and extent of adhesions [29], while data from an initial clinical study were encouraging [30]. More recently, efficacy has been fully established in a large double-blind randomised US multicentre study in gynaecological laparoscopy (PAMELA) [31,32]. The data from this study are in final analysis and already indicate a significant reduction in the incidence of adhesions. Adept is not a site-specific agent, and efficacy has been shown throughout the peritoneal cavity [31,32]. Furthermore, data from a major European registry documenting clinical experience with the agent (ARIEL; Adept® Registry for Clinical Evaluation) have shown that, for both open and laparoscopic surgery, the majority of general surgeons rated Adept's ease of use as 'good' or 'excellent' in terms of its lack of effect on the viewing of the surgical field and the handling of tissues [33, 34]. The results also indicated that Adept has a good safety profile, with a low incidence of adverse events and no deleterious effects on anastomotic healing [35]. These results are clearly encouraging and we await the full publication of the US PAMELA study as well as the findings from a large European double-blind multicentre study (GENEVA).

Where are we going?

Reducing the burden

Adhesions continue to present a considerable burden to patients and surgical teams, and that burden is likely to rise with the growing use of increasingly complex surgical procedures. For many reasons - including the fact that adhesion-related problems often occur years after surgery and may be treated by clinicians other than the initial surgeon - it is a burden that is incompletely understood and largely underestimated. This lack of awareness means that surgeons may not always appreciate the need to act.

The implications of doing nothing have been highlighted in the previous sections of this chapter: patients are at risk of numerous problems, including small bowel obstruction, female secondary infertility, chronic and recurrent pelvic pain and re-operative complications, while surgical teams face ever-increasing workloads. We should endeavour to increase awareness of the burden of adhesions, so that all of us involved in colorectal surgery take a stringent approach to adhesion prevention; this should include consideration of the use of anti-adhesion adjuvants, particularly in high risk procedures.

Identifying high risk procedures

The SCAR-3 study

If the surgical procedures associated with the greatest risks of adhesion-related complications can be identified, then adhesion-reduction strategies may be targeted to these procedures and patients may be better informed of the risks involved. It is for this reason that a third SCAR study - established to identify specific high risk procedures - was recently initiated.

The SCAR-3 study used patient data from the 1996-97 cohort of the earlier SCAR-2 study; patients were followed-up for 5 years [36,37]. While 3.8% of all patients undergoing open lower abdominal surgical procedures (n=12,756) were readmitted as a direct consequence of adhesions within 5 years, the risk of a directly-related readmission increased to 5.0% and 5.2% in patients undergoing surgery on the colon or rectum, respectively (p=0.681) and represented approximately a one in 20 risk of a direct adhesion-related readmission following surgery at each of these sites after 5 years (Table 3). For procedures on the colon, the highest risk of readmission occurred in the subgroups of patients who underwent panprocto-colectomy (15.4%) or total colectomy (8.8%). The most common surgical procedure of the colon was hemicolectomy (7.1%); the risk of readmission ranged from 3.8% for a right-sided hemicolectomy to 4.9% for a left-sided operation (p=0.091). Colostomy procedures were associated with a risk of 5.8%. A similar readmission risk was also found for abdominal wall procedures (5.4%). The large majority of rectal procedures were for excision of the rectum and had a readmission risk of 5.6%. In contrast, abdominal procedures for rectal prolapse carried a readmission risk of 1.4%.

Previous surgery was found to increase risk; patients who had undergone abdominal or pelvic surgery within the previous 5 years faced a readmission risk of 5.8%, compared with 2.5% of patients who had not undergone surgery (p<0.001). Age was found to be an important factor in readmission risk; overall, patients <60 years old had a much greater risk than those ≥60 years old (p<0.001). This trend was supported by data on each individual site of surgery. In those patients who had not had surgery within the previous 5 years, the directly related risk of readmission was higher for patients <60 years old who underwent procedures on the colon (p=0.210), rectum (p=0.101) or abdominal wall (p=0.772) (Table 3).

In those patients having had previous surgery, the risk was higher for patients <60 years old who had undergone procedures on the colon (p<0.001), rectum (p=0.022) or abdominal wall (p<0.001) (Table 3). Again, the risk of readmission in patients <60 years old following procedures on the colon was approximately three times that reported for patients ≥60 years old (colon, 9.8% vs. 3.4 %, respectively).

Developments in anti-adhesion strategies

Due to a greater understanding of the extent of adhesion-related complications in recent years and the continuing need for effective and easy-to-use strategies, a number of anti-adhesion agents are currently in development. These include barrier agents, such as a polypropylene mesh implant that acts as a biodegradable tissue scaffold [38] and an N,O-carboxymethylchitosan-based gel, which was

Table 3. Directly adhesion-related readmission risk 5 years after colorectal or abdominal wall surgical procedures (n R, total number of patients readmitted; total n, total number of procedures) [36,37].

Site and type of surgery	All % (n R/total n)	No previous surgery within 5 years		Previous surgery within 5 years	
		<60 years % (n R/total n)	≥60 years % (n R/total n)	<60 years % (n R/total n)	≥60 years % (n R/total n)
Colon	5.0 (158/3176)	5.0 (18/364)	3.5 (33/945)	9.8 (67/685)	3.4 (40/1182)
Panproctocolectomy	15.4 (19/123)	11.1 (1/9)	11.1 (1/9)	19.3 (16/83)	4.5 (1/22)
Total colectomy	8.8 (14/160)	6.7 (1/15)	9.1 (3/33)	11.0 (8/73)	5.1 (2/39)
Right hemicolectomy	3.8 (47/1235)	6.5 (11/169)	2.8 (13/463)	7.7 (13/169)	2.3 (10/434)
Left hemicolectomy	4.9 (50/1023)	1.8 (2/110)	5.1 (16/314)	8.9 (15/169)	4.0 (17/430)
sigmoid hemicolectomy	4.7 (37/779)	1.3 (1/78)	4.3 (10/233)	9.5 (13/137)	3.9 (13/331)
Colostomy	5.8 (24/416)	7.1 (2/28)	0.0 (0/62)	9.1 (13/143)	4.9 (9/183)
Rectum	5.2 (88/1690)	8.4 (14/167)	5.2 (30/573)	7.4 (18/245)	3.7 (26/705)
Excision of rectum	5.6 (86/1539)	9.2 (14/152)	5.7 (30/522)	7.7 (17/222)	3.9 (25/643)
Prolapse of rectum	1.4 (2/140)	0.0 (0/14)	0.0 (0/46)	4.3 (1/23)	1.8 (1/57)
Abdominal wall	5.4 (118/2180)	4.2 (26/624)	3.9 (22/564)	9.7 (50/514)	4.2 (20/478)

shown to reduce the extent and severity of adhesion recurrence in patients undergoing surgery [39]. In addition, a polyhydroxybutyrate-co-hydroxyvalerate membrane loaded with streptokinase has been shown successfully to prevent adhesion formation in preclinical studies [40].

The selective suppression of the inflammatory cascade is a novel mechanism that has recently been targeted as a possible treatment for the prevention of adhesion formation. Previous studies have indicated that non-steroidal anti-inflammatory drugs (NSAIDs) may prevent adhesion formation following surgical trauma to the epithelium [41]. This is supported by the results of a recent study in which treatment with rofecoxib, an NSAID (now withdrawn) commonly used to relieve the pain and inflammation of osteoarthritis, was found effectively to prevent the development of postoperative peritoneal adhesions following midline laparotomy in rats [42].

These and other promising therapies aim to reduce the burden of adhesions in patients undergoing lower abdominal surgery; however, they are currently in the early stages of development and require further clinical investigation in order to fully evaluate treatment, efficacy and safety.

Medicolegal considerations

Recent years have seen a rise in the number of legal claims relating to post-surgical adhesions. Between 1995 and 1999, the UK Medical Defence Union - one of several insurers for the private sector - received 77 adhesion-related claims, with average settlements of £50,765 (€74,625). The most common claims of negligence were failure/delay of diagnosis, bowel damage at adhesiolysis, chronic abdominal/pelvic pain, infertility/risk of infertility, starch granuloma caused by the use of starch-powdered gloves and failure to take precautions to prevent adhesion formation [43]. With increasing numbers of patients undergoing surgery, the incidence of adhesions and therefore, the possibility of litigious claims are likely to increase.

Informed consent initiatives and the duty of care

Surgeons have a duty of care to provide advice and information to patients, enabling them to make rational and informed decisions on whether to accept or refuse treatment. However, a patient survey by the International Adhesions Society [44,45] found that adhesions were mentioned as part of the informed consent process in only 10.4% of cases, in which only 54% of adhesiolysis patients were given some information about adhesions prior to surgery.

A lack of patient education is often linked to cases of negligence, with many patients claiming that, with sufficient information, consent would not have been granted. By informing patients of the risks of adhesion formation before surgery, surgical teams can satisfy the duty of care in providing patients with sufficient information on which to make informed decisions. In addition, claims of negligence relating to adhesion-induced complications and thus the financial burden on healthcare systems, may be reduced.

Recommendations have recently been developed in gynaecological surgery to advise patients of the risk of adhesions as a part of the consent process and to consider the use of anti-adhesion agents in high risk surgery [46]. Similar recommendations could usefully be adopted within the arena of general and specifically colorectal surgery in order to minimise the ongoing and costly burden of adhesions and adhesion-related complications.

Conclusions

Adhesions are a widespread problem following abdominopelvic surgery and are associated with numerous complications. Despite advances in surgical practice, adhesions continue to represent a significant burden for patients, surgeons and healthcare systems. At present, surgeons are advised to employ good surgical practice to prevent adhesion formation. In addition, increasing evidence is becoming available to support the efficacy of anti-adhesion adjuvants to complement good surgical technique, including agents that are relatively inexpensive and simple to use.

It is becoming apparent that we need to increase awareness of post-surgical adhesions in order to reduce the burden of adhesive disease. A recent study has identified procedures that are associated with particularly high risks of adhesions and it is critical that surgeons should be made aware of these procedures, so that they can advise patients of the risks involved and utilise anti-adhesion strategies in these cases. Failure of surgeons to warn patients of the risks of adhesions can result in claims of negligence - a situation that is becoming increasingly common. Surgeons have a duty of care to protect their patients by providing the best possible standard of care in order to prevent adhesion formation. The implementation of simple to use and relatively inexpensive anti-adhesive agents, particularly in procedures with a high risk of adhesion formation, may help to protect patients from the complications associated with surgical adhesions and meets the demands of duty of care.

References

1. Holmdahl L, Risberg B, Beck DE, et al. Adhesions: pathogenesis and prevention-panel discussion and summary. *Eur J Surg* Suppl 577 1997; 163: 56-62.
2. Holmdahl L, Risberg B. Adhesions: prevention and complications in general surgery. *Eur J Surg* 1997; 163: 169-74.
3. Diamond MP, Freeman ML. Clinical implications of postsurgical adhesions. *Hum Reprod Update* 2001; 7: 567-76.
4. Monk BJ, Berman ML, Montz FJ. Adhesions after extensive gynecologic surgery: clinical significance, etiology, and prevention. *Am J Obstet Gynecol* 1994; 170: 1396-403.
5. Holmdahl L. Making and covering of surgical footprints. *Lancet* 1999; 353: 1456-7.
6. Menzies D, Ellis H. Intestinal obstruction from adhesions - how big is the problem? *Ann R Coll Surg Engl* 1990; 72: 60-3.
7. Ellis H. The magnitude of adhesion related problems. *Ann Chir Gynaecol* 1998; 87: 9-11.
8. diZerega GS. Biochemical events in peritoneal tissue repair. *Eur J Surg* Suppl 1997; 577: 10-6.
9. Hershlag A, Diamond MP, Decherney AH. Adhesiolysis. *Clin Obstet Gynecol* 1991; 34: 395-402.
10. Mishell DR, Davajan V. Evaluation of the infertile couple. In: *Infertility Contraception & Reproductive Endocrinology*, 3rd edition. Mishell DR, Davajan V, Lobo RA, Eds. Blackwell Scientific Publications Inc., Massachusetts, 1991: 557-70.
11. Ellis H, Moran BJ, Thompson JN, et al. Adhesion-related hospital readmissions after abdominal and pelvic surgery: a retrospective cohort study. *Lancet* 1999; 353: 1476-80.

12. Coleman MG, McLain AD, Moran BJ. Impact of previous surgery on time taken for incision and division of adhesions during laparotomy. *Dis Colon Rectum* 2000; 43: 1297-9.
13. van der Krabben AA, Dijkstra FR, Nieuwenhuijzen M, Reijnen MM, Schaapveld M, van Goor H. Morbidity and mortality of inadvertent enterotomy during adhesiotomy. *Br J Surg* 2000; 87: 467-71.
14. Swank DJ, Swank B, Hop WC, *et al*. Laparoscopic adhesiolysis in patients with chronic abdominal pain: a blinded randomised controlled multi-centre trial. *Lancet* 2003; 361: 1247-51.
15. Lower AM, Hawthorn RJ, Ellis H, Brien F, Buchan S, Crowe AM. The impact of adhesions on hospital readmissions over ten years after 8849 open gynaecological operations: an assessment from the Surgical and Clinical Adhesions Research Study. *BJOG* 2000; 107: 855-62.
16. Parker MC, Ellis H, Moran BJ, *et al*. Postoperative adhesions: ten-year follow-up of 12,584 patients undergoing lower abdominal surgery. *Dis Colon Rectum* 2001; 44: 822-9.
17. Sunderland G. SCAR2 - The risk of adhesions following colorectal surgery. *Colorectal Dis* 2003; 5: 598.
18. Parker MC, Wilson MS, Menzies D, *et al*. Colorectal surgery: the risk and burden of adhesion-related complications. *Colorectal Dis* 2004; 6: 506-11.
19. Ivarsson ML, Holmdahl L, Franzen G, Risberg B. Cost of bowel obstruction resulting from adhesions. *Eur J Surg* 1997; 163: 679-84.
20. Wilson MS, Menzies D, Knight A, Crowe AM. Demonstrating the clinical and cost effectiveness of adhesion reduction strategies. *Colorectal Dis* 2002; 4: 355-60.
21. Menzies D, Parker M, Hoare R, Knight A. Small bowel obstruction due to postoperative adhesions: treatment patterns and associated costs in 110 hospital admissions. *Ann R Coll Surg Engl* 2001; 83: 40-6.
22. Interceed (TC7) Adhesion Barrier Study Group. Prevention of postsurgical adhesions by INTERCEED(TC7), an absorbable adhesion barrier: a prospective randomized multicenter clinical study. *Fertil Steril* 1989; 51: 933-8.
23. Wiseman DM, Trout JR, Franklin RR, Diamond MP. Meta-analysis of the safety and efficacy of an adhesion barrier (Interceed TC7) in laparotomy. *J Reprod Med* 1999; 44: 325-31.
24. Becker JM, Dayton MT, Fazio VW, *et al*. Prevention of postoperative abdominal adhesions by a sodium hyaluronate-based bioresorbable membrane: a prospective, randomized, double-blind multicenter study. *J Am Coll Surg* 1996; 183: 297-306.
25. Beck DE, Cohen Z, Fleshman JW, *et al*. A prospective, randomized, multicenter, controlled study of the safety of Seprafilm adhesion barrier in abdominopelvic surgery of the intestine. *Dis Colon Rectum* 2003; 46: 1310-9.
26. Mettler L, Audebert A, Lehmann W, Schive K, Jacobs VR. Prospective clinical trial of SprayGel as a barrier to adhesion formation: an interim analysis. *J Am Assoc Gynecol Laparosc* 2003; 10: 339-44.
27. Johns DA, Ferland R, Dunn R. Initial feasibility study of a sprayable hydrogel adhesion barrier system in patients undergoing laparoscopic ovarian surgery. *J Am Assoc Gynecol Laparosc* 2003; 10: 334-8.
28. Hosie K, Gilbert JA, Kerr D, Brown CB, Peers EM. Fluid dynamics in man of an intraperitoneal drug delivery solution: 4% icodextrin. *Drug Deliv* 2001; 8: 9-12.
29. Verco SJ, Peers EM, Brown CB, Rodgers KE, Roda N, diZerega G. Development of a novel glucose polymer solution (icodextrin) for adhesion prevention: pre-clinical studies. *Hum Reprod* 2000; 15: 1764-72.
30. diZerega GS, Verco SJ, Young P, *et al*. A randomized, controlled pilot study of the safety and efficacy of 4% icodextrin solution in the reduction of adhesions following laparoscopic gynaecological surgery. *Hum Reprod* 2002; 17: 1031-8.
31. Peers E, Brown CB, Adept Adhesion Study Group. Adept (4% icodextrin): change in American Fertility Society score in a large, multicentre, randomised, double-blind clinical trial. Abstract F11.02 presented at the 14th Annual Congress of the International Society for Gynecologic Endoscopy. 3rd-6th April 2005, London.
32. Peers E, Brown CB, Adept Adhesion Study Group. Adept (4% icodextrin): significantly reduces post-surgical adhesion incidence in a large, randomised, double-blind clinical trial. Abstract F13.05 presented at the 14th Annual Congress of the International Society for Gynecologic Endoscopy. 3rd-6th April 2005, London.
33. Menzies D, Hidalgo M, Walz MK, Duron JJ, Tonelli F. Ease of use and safety of icodextrin 4% solution in the prevention of adhesion formation following general surgery: experience from the multicentre ARIEL registry. Abstract presented at the 5th EACP, Geneva, Switzerland, 2004. *Colorectal Dis* 2004; 6 (Suppl 2): 18 (P31).
34. Ommer A, Walz MK. Clinical experiences with icodextrin 4% solution in open and laparoscopic general surgery in the multicentre ARIEL Registry. Abstract presented at the 5th EACP, Geneva, Switzerland, 2004. *Colorectal Dis* 2004; 6 (Suppl 2): 10 (O34).
35. Rogers KE, Verco SJS, diZerega GS. Effects of intraperitoneal 4% icodextrin solution on the healing of bowel anastomoses and laparotomy incisions in rabbits. *Colorectal Dis* 2003; 5: 324-30.
36. Wilson M, on behalf of the Surgical and Clinical Adhesions Research (SCAR) Group. The risks of post-operative adhesions in colorectal surgery. Oral presentation at the European Association of Coloproctology 5th Annual Meeting, Geneva, Switzerland, 16th-18th September 2004. *Colorectal Dis* 2004; 6 (Suppl 2): 10 (O35).
37. Parker MC, Wilson MS, Menzies D, *et al*. The SCAR-3 study: 5-year adhesion-related readmission risk following lower abdominal surgical procedures. *Colorectal Dis* 2005; in press.
38. Butler CE, Prieto VG. Reduction of adhesions with composite AlloDerm/polypropylene mesh implants for abdominal wall reconstruction. *Plast Reconstr Surg* 2004; 114: 464-73.
39. Diamond MP, Luciano A, Johns DA, Dunn R, Young P, Bieber E. Reduction of postoperative adhesions by N,O-carboxymethylchitosan: a pilot study. *Fertil Steril* 2003; 80: 631-6.
40. Yagmurlu A, Barlas M, Gursel I, Gokcora IH. Reduction of surgery-induced peritoneal adhesions by continuous release of streptokinase from a drug delivery system. *Eur Surg Res* 2003; 35: 46-9.

41. Eggleston RB, Mueller PO. Prevention and treatment of gastrointestinal adhesions. *Vet Clin North Am Equine Pract* 2003; 19: 741-63.
42. Aldemir M, Ozturk H, Erten C, Buyukbayram H. The preventive effect of rofecoxib in postoperative intraperitoneal adhesions. *Acta Chir Belg* 2004; 104: 97-100.
43. Ellis H. Medicolegal consequences of postoperative intra-abdominal adhesions. *J R Soc Med* 2001; 94: 331-2.
44. Wiseman DM. Adhesions and informed consent: patient awareness of adhesions prior to surgery. Oral presentation at VIth International Symposium on Peritoneum, 2003.
45. Wiseman DM. Obtaining informed consent: patient awareness of adhesions. *Adhesions New & Views* 2003; 4: 10-12. Available at www.adept-and-adhesions.co.uk/anv/04Obtaining_informed.pdf.
46. Trew G. Consensus in adhesion reduction management. *The Obstetrician and Gynecologist* 2004; 6 (Suppl): 1-6.
47. Risberg B. Adhesions: preventive strategies. *Eur J Surg* Suppl 1997; 577: 32-9.
48. Wiseman DM, Gottlick-Iarkowski L, Kamp L. Effect of different barriers of oxidized regenerated cellulose (ORC) on cecal and sidewall adhesions in the presence and absence of bleeding. *J Invest Surg* 1999;12:141-6.
49. Gynecare Worldwide. http://www.gynecare.com/active/ethus/en_US/html/gynecare/patient/PDF/INTERCEED_Essential_Product_Information.pdf. 2004.
50. Anon. http://www.fda.gov/medwatch/SAFETY/2003/intergel.htm. 2003.
51. Rosenberg SM, Board JA. High-molecular weight dextran in human infertility surgery. *Am J Obstet Gynecol* 1984; 148: 380-5.
52. Gauwerky JF, Heinrich D, Kubli F. Complications of intraperitoneal dextran application for prevention of adhesions. *Biol Res Pregnancy Perinatol* 1986; 7: 93-7.
53. Shear L, Swartz C, Shinaberger JA, Barry KG. Kinetics of peritoneal fluid absorption in adult man. *N Engl J Med* 1965; 272: 123-7.
54. Hart R, Magos A. Laparoscopically instilled fluid: the rate of absorption amd the effects on patient discomfort and fluid balance. *Gynaecol Endos* 1996; 5: 287-91.

Chapter 23

Should we sub-specialise further?

Omer Aziz BSc MRCS, Research Fellow, Surgical Oncology
Paris P Tekkis MD FRCS, Senior Lecturer, Surgical Oncology
Imperial College, St. Mary's Hospital, London, UK

What are the issues?

Sub-specialisation in colorectal surgery

Since the late 1970s, there has been evidence to suggest that for certain procedures "low volume" hospitals are associated with higher rates of operative mortality [1, 2]. This has led to a closer examination of the relationship between volume and postoperative outcome, with complications, mortality, and utilisation of resources being shown to be lower for "high volume" hospitals and surgeons [3-5]. In parallel with this, there has also been a debate on the role of sub-specialisation in surgery, with the same authors suggesting that this too will result in a reduction in postoperative mortality, and in the context of solid tumour surgery, longer recurrence-free survival.

The debate on sub-specialisation has not surprisingly also landed on the doorstep of colorectal surgery, and in particular, surgery for colorectal cancer. The management of this, like most tumours, requires a multidisciplinary approach, with institutional factors likely to be very important in determining outcome. In the case of colorectal cancer, however, the surgeon is usually the first person to see the patient and is often responsible for deciding the initial management strategy. It has even been suggested that the surgeon is the single most important "external" factor to consider when investigating variations in outcome following colorectal cancer surgery [6]. This chapter aims to provide an up-to-date outline of the arguments for and against sub-specialisation in colorectal surgery.

Further sub-specialisation in colorectal cancer surgery

Variability in outcome from colorectal cancer surgery, as reported by studies such as the German Study Group for Colorectal Carcinoma [7] and the Wessex Cancer Registry [8], suggests that patient-related factors (such as age and stage of cancer at presentation), and institution-related factors are associated with adverse surgical outcomes. This has in turn resulted in closer investigation of the effects of "surgical performance" on outcome from colorectal cancer surgery [9].

The publication of guidelines on improving outcome from colorectal cancer, such as those by the NHS Executive in 1997, has resulted in an intuitive drive towards specialisation, despite inconclusive evidence on what effect this will actually have on outcome [10]. Although published evidence of the effects of sub-specialisation in countries such as Sweden has supported this move, it is circumstantial and therefore must be treated with caution [11]. The question that remains unanswered therefore is: what aspects of specialisation should be present to improve survival from colorectal cancer, and how should this be monitored?

Defining a specialist colorectal surgeon

There is, until now, no consensus on how best to define a "specialist" colorectal surgeon. This is mainly due to geographical variations in colorectal surgical training, varying health systems, and memberships of differing specialist organisations. The resulting variability in this definition has made it difficult to compare much of the research on sub-specialisation in colorectal surgery.

Defining the volume of colorectal surgery performed by a surgeon

The mode of quantifying the volume of surgery undertaken by a surgeon has also varied between studies, with some using rankings of "high", "intermediate" and "low" to describe this, while others have used numerical ranges (0-20, 21-40, and >41 cases per annum). Comparison of these data has therefore also been difficult.

Defining the volume of colorectal surgery performed by a hospital

The management of colorectal cancer is dependent on radiology, nursing, oncology, and colorectal services within a hospital. It is therefore not inconceivable that in centres where higher volume colorectal surgery is undertaken, management may be better organised and more efficient. Quantifying what makes a centre high volume has had the same problems and limitations as defining a high volume surgeon, and similarly requires a well thought-out and universally transferable definition.

What outcome measures define success from colorectal surgery?

In measuring success from any procedure, firm and comparable measures of outcome (endpoints) are required to help reduce heterogeneity in reporting between studies. This is particularly so when trying to assess the effect of surgeon- and institution-related factors on success from colorectal surgery. These include postoperative mortality, anastomotic leak rates, and incidence of stoma formation. With regards to colorectal cancer, however, long-term recurrence and curative resection rates are probably the best measures of success.

Emergency colorectal surgery and specialisation

Emergency colorectal surgery accounts for a significant amount of colorectal operative workload, and is therefore an important aspect for the specialty to address. Surgery for malignant bowel obstruction is a good example of an emergency colorectal operation that carries significant risk to the patient, with some suggesting it may account for over 20% of all postoperative deaths after bowel cancer surgery [12].

The management of left-sided bowel emergencies also highlights the variability in practice between surgeons, with some preferring to perform a resection and primary anastomosis, whereas others prefer a staged procedure. This decision is based on individual surgeon experience and judgment, and it is not inconceivable that specialist delivery of care in these circumstances may lead to a better outcome. Add to this the fact that at present in the UK much of this emergency surgery is carried out by "general surgeons" who would not perform this operation as part of their elective workload, and it becomes clear that the question of whether specialisation in colorectal emergency surgery improves outcomes from these operations is an important one to answer.

Where are we now?

Sub-specialisation in colorectal cancer surgery

Table 1 summarises recent evidence on the effects of volume of surgery and sub-specialisation on outcome from colorectal cancer surgery. This includes nine studies published between 1996 and 2004 [5, 9, 13-19], and with a sample group ranging from 384 to 304,285 patients. Table 2 shows the large number of definitions of specialisation and volume that have been used, making definite comparisons between studies difficult.

Initial reports suggested sub-specialisation does not affect outcome

In 1997, the Trent and Wales Colorectal Cancer Audit [12] failed to identify any improvement in postoperative mortality for operations performed by "self-declared" specialist surgeons, although an obvious limitation of this study was the relatively ambiguous definition of specialisation. With regards to outcomes from higher volume surgery, a study based in Northern Ireland in 1999 [15] failed to identify benefit associated with colorectal surgeons who performed more operations per annum. In the same year, a study of patients on the North Western Regional Cancer Registry [16] also could not show a benefit in outcome for surgeons with a volume of colorectal cancer operations of more than three cases per month.

Research suggesting surgeon as a prognostic factor

In a study comparing surgeons performing over 15 resections in 15 months to those performing a smaller number, Hermanek et al identified a higher local recurrence for the low volume surgeons [20]. These results were mirrored by others who found a lower risk of local recurrence and death from rectal cancer with surgeons who had been specialists for at least 10 years [14]. Interestingly, this risk was also lower for patients operated on in university compared with community hospitals, although it must be noted that some community hospitals did just as well as the university hospitals. These findings have led to the suggestion of the surgeon as an important prognostic factor in the treatment of colorectal cancer [21].

More recently the case for sub-specialisation has been strengthened

In a large study of 4,562 patients undergoing operations for colorectal cancer in the Wessex region, Smith et al [9] investigated the effects of surgeon specialisation and volume in outcome from colorectal cancer surgery (both emergency and elective). A specialist was defined as, "a member of the Association of Coloproctology of Great Britain and Ireland (ACPGBI) with a commitment to and special interest in coloproctology". In this study, specialists had a significantly lower postoperative mortality (6.4% versus 10.2%), lower anastomotic leak rate (2.4% versus 4.7%), higher local recurrence-free survival (89.8% versus 83.2%), and better long-term survival (45.9% versus 36.8%) than non-specialists. Importantly, local recurrence-free survival rates were higher for specialists than non-specialists for both colonic and rectal surgery. Figure 1 shows the overall Kaplan-Meier survival rate for all patients operated on by specialists versus non-specialists. The authors noted that observed variations of treatment outcome may have been related to case mix, with specialist surgeons tending to see younger, fitter patients without severe comorbidity. The non-specialist on the other hand tended to see a higher proportion of elderly patients presenting as an emergency. Adjusting for case-mix factors, however, still resulted in improved outcome following specialist intervention. Finally, with regards to case volume, surgeon workload was divided into the following groups: <5, 5-9, 10-19, 20-29, 30-49, >50 cases per annum. A highly significant association between specialisation and volume was also identified.

A much larger retrospective study by Callahan et al [18] identified 48,582 colectomies (both emergency and elective) from a statewide database in New York. Using a multivariate model, they evaluated the independent effect of having surgical sub-specialty training or a specialist surgical interest on treatment-related mortality. Specialists were defined as surgeons who were members of the Society of Surgical Oncology or Society of Colorectal Surgery,

Table 1. Effect of sub-specialisation on outcome from colorectal cancer surgery.

Author (et al)	Year	Patients	Definition S	Definition V	Findings
Rosen	1996	1,753	1	-	Specialists had an 8-year mean in-hospital mortality rate of 1.4% compared with 7.3% by other institutional surgeons (p=0.0001). Specialist colorectal surgeons also had a lower in-hospital mortality rate than other institutional surgeons as patients' severity of illness increased.
Holm	1997	1,399	2	1	Patients operated on by specialists had a lower risk of local recurrence and death from rectal cancer. The risk was also lower for patients operated on in university hospitals compared with community hospitals, although the results in some community hospitals were similar to those in university hospitals. There was no significant association between volume of surgery and outcome.
Kee	1999	3,217	3	2	Multi-level model analysis revealed a surgeon's workload or experience had no significant effect on mortality at 2 years. Survival of patients treated in hospitals with over 33 cases per annum was slightly worse than for those treated in hospitals with lower caseloads.
Parry	1999	927	4	3	Neither operator grade (consultant vs junior), consultant workload nor hospital throughput were identified as independently influencing patient survival.
Birkmeyer	2002	304,285	-	4	Postoperative mortality was significantly lower in very high volume as compared to very low volume hospitals with regards to colectomy (5.4% vs 7.4%), but for other procedures, such as oesophagectomy, this difference was much greater (8.1% versus 23.1%). Adjusted mortality for colectomy was calculated as 4.5% for very high versus 5.6% for very low volume hospitals.
Read	2002	384	3	-	Actuarial disease-free survival and local control rates at 5 years were 77% and 93% for colorectal surgeons versus non-colorectal surgeons (p<0.005). Multi-variate analysis showed the surgeon was an independent predictor of disease-free survival (p<0.006) and local control (p<0.02).
Smith	2003	4,562	5	5	Specialist figures showed significantly lower postoperative mortality, anastomotic leak rates, higher local recurrence-free survival, and better long-term survival. There was a highly significant association between specialisation and volume (>50 cases per annum).
Callahan	2003	48,582	6	6	Risk-adjusted mortality rate from colectomy for the specialist versus non-specialist was 2.4% versus 4.8% (p<0.001), even after accounting for hospital and surgeon volume and patient characteristics. Observed mortality rates decreased with increasing quartiles of both hospital (5.8% to 3%, p<0.0001) and surgeon volume (6.3% to 2.8%, p<0.0001).
McArdle	2004	3,200	7	7	Cancer-specific survival rate at 5 years was 72.7% for specialists and 63.8% for non-specialists. Adjusted hazard ratio for non-specialists was 1.35 (95% CI=1.13-1.62, p=0.01). There were no consistent differences in hazard ratios adjusted by volume.

S=Definition of 'specialisation'
V=Definition of 'volume'
See Table 2

Table 2. Definitions of sub-specialisation and volume of surgery used.

Definition of specialist used

1. Board-certified colorectal surgeon
2. Surgeons who were board-certified specialists for over 10 years
3. Number of years qualified: (Q1=<13years, Q2=14-17, Q3=18-22 years, Q4=23-30 years, Q5=>31 years)
4. Consultant surgeon
5. Member of Association of Coloproctology of Great Britain and Ireland with commitment to and special interest in coloproctology
6. Member of the Society of Surgical Oncology or Society of Colorectal Surgery
7. Surgeons defined as specialists by a panel of six senior consultants on the basis of personal knowledge, and reputation

Definition of volume of surgery used

1. Surgeon volume groups: 1-3 operations per year, >3 operations per year
2. Surgeon volume groups: 9.8-12.7, 12.8-16.1, 16.2-24.9, >25 (workload per year)
   Hospital volume groups: 24-32, 33-46, 47-54, >55 (cases per year)
3. Surgeon volume groups: 1-6, 7-12, 13-18, >19 (no of procedures)
   Hospital volume groups: 1-30, 31-44, 45-55, >56 (admissions)
4. Surgeon volume groups: very low (<33), low (33-56), medium (57-84), high (85-124), very high (>124). Brackets show cases per annum.
5. Surgeon volume groups: <5, 5-9, 10-19, 20-29, 30-49, >50 (cases per annum)
6. Surgeon volume groups: 1-27, 28-41, 48-78, 79+ (no of procedures)
   Hospital volume groups: 2-191, 192-344, 345-551, 552+ (no of procedures)
7. Surgeon volume groups: high (>60 cases), medium (30-60 cases), and low (<30 cases)

with their trial including 61 specialists and 2590 non-specialist surgeons. They found that, in general, specialists treated patients with lower comorbidity rates as compared to non-specialists, and had a significantly shorter postoperative length of hospital stay. Interestingly, specialists also treated significantly fewer patients on Medicaid (3.1% versus 6.2%), a federally funded health insurance programme for low-income families in the USA. The risk-adjusted mortality rate from colectomy for specialist versus non-specialist was 2.4% versus 4.8%, having accounted for hospital and surgeon volume and patient characteristics. Observed mortality rates decreased with increasing quartiles of both hospital (5.8% to 3%) and surgeon volume (6.3% to 2.8%). The authors boldly concluded that if all eligible patients for the studied procedures could have obtained care from sub-specialists, then 1073 deaths after colectomy could potentially have been avoided during the 4-year study period.

Although all these studies suggest that surgical mortality from colorectal surgery is inversely related to volume, the largest study aiming to answer this question is by Birkmeyer et al [5]. Using a national Medicare database (a USA federal healthcare insurance programme for people age 65 and over, and for the disabled), mortality associated with several procedures was examined, including after 304,285 colectomies. Using regression analysis, the authors attempted to describe the relationship between hospital volume and mortality, taking into account patient characteristics. Hospital volume of surgery was divided into groups of "very low" (<33), "low" (33-56), "medium" (57-84), "high" (85-124), and "very high" (>124). They found that although postoperative mortality was significantly lower in very high volume as compared to very low volume hospitals with regards to colectomy (5.4% versus 7.4%), for other procedures, such as oesophagectomy, the magnitude of this

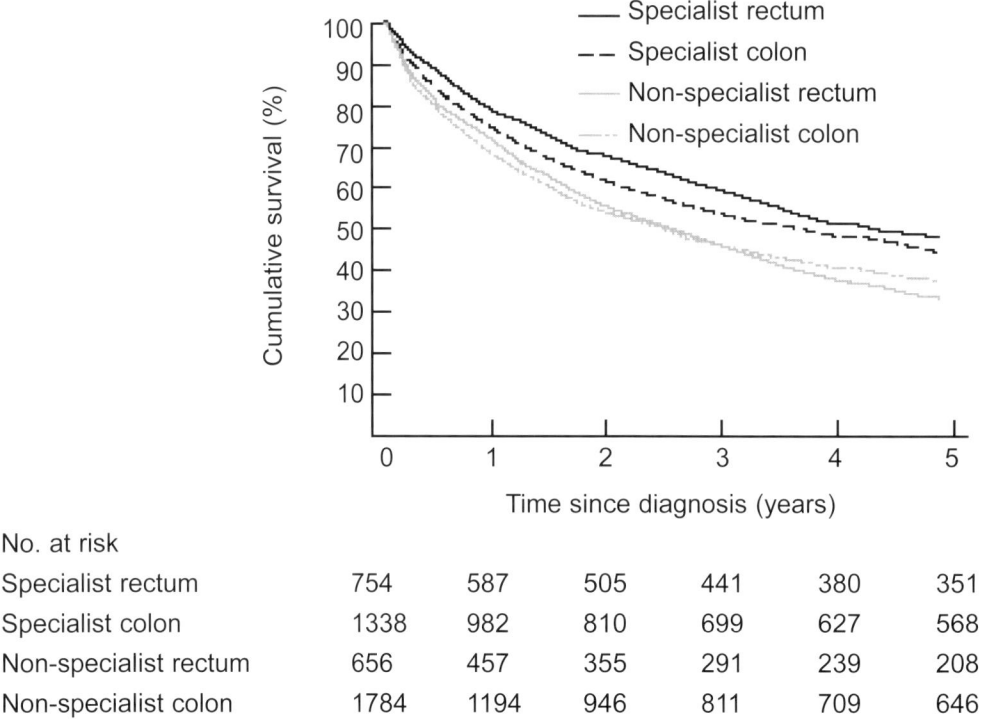

Figure 1. Five-year Kaplan-Meier survival by specialist versus non-specialist according to site (from Smith et al, 2003 [9]).

difference was much higher (8.1% versus 23.1%). The adjusted mortality for colectomy was calculated as 4.5% for very high versus 5.6% for very low volume hospitals. They concluded that this effect was too large to be attributed to chance or confounding variables, and that mortality at very low volume centres was considerably higher. Although this study was impressive in size, the authors acknowledge that a major limitation was their use of administrative data. Although the mechanisms underlying relations between volume and outcome could not be defined, authors suggested that high volume hospitals have more surgeons who specialise in specific procedures, more consistent processes for postoperative care, and better staffing and general resources for dealing with complications.

Finally, a recent study by McArdle et al [19] reported on the outcomes of 3200 consecutive colorectal cancer resections between 1991 and 1994, with particular regards to caseload and degree of surgeon specialisation. Surgeons carrying out more than 30 curative resections during the course of the study were analysed, with those who were "specialists" being selected by a panel of six senior consultants on the basis of personal knowledge and reputation. Consultants were also divided into three groups: those obtaining surgical fellowship before 1970, those between 1971 and 1980, and those after 1980. The results from comparing cancer-specific survival between specialists and non-specialists are shown in Figure 2. There was no difference in survival for the first 2 years, but between 2 and 5 years there was a significant survival improvement for those treated by specialists and especially for those with rectal cancer. The cancer-specific survival rate at 5 years was 72.7% for specialists and 63.8% for non-specialists. The adjusted hazard ratio for non-specialists was 1.35 (95% CI=1.13-1.62, p=0.01). There were no differences in outcome between the three groups according to length of experience. Although these findings are important, this study once again highlights the difficulty in defining a specialist colorectal surgeon. There were no consistent differences in

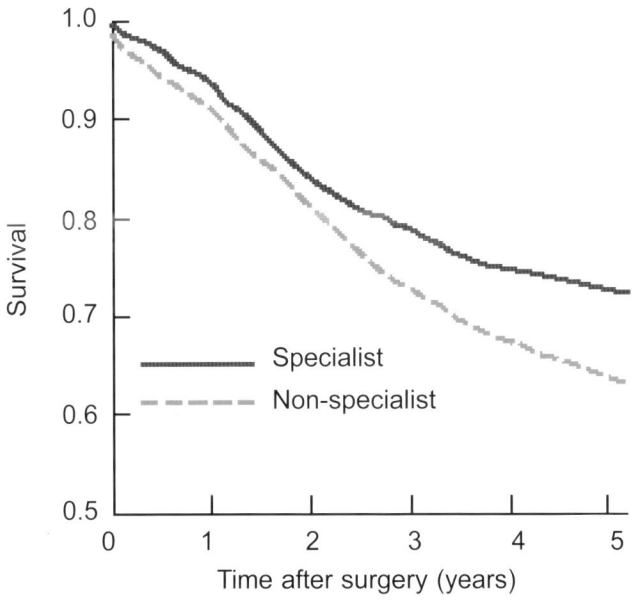

Figure 2. Cancer-specific survival in patients who had curative resection, according to specialist interest (from McArdle et al, 2004 [19]).

hazard ratios adjusted by volume (high volume surgeons performing more than 60 cases, medium volume 30-60 cases, and low volume less than 30 cases), although they did find that surgeons with a high volume of cases treated a significantly greater number of patients with rectal cancer, whereas lower volume surgeons operated on a significantly greater number of emergency patients and those presenting with metastatic disease. The authors concluded that it was specialisation rather than volume that was likely to improve outcome from curative resection for colorectal cancer.

Emergency colorectal surgery and specialisation

An audit by Darby et al in 1992 [22] revealed significant differences in the management of patients with colorectal emergencies between firms headed by specialist and non-specialist consultants. Identifying this as an important finding, they suggested that in order to minimise these differences, recent advances in emergency colorectal practice should be included in the training of all surgeons.

In 2003, Zorcolo et al retrospectively examined the results from a series of 336 emergency colorectal operations performed over a decade for cancer and diverticular disease, comparing specialist with non-specialist surgeons with regards to the outcome of surgery, postoperative morbidity, and mortality [23]. They defined a specialist as a surgeon with a specific interest in colorectal surgery, and a non-specialist as a surgeon specialised in upper gastrointestinal surgery. With both groups, matched for the severity of presentation and presence of comorbidity, they found that specialists were significantly more likely to perform primary anastomosis (64% versus 37%) and had significantly lower overall morbidity (15% versus

24%). Mortality rates were lower also for the specialist group (10.4 versus 17.4%), but this finding was not significant. The limitations of this study included its small sample size, retrospective design, and imprecise definitions of specialist surgeons, but the findings have raised some new questions. The fact that primary anastomosis was performed more frequently by the specialist colorectal surgeon highlights the potential difference between the two groups. It has been shown that in appropriately selected patients presenting with acute obstruction and sepsis, one-stage resection and primary anastomosis carries considerable advantages [24, 25], with faecal peritonitis no longer an absolute contra-indication [26]. In this study the overall incidence of anastomotic leak in patients with generalised peritonitis was 6.3%, and 30-day mortality was 6% for patients undergoing primary anastomosis versus 21% for those who had undergone a Hartmann's procedure.

More recently, Tekkis et al [27] have investigated the early outcome following surgery for malignant large bowel obstruction, with data collected prospectively for 1046 patients in 148 UK hospitals during a 12-month period. Using a 3-level Bayesian logistic regression analysis, a predictive model of in-hospital mortality was developed. Although the authors identified significant inter-hospital variability in operative mortality evident with increasing age (variance=0.04, SE=0.001, p<0.001), no difference could be detected in adjusted operative mortality between specialist colorectal surgeons (member of ACPGBI) and non-specialists (general surgeons who were not ACPGBI members).

Where are we going?

Sub-specialisation in colorectal cancer surgery

Although the evidence regarding the importance of sub-specialisation in colorectal and in particular colorectal cancer surgery does appear to suggest better outcomes with specialisation, there are at present several issues that need to be resolved.

The first is better definition and measurement of specialisation and as a result the subsidiary question: what it is that characterises a good surgeon? There is at present no national or internationally agreed definition of a specialist in coloproctology, with several examples highlighted in Table 2. It has previously been suggested that the definition of a specialist should reflect more than the current workload and should include participation in a relevant programme of continuing professional development [9]. Memberships of organisations such as the ACPGBI have been used in an attempt to try and identify such a specialist, although it is clear that this guarantees neither a practising specialist nor someone with sufficient experience to be deemed one.

Defining what volume of surgery a surgeon needs to perform rightly to be deemed a specialist is another issue that requires further definition. The cut-off point that determines how many cases per year are adequate needs to be based on evidence. This in turn highlights the need for further high quality research. Although retrospective observational studies have provided us with important insights into the potential benefits of specialisation, they do not have the power to draw definite conclusions about the cause and effect of this. Having said this, it is very unlikely that a randomised controlled trial of treatment by specialists versus non-specialists could ever be carried out, suggesting the need for further prospective research.

Although the outcome from colorectal cancer surgery has been shown to be surgeon-dependent, we must not forget several other factors that also determine survival - even for patients who are matched for severity of disease. These include the level and provision of radiology, pathology, oncology, and nursing services, all of which would have a part to play in improving outcome from colorectal cancer surgery. The contribution of surgical technique to survival is likely to vary according to cancer site, as well as depending to some extent on the technical ability and experience of the operating surgeon. Results from studies such as that by McArdle et al [19] suggest that within colorectal cancer surgery it is rectal cancer resections that benefit most from specialisation. This would seem logical given that most surgeons would agree that anterior or abdominoperineal resection are more demanding operations than surgery for more proximal colonic tumours, mainly because of the need for preservation of both sphincter and innervation, whilst at the same time obtaining adequate clearance with total mesorectal excision. The former are likely to require a higher degree of experience and judgment that will come with specialisation and increased caseload, making this an important point for further research and moves towards colorectal sub-specialisation to focus on.

Establishing a specialist colorectal service

A study by Shankar et al [28] examined the effects of establishing a specialist colorectal service at their district general hospital (DGH). They prospectively collected data on postoperative outcome for colorectal cancer surgery over a 3-year period and compared this to results achieved by their hospital in the Trent and Wales audit of 1993, which had been an independent population-based audit of all patients in those regions presenting to hospital with colorectal cancer. The specialist unit consisted of a one-stop colorectal clinic along with a multidisciplinary team consisting of surgeons, radiologists, pathologists, oncologists and specialist nurses. They identified that the percentage of patients with Dukes' stage A increased from 11% to 23%, the rates of emergency colorectal cancer operations fell from 29% to 8.2%, and the rate of permanent stoma formation fell from 52% to 32%. Their results suggest therefore that the establishment of a specialist service with judicious use of adjuvant treatment in their DGH resulted in earlier diagnosis and shorter waiting periods for patients, thereby supporting an integrated multi-disciplinary approach. This is possibly an indication not only of the fact that a specialist colorectal service can be set up in the DGH setting, but also that it may indeed significantly improve the standard of care for the majority of patients with colorectal cancer who are managed in district hospitals. They calculated that the additional cost of £22 per patient required in this specialist unit was justified by their improved results.

Outcome measures used to gauge success

In an attempt to reduce recurrence and achieve better survival rates, a surgeon may be more aggressive, thereby trading seemingly higher early postoperative morbidity in exchange for better long-term survival. For this reason overall long-term survival and recurrence rates are better indices of success, particularly with regards to colorectal cancer surgery. Quality of life is also an important outcome, yet there is at present little published in the literature on this.

The future

Although relations between volume and outcome have long been recognised, large-scale efforts to reduce surgical mortality by concentrating selected procedures in high volume hospitals are only now beginning to gain momentum. A visible example in the USA is the previously mentioned Leapfrog Group (insuring over 25 million people), which encourages selection of hospitals that meet their own minimum per annum volume criteria for CABG (500 cases), coronary angioplasty (400), CEA (carotid endarter-ectomy - 100), AAA repair (abdominal aortic aneurysm - 30), and oesophagectomy for cancer (6). Although there is no evidence to suggest that these specific thresholds carry any significance, they are an example of how standards may be set in the future for colorectal surgery.

Emergency colorectal surgery and specialisation

Whether the ability to offer specialist emergency colorectal surgery on a national scale is feasible remains to be seen. At present this would depend largely on whether patients live within a reasonable radius of high volume or sub-specialist hospitals. With emergency surgery, transport to such units would usually be possible, making sub-specialisation at the district hospital level even more important. Studies such as that by Tekkis et al [27] have helped to identify risk factors that determine postoperative survival following emergency surgery (for malignant bowel obstruction) and have developed a risk stratification system to be used as an adjunct to the process of informed consent. The effect of surgeon experience on this latter system has yet to be included, but is likely to form an important part of such risk stratification.

References

1. Luft HS. The relation between surgical volume and mortality: an exploration of causal factors and alternative models. *Med Care* 1980; 18(9): 940-59.
2. Begg CB, Cramer LD, Hoskins WJ, Brennan MF. Impact of hospital volume on operative mortality for major cancer surgery. *JAMA* 1998; 280(20): 1747-51.
3. Halm EA, Lee C, Chassin MR. Is volume related to outcome in health care? A systematic review and methodologic critique of the literature. *Ann Intern Med* 2002; 137(6): 511-20.
4. Pearce WH, Parker MA, Feinglass J, et al. The importance of surgeon volume and training in outcomes for vascular surgical procedures. *J Vasc Surg* 1999; 29(5): 768-76; discussion 777-8.
5. Birkmeyer JD, Siewers AE, Finlayson EV, et al. Hospital volume and surgical mortality in the United States. *N Engl J Med* 2002; 346(15): 1128-37.
6. Steele RJ. The influence of surgeon case volume on outcome in site-specific cancer surgery. *Eur J Surg Oncol* 1996; 22(3): 211-3.
7. Kessler H, Hermanek P, Jr., Wiebelt H. Operative mortality in carcinoma of the rectum. Results of the German Multicentre Study. *Int J Colorectal Dis* 1993; 8(3): 158-66.
8. Pickering RM, Chadwell IR, Mountney L. Importance of district of residence and known primary site for bowel cancer survival: analysis of data from Wessex Cancer Registry. *J Epidemiol Community Health* 1992; 46(3): 266-70.
9. Smith JA, King PM, Lane RH, Thompson MR. Evidence of the effect of "specialization" on the management, surgical outcome and survival from colorectal cancer in Wessex. *Br J Surg* 2003; 90(5): 583-92.
10. Guidance on commisioning cancer services. Improving outcomes in colorectal cancer. NHS Executive, 1997.
11. Dahlberg M, Glimelius B, Pahlman L. Changing strategy for rectal cancer is associated with improved outcome. *Br J Surg* 1999; 86(3): 379-84.
12. Mella J, Biffin A, Radcliffe AG, et al. Population-based audit of colorectal cancer management in two UK health regions. Colorectal Cancer Working Group, Royal College of Surgeons of England Clinical Epidemiology and Audit Unit. *Br J Surg* 1997; 84(12): 1731-6.
13. Rosen L, Stasik JJ, Jr., Reed JF, 3rd, et al. Variations in colon and rectal surgical mortality. Comparison of specialties with a state-legislated database. *Dis Colon Rectum* 1996; 39(2): 129-35.
14. Holm T, Johansson H, Cedermark B, et al. Influence of hospital- and surgeon-related factors on outcome after treatment of rectal cancer with or without preoperative radiotherapy. *Br J Surg* 1997; 84(5): 657-63.
15. Kee F. Number of cases operated on is important in volume-outcome debate for colorectal cancer. *BMJ* 1999; 319(7209): 576-7.
16. Parry JM, Collins S, Mathers J, et al. Influence of volume of work on the outcome of treatment for patients with colorectal cancer. *Br J Surg* 1999; 86(4): 475-81.
17. Read TE, Myerson RJ, Fleshman JW, et al. Surgeon specialty is associated with outcome in rectal cancer treatment. *Dis Colon Rectum* 2002; 45(7): 904-14.
18. Callahan MA, Christos PJ, Gold HT, et al. Influence of surgical subspecialty training on in-hospital mortality for gastrectomy and colectomy patients. *Ann Surg* 2003; 238(4): 629-36.
19. McArdle CS, Hole DJ. Influence of volume and specialization on survival following surgery for colorectal cancer. *Br J Surg* 2004; 91(5): 610-7.
20. Hermanek P, Wiebelt H, Staimmer D, Riedl S. Prognostic factors of rectum carcinoma - experience of the German Multicentre Study SGCRC. German Study Group Colo-Rectal Carcinoma. *Tumori* 1995; 81(3 Suppl): 60-4.
21. Meagher AP. Colorectal cancer: is the surgeon a prognostic factor? A systematic review. *Med J Aust* 1999; 171(6): 308-10.
22. Darby CR, Berry AR, Mortensen N. Management variability in surgery for colorectal emergencies. *Br J Surg* 1992; 79(3): 206-10.
23. Zorcolo L, Covotta L, Carlomagno N, Bartolo DC. Toward lowering morbidity, mortality, and stoma formation in emergency colorectal surgery: the role of specialization. *Dis Colon Rectum* 2003; 46(11): 1461-7.
24. Mealy K, Salman A, Arthur G. Definitive one-stage emergency large bowel surgery. *Br J Surg* 1988; 75(12): 1216-9.
25. Alanis A, Papanicolaou GK, Tadros RR, Fielding LP. Primary resection and anastomosis for treatment of acute diverticulitis. *Dis Colon Rectum* 1989; 32(11): 933-9.
26. Biondo S, Jaurrieta E, Marti Rague J, et al. Role of resection and primary anastomosis of the left colon in the presence of peritonitis. *Br J Surg* 2000; 87(11): 1580-4.
27. Tekkis PP, Kinsman R, Thompson MR, Stamatakis JD. The Association of Coloproctology of Great Britain and Ireland study of large bowel obstruction caused by colorectal cancer. *Ann Surg* 2004; 240(1): 76-81.
28. Shankar PJ, Achuthan R, Haray PN. Colorectal subspecialization in a DGH. The way forward! *Colorectal Dis* 2001; 3(6): 396-401.

Chapter 24

Fertility after pouch surgery

Kasper Ørding Olsen MD PhD, Research Fellow, Colorectal Surgery
University Hospital of Aarhus, Aarhus C, Denmark

What is the problem?

Pouch surgery (ileal pouch-anal anastomosis) is often carried out in women who are still in their fertile years and of whom many have not given birth at the time of surgery. Thus, many of these women have not made use of their reproductive potential and may still want children of their own. How should we inform these patients before surgery about the potential effect it might have on their fertility? Are there individual needs that should be taken into account and will they change our therapeutic (surgical) strategy? Attention must be paid to the differences between ulcerative colitis (UC) and familial adenomatous polyposis (FAP) when counselling patients. Crohn's disease will not be dealt with in this chapter because only a few centres are prepared deliberately to perform pouch surgery in patients with this disease.

Where are we now?

Considering fertility after pouch surgery, it is important to know whether women suffering from either UC or FAP have normal fertility before they start out having surgery, or if their fertility from the beginning is impaired compared to other women.

This matter will be dealt with below, where the two diseases will be discussed separately. The second and third issues are whether it is safe to get pregnant and continue a pregnancy having a pouch and to what extent a pregnancy and delivery affects pouch function.

It is indeed safe to get pregnant and carry through a pregnancy for both mother and child [1-5]; moreover, the deterioration in pouch function observed during pregnancy returns to normal for most patients shortly after delivery, irrespective of whether the child was delivered by a vaginal delivery or a Caesarean section, indicating that the method of delivery should be dictated by obstetrical considerations [2-5]. Regardless of these findings, many centres still recommend Caesarean section as the mode of delivery.

The next issue is if the postoperative functional outcome and quality of life with a pouch is of a standard high enough to give the improvement in daily life expected for females wanting to reproduce and thus having the willingness to carry through a pregnancy.

Functional outcome is generally reported as acceptable to excellent [6-9] and quality of life with a pouch is preferred to living with a stoma [6,10,11], patient satisfaction is high [6,7] and postoperative quality of life is

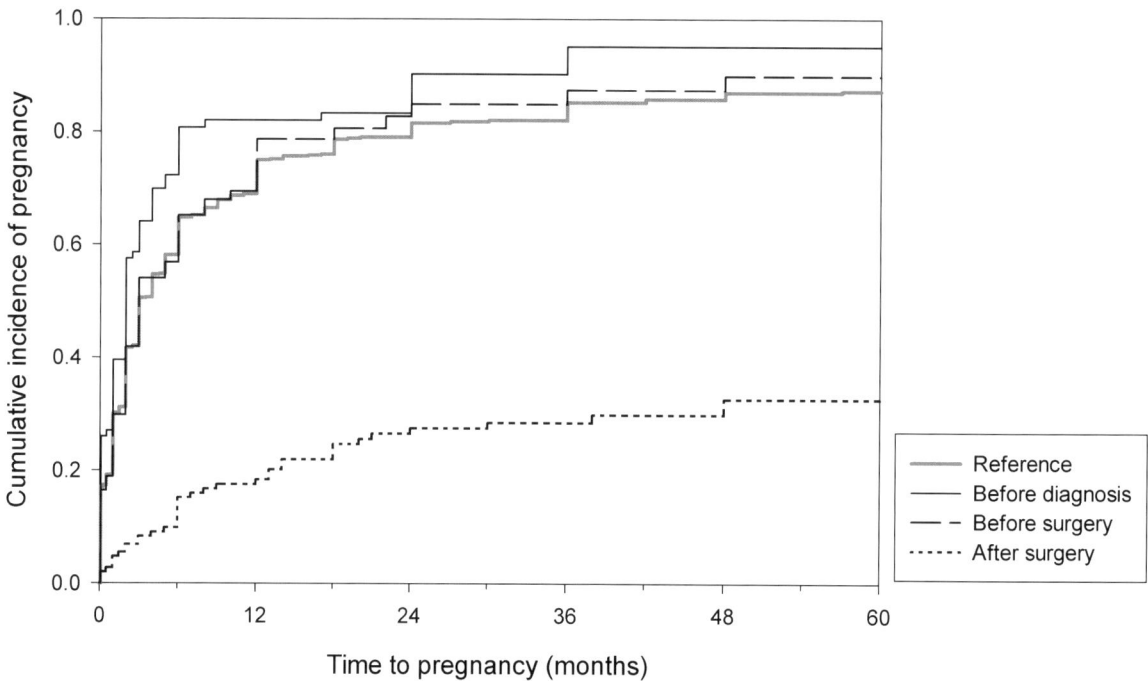

Figure 1. Cumulative incidence of pregnancy within 5 years. Patients and reference population. Reproduced with permission from the American Gastroenterological Association. Olsen KØ, Juul S, Berndtsson I, *et al*. Ulcerative colitis: female fecundity before diagnosis, during disease, and after surgery compared with a population sample. *Gastroenterology* 2002; 122(1): 15-9.

Table 1. Age-adjusted fecundability ratios. Cox regression analysis. Reproduced with permission from the American Gastroenterological Association. Olsen KØ, Juul S, Berndtsson I, *et al*. Ulcerative colitis: female fecundity before diagnosis, during disease, and after surgery compared with a population sample. *Gastroenterology* 2002; 122(1): 15-9.

	Denmark Fecundability ratio (95% CI)	n	Sweden Fecundability ratio (95% CI)	n	Pooled data* Fecundability ratio (95% CI)	n	P
Reference population	1	511	1	403	1	914	-
Patients before diagnosis	1.33 (0.98-1.79)	63	1.75 (1.18-2.56)	35	1.46 (1.16-1.85)	98	0.002
Patients before colectomy	1.01 (0.71-1.42)	46	1.04 (0.71-1.51)	38	1.01 (0.79-1.31)	84	0.92
Patients after IPAA	0.25 (0.17-0.37)	92	0.14 (0.08-0.25)	57	0.20 (0.15-0.28)	149	<0.001

n=number of periods observed (TTP); * adjusted for age and country

Analyses adjusting for smoking status only changed ratios in the second digit and are therefore not shown reported as good [12,13] to excellent and comparable to quality of life in the general US population [9,14], results being good also in selected older individuals [15]. However, in the Netherlands it was found that FAP patients' quality of life after surgery scored significantly lower than in the general population [16].

Given this generally good quality of life, what about their sexual life: is that of a quality that will allow for pregnancy to occur? Although increase in vaginal dryness, dyspareunia and fear of stool leakage are observed quite often after pouch surgery, most patients are satisfied with their sexual life [7,17-22], and thus there seems to be no sexual reason for a potential postoperative reduced fertility.

There are studies indicating that fertility will be influenced by pelvic surgery. After conventional proctocolectomy, the occurrence of distressing vaginal discharge and dyspareunia increased significantly; only 37% of women who attempted to become pregnant succeeded within 5 years' follow-up [23]; and in another study, 17 of 21 women had postoperative pathological fallopian tube anatomy [24]. In a study of pouch patients, only one out of 14 who attempted to become pregnant succeeded and only seven of 21 had normal fallopian tube anatomy when examined by hysterosalpingography [18]. These are small but important studies making fertility an issue to be dealt with when counselling patients before pouch surgery.

Ulcerative colitis

Fertility before surgery

In their work from 1980, Willoughby and Truelove found that the fertility amongst 147 UC patients was normal and that only 6.8% reported involuntarily infertility [25]. Baird et al found a reduced number of pregnancies in women suffering from inflammatory bowel disease (IBD), but measures of methods of birth control, infertility and fecundability ratios indicated that the reduced fertility was due to choices made by the patients rather than the disease [26]. In Scotland, Hudson et al found that women with UC had fertility similar to the general population [27], findings confirmed for Denmark and Sweden (Figure 1 and Table 1) by our study from 2002 [28] and from Canada by Johnson et al [29]; thus, before surgery these patients are comparable to the general population concerning fertility.

Fertility after surgery

At first, optimistic reports like Metcalf et al from 1986 found minimally impaired fertility, but judged on small numbers where six out of eight were successful in getting pregnant [17]. Later in 1994, Öresland et al published data where only one out of 14 who attempted eventually got pregnant [18]. They rightfully warned caution in the interpretation due to the small numbers, but also stated that in their experience the majority of these patients could be helped by the advancement of assisted reproduction, and emphasised the importance of the fertility aspect being part of the pre-operative information to these patients. Hudson et al found that only five out 11 surgically treated patients conceived within 2 years [27]; in contrast to this Tiainen et al reported that eight out of ten who tried got pregnant within 1 year [30].

In 1999, we published a study of 237 women who had had pouch surgery [31]. We found that after surgery these women had less than half the expected number of children compared to the general population and, if children born following in vitro fertilization were excluded, the number of children was only 35% of the expected. The weakness of this study was that it did not take into account whether there was a desire for children or not and thus the study was unable to tell if it was voluntary birth control rather than a fertility problem.

Recently, two good studies throwing more light on the subject have been published: our co-operate Danish/Swedish study from 2002 [28] and a Canadian study by Johnson et al from 2004 [29], results from both pointing in the same direction. In the Danish/Swedish study, a reference population of 661 participants from the general population and 290 patients having had pouch surgery gave information on their reproductive history. The data concerning reproduction were collected by interview, the main measure being time intervals of unprotected intercourse (ending in a pregnancy or a censored observation) which in a Cox proportional hazards model was used to calculate

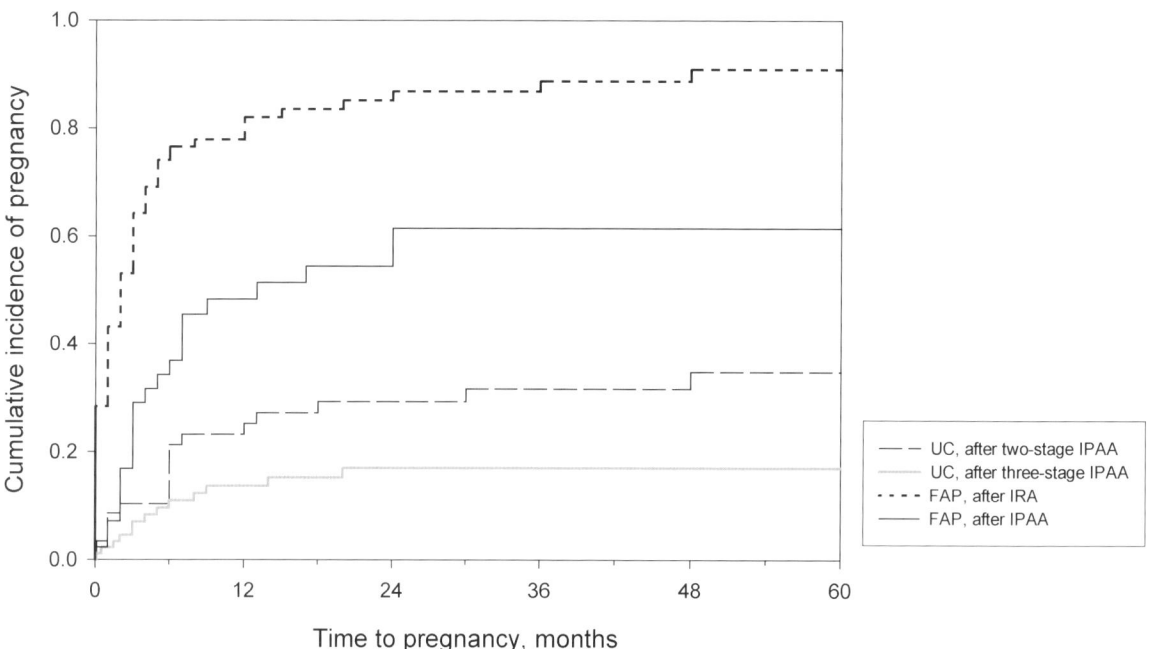

Figure 2. Cumulative incidence of pregnancy within 5 years. FAP patients after IRA and after IPAA, and UC patients after two-stage and three-stage IPAA. Reproduced with permission from the author, Olsen KØ. The effect of ulcerative colitis and familial adenomatous polyposis on female reproduction. Ph. D. Thesis. Faculty of Health Sciences, University of Aarhus, Denmark, 2001.

fecundability ratios between groups, the model adjusting for age and country at the beginning of each time interval of unprotected intercourse. The results are shown graphically in Figure 1 and the fecundability ratios from the Cox regression model in Table 1. The numbers speak for themselves; normal fertility before surgery, severely reduced fertility after pouch surgery. Before diagnosis, 95% got pregnant within 5 years, after diagnosis but before surgery the number was 90%, but after pouch surgery only 36% of the patients succeeded in getting pregnant within 5 years and 30% of these pregnancies were after *in vitro* fertilization compared to only 1.3% in the reference population. An interesting but non-significant finding was that fertility after three-stage pouch surgery was more reduced than after two-stage procedures (Figure 2) [32]. In the Canadian study [29], 153 women with an ileo-anal pouch gave information both on episodes of infertility, defined as failure to become pregnant during 12 months of unprotected intercourse, and data of their reproductive history. The infertility rate of 38.6% in pouch patients was significantly higher than in patients managed non-operatively where the rate was 13.3%. Patients managed non-operatively, and pouch patients before surgery, had success rates of achieving pregnancy from 95.8%-97.5%, but after surgery the success rate was down to 56.1%, and 30.3% who attempted pregnancy postoperatively used fertility treatment as opposed to 0-6.3% in the other groups.

Summing up, fertility is severely reduced after pouch surgery, with success rates for achieving pregnancy somewhere in the range of 36% [28] to 56% [29] and with a large proportion succeeding only because they are assisted by fertility treatment.

Familial adenomatous polyposis

Fertility before surgery

In 1990, Johansen *et al* found the accumulated rate of deliveries amongst 58 females with FAP to be no different to the general population [33]. In another study,

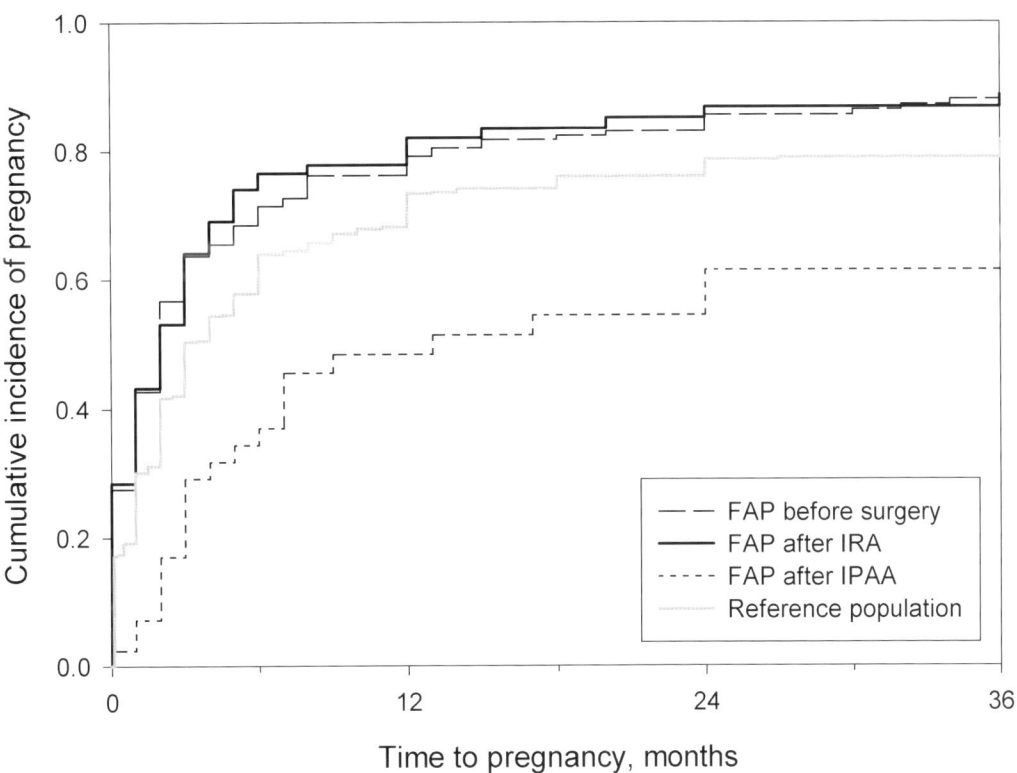

Figure 3. Cumulative incidence of pregnancy within 3 years. FAP patients before surgery, after IRA or IPAA and reference population. Reproduced with permission from John Wiley & Sons Ltd, on behalf of the BJSS Ltd. Olsen KØ, Juul S, Bulow S, et al. Female fecundity before and after operation for familial adenomatous polyposis, Br J Surg 2003; 90(2): 227-31. © British Journal of Surgery Society Ltd.

the reproductive fitness was found to be close to one, indicating that these women reproduce without problems [34]. Using time of unprotected intercourse as a fertility measure, in 2003 we found the fertility of women with FAP to be comparable to or even better than a reference population (Figure 3) [35]. Thus, before surgery females with FAP have normal fertility.

Fertility after surgery

Data for this group of patients are very limited. The best estimates so far are given by us in the above mentioned co-operative study from the Nordic Polyposis registers [35]. In this study we found that fertility after colectomy with ileorectal anastomosis (IRA) was normal, but after pouch surgery it was significantly reduced when measured as time to pregnancy (Figure 3) and as fecundability ratios using a Cox regression model adjusting for age and country at the beginning of each time interval of unprotected intercourse (Table 2). After 24 months of unprotected intercourse the success rate of becoming pregnant was 86% before surgery, 87% after IRA but only 61% after pouch surgery, showing that also in FAP patients pouch surgery has a marked effect on fertility, thereby making it an issue to inform the patients before surgery.

Summary

Pouch surgery has a detrimental effect on postoperative fertility with significant differences between UC and FAP populations and with marked but non-significant differences between two- and three-stage procedures in the UC population. Success rates for UC patients achieving pregnancy are in the range of 36% [28] to 56.1% [29] with a large proportion succeeding only because they are assisted by fertility treatment, while for FAP patients the equivalent success rate is about 61% [35].

Table 2. Fecundability ratios adjusted for age and country. Reproduced with permission from John Wiley & Sons Ltd, on behalf of the BJSS Ltd. Olsen KØ, Juul S, Bulow S, et al. Female fecundity before and after operation for familial adenomatous polyposis, Br J Surg 2003; 90(2): 227-31. © British Journal of Surgery Society Ltd.

	Number of time to pregnancy periods	Fecundability ratios (95% CI)	P value
FAP before surgery as reference			
FAP pre-operative	171	1	-
FAP after IRA	81	1.05 (0.79-1.40)	0.79
FAP after IPAA	42	0.46 (0.29-0.73)	0.001
The database reference population as reference			
Reference population	914	1	-
FAP pre-operative	171	1.34 (1.03-1.74)	0.027
FAP after IRA	81	1.39 (1.07-1.81)	0.015
FAP after IPAA	42	0.54 (0.35-0.82)	0.004
UC after IPAA	149	0.17 (0.12-0.25)	<0.001
FAP after IPAA as reference			
FAP after IPAA	42	1	-
UC after IPAA two-stage	58	0.49 (0.22-1.06)	0.07
UC after IPAA all	149	0.33 (0.16-0.65)	0.001

Where are we going?

First of all, postoperative fertility has become an issue that needs to be discussed with patients when obtaining their informed consent before surgery. Though it is an issue of importance for patients, it would most likely be incorrect to suggest withholding surgery where there is no other available choice. This is applicable for both UC, where most females require surgery for acute non-responsive or chronic disease and often are very sick or suffer from side effects to medical treatment, as well as for FAP, where some sort of surgery clearly is needed to prevent cancer from developing.

For UC patients the finding that an ileostomy in well educated patients gives good quality of life with much less complications than pouch surgery [36] could in selected compliant individuals make it an option to perform a subtotal colectomy with an end ileostomy and delay the pouch procedure until reproduction has taken place. If it is possible to get really good disease control in the rectal remnant, there might also be a possibility of a revival of performing subtotal colectomy and IRA for UC - at least for females who have not yet had their children at the time of surgery. A trial/study of the possibilities for IRA in just those circumstances has been taken on in Sweden (personal communication Tom Öresland).

For FAP patients there seems to be a real possibility to select more low risk patients for IRA procedures [37,38], thereby rendering them with much better postoperative fertility. In cases of very compliant patients, who are aware of the cancer risk and where it seems possible to gain control of the rectal polyps, at least for some time, it might also be a possibility to perform IRA to allow childbearing and then later convert to a pouch as this can be done with good functional results [39,40].

Individualising the surgical strategy is one option; another option would be to find measures to preserve tubal patency and normal anatomical relationships in the pelvis in spite of the surgery we perform. Various materials to prevent pelvic adhesions are available [41], but so far there are no data supporting any effectiveness to improve post-surgical fertility, so clearly more research is needed in this area.

Until we have come further, the best we can do is to be honest with patients about the post-surgical fertility problem and ensure that the ones who have a problem and who want help obtain an early offer of fertility treatment/assisted reproduction.

References

1. Pezim ME. Successful childbirth after restorative proctocolectomy with pelvic ileal reservoir. *Br J Surg* 1984; 71(4): 292.
2. Nelson H, Dozois RR, Kelly KA, Malkasian GD, Wolff BG, Ilstrup DM. The effect of pregnancy and delivery on the ileal pouch-anal anastomosis functions. *Dis Colon Rectum* 1989; 32(5): 384-8.
3. Scott HJ, McLeod RS, Blair J, O'Connor B, Cohen Z. Ileal pouch-anal anastomosis: pregnancy, delivery and pouch function. *Int J Colorectal Dis* 1996; 11(2): 84-7.
4. Ravid A, Richard CS, Spencer LM, O'Connor BI, Kennedy ED, MacRae HM, et al. Pregnancy, delivery, and pouch function after ileal pouch-anal anastomosis for ulcerative colitis. *Dis Colon Rectum* 2002; 45(10): 1283-8.
5. Hahnloser D, Pemberton JH, Wolff BG, Larson D, Harrington J, Farouk R, et al. Pregnancy and delivery before and after ileal pouch-anal anastomosis for inflammatory bowel disease: immediate and long-term consequences and outcomes. *Dis Colon Rectum* 2004; 47(7): 1127-35.
6. Nicholls J, Pescatori M, Motson RW, Pezim ME. Restorative proctocolectomy with a three-loop ileal reservoir for ulcerative colitis and familial adenomatous polyposis. Clinical results in 66 patients followed for up to 6 years. *Ann Surg* 1984; 199(4): 383-8.
7. Öresland T, Fasth S, Nordgren S, Hulten L. The clinical and functional outcome after restorative proctocolectomy. A prospective study in 100 patients. *Int J Colorectal Dis* 1989; 4: 50-6.
8. Bone J, Sorensen FH, Kraglund K, Laurberg S, Petersen OB. [Results of ileoanal reservoir surgery] Resultat af ileoanalt reservoir-kirurgi. *Ugeskr Laeger* 1996; 158(15): 2105-8.
9. Fazio VW, O'Riordain MG, Lavery IC, Church JM, Lau P, Strong SA, et al. Long-term functional outcome and quality of life after stapled restorative proctocolectomy. *Ann Surg* 1999; 230(4): 575-84.
10. Pemberton JH, Phillips SF, Ready RR, Zinsmeister AR, Beahrs OH. Quality of life after Brooke ileostomy and ileal pouch-anal anastomosis. Comparison of performance status. *Ann Surg* 1989; 209(5): 620-6.
11. Kohler LW, Pemberton JH, Zinsmeister AR, Kelly KA. Quality of life after proctocolectomy. A comparison of Brooke ileostomy, Kock pouch, and ileal pouch-anal anastomosis [see comments]. *Gastroenterology* 1991; 101(3): 679-84.
12. McLeod RS, Churchill DN, Lock AM, Vanderburgh S, Cohen Z. Quality of life of patients with ulcerative colitis preoperatively and postoperatively. *Gastroenterology* 1991; 101(5): 1307-13.
13. Berndtsson I, Öresland T. Quality of life before and after proctocolectomy and IPAA in patients with ulcerative proctocolitis - a prospective study. *Colorectal Dis* 2003; 5(2): 173-9.
14. Thirlby RC, Land JC, Fenster LF, Lonborg R. Effect of surgery on health-related quality of life in patients with inflammatory bowel disease: a prospective study. *Arch Surg* 1998; 133(8): 826-32.
15. Delaney CP, Fazio VW, Remzi FH, Hammel J, Church JM, Hull TL, et al. Prospective, age-related analysis of surgical results, functional outcome, and quality of life after ileal pouch-anal anastomosis. *Ann Surg* 2003; 238(2): 221-8.
16. Van Duijvendijk P, Slors JF, Taat CW, Oosterveld P, Sprangers MA, Obertop H, et al. Quality of life after total colectomy with ileorectal anastomosis or proctocolectomy and ileal pouch-anal anastomosis for familial adenomatous polyposis. *Br J Surg* 2000; 87(5): 590-6.
17. Metcalf AM, Dozois RR, Kelly KA. Sexual function in women after proctocolectomy. *Ann Surg* 1986; 204(6): 624-7.
18. Öresland T, Palmblad S, Ellstrom M, Berndtsson I, Crona N, Hulten L. Gynaecological and sexual function related to anatomical changes in the female pelvis after restorative proctocolectomy. *Int J Colorectal Dis* 1994; 9(2): 77-81.
19. Damgaard B, Wettergren A, Kirkegaard P. Social and sexual function following ileal pouch-anal anastomosis. *Dis Colon Rectum* 1995; 38(3): 286-9.
20. Bambrick M, Fazio VW, Hull TL, Pucel G. Sexual function following restorative proctocolectomy in women. *Dis Colon Rectum* 1996; 39(6): 610-4.
21. Sjogren B, Poppen B. Sexual life in women after colectomy-proctomucosectomy with S-pouch. *Acta Obstet Gynecol Scand* 1995; 74(1): 51-5.
22. Berndtsson I, Öresland T, Hulten L. Sexuality in patients with ulcerative colitis before and after restorative proctocolectomy: a prospective study. *Scand J Gastroenterol* 2004; 39(4): 374-9.
23. Wikland M, Jansson I, Asztely M, Palselius I, Svaninger G, Magnusson O, et al. Gynaecological problems related to

23. anatomical changes after conventional proctocolectomy and ileostomy. *Int J Colorectal Dis* 1990; 5(1): 49-52.
24. Asztely M, Palmblad S, Wikland M, Hulten L. Radiological study of changes in the pelvis in women following proctocolectomy. *Int J Colorectal Dis* 1991; 6(2): 103-7.
25. Willoughby CP, Truelove SC. Ulcerative colitis and pregnancy. *Gut* 1980; 21(6): 469-74.
26. Baird DD, Narendranathan M, Sandler RS. Increased risk of preterm birth for women with inflammatory bowel disease. *Gastroenterology* 1990; 99(4): 987-94.
27. Hudson M, Flett G, Sinclair TS, Brunt PW, Templeton A, Mowat NA. Fertility and pregnancy in inflammatory bowel disease. *Int J Gynaecol Obstet* 1997; 58(2): 229-37.
28. Olsen KØ, Juul S, Berndtsson I, Öresland T, Laurberg S. Ulcerative colitis: female fecundity before diagnosis, during disease, and after surgery compared with a population sample. *Gastroenterology* 2002; 122(1): 15-9.
29. Johnson P, Richard C, Ravid A, Spencer L, Pinto E, Hanna M, et al. Female infertility after ileal pouch-anal anastomosis for ulcerative colitis. *Dis Colon Rectum* 2004; 47(7): 1119-26.
30. Tiainen J, Matikainen M, Hiltunen KM. Ileal J-pouch - anal anastomosis, sexual dysfunction, and fertility. *Scand J Gastroenterol* 1999; 34(2): 185-8.
31. Olsen KØ, Joelsson M, Laurberg S, Öresland T. Fertility after ileal pouch-anal anastomosis in women with ulcerative colitis. *Br J Surg* 1999; 86(4): 493-5.
32. Olsen KØ. The effect of ulcerative colitis and familial adenomatous polyposis on female reproduction. Faculty of Health Sciences, University of Aarhus, Denmark, 2001.
33. Johansen C, Bitsch M, Bulow S. Fertility and pregnancy in women with familial adenomatous polyposis. *Int J Colorectal Dis* 1990; 5(4): 203-6.
34. Bisgaard ML, Fenger K, Bulow S, Niebuhr E, Mohr J. Familial adenomatous polyposis (FAP): frequency, penetrance, and mutation rate. *Hum Mutat* 1994; 3(2): 121-5.
35. Olsen KØ, Juul S, Bulow S, Jarvinen HJ, Bakka A, Bjork J, et al. Female fecundity before and after operation for familial adenomatous polyposis. *Br J Surg* 2003; 90(2): 227-31.
36. Jimmo B, Hyman NH. Is ileal pouch-anal anastomosis really the procedure of choice for patients with ulcerative colitis? *Dis Colon Rectum* 1998; 41(1): 41-5.
37. Vasen HF, van der Luijt RB, Slors JF, Buskens E, de Ruiter P, Baeten CG, et al. Molecular genetic tests as a guide to surgical management of familial adenomatous polyposis. *Lancet* 1996; 348(9025): 433-5.
38. Bulow C, Vasen H, Jarvinen H, Bjork J, Bisgaard ML, Bulow S. Ileorectal anastomosis is appropriate for a subset of patients with familial adenomatous polyposis [In Process Citation]. *Gastroenterology* 2000; 119(6): 1454-60.
39. Bjork J, Akerbrant H, Iselius L, Svenberg T, Öresland T, Pahlman L, et al. Outcome of primary and secondary ileal pouch-anal anastomosis and ileorectal anastomosis in patients with familial adenomatous polyposis. *Dis Colon Rectum* 2001; 44(7): 984-92.
40. Soravia C, O'Connor BI, Berk T, McLeod RS, Cohen Z. Functional outcome of conversion of ileorectal anastomosis to ileal pouch-anal anastomosis in patients with familial adenomatous polyposis and ulcerative colitis. *Dis Colon Rectum* 1999; 42(7): 903-8.
41. Farquhar C, Vandekerckhove P, Watson A, Vail A, Wiseman D. Barrier agents for preventing adhesions after surgery for subfertility. *Cochrane Database Syst Rev* 2000; (2): CD000475.

Chapter 25

Erectile dysfunction

Ian Lindsey FRACS, Consultant Colorectal Surgeon
John Radcliffe Hospital, Oxford, UK

What is the issue?

Incidence and pre-operative counselling

Impotence occurs in about 25% after rectal excision for cancer and about 2% for inflammatory bowel disease (IBD), and can be a devastating complication particularly for young male patients. It is important medico-legally to be aware of the risks of impotence and communicate these risks to patients in an appropriate fashion. It can be difficult to discuss this issue with patients, particularly in the rectal cancer setting when there is much other important information to deal with.

Aetiology: the role of pelvic nerve injury

It has been difficult to ascertain the cause of impotence after proctectomy. In the past, impotence was often attributed to psychological factors surrounding the surgery. Patients are often elderly, have concerns about cancer, and undergo major invasive and disfiguring surgery which frequently leaves them with a stoma. It is easy to imagine erectile difficulties in such patients, yet increased impotence rates have never been demonstrated among ileostomists. It is important that poor functional outcomes are not solely attributed to these psychological factors.

A better awareness of the anatomy of the nerves in the pelvis which govern sexual function has lead to an emerging consensus regarding the major role surgical neural injury plays in the aetiology of post-proctectomy impotence. However, it has been difficult to confirm this objectively because most studies have only employed subjective questionnaires, and the response rate to these questionnaires is typically poor. An objective means of evaluating the role of neural injury would prove extremely helpful.

Anatomy: the site of nerve injury

If agreement can be reached on the principal role of nerve injury, the question of the possible site of injury can be addressed. The parasympathetic nerves may be damaged laterally at the pelvic plexus, or more anteriorly, where the smaller cavernous nerves have issued to run at the postero-lateral borders of the prostate. A greater understanding of these nerves has emerged largely through urological research surrounding radical prostate surgery.

Prevention: influence of the surgeon and the choice of surgical planes

If the site of injury can be localised, steps can be taken to minimise or prevent this damage. A full understanding of the anatomical structures relevant to anterior rectal mobilisation, including the planes available to the surgeon, both in the malignant and inflammatory setting, is important. The surgeon and the choices made during anterior mobilisation may be a significant variable influencing the risks of nerve injury and impotence.

Treatment

Until recently, available treatments for erectile dysfunction were limited to vacuum-constriction devices, intracavernosal injection or transurethral delivery of vasoactive agents, penile prosthetic implantation or vascular reconstructive surgery. Most of these options have variable efficacy and satisfaction rates, with decline in compliance over time.

There has been a significant change in the treatment of impotence with the development of the selective type-5 phosphodiesterase inhibitor, sildenafil (Viagra). Sildenafil is administered in tablet form and is well tolerated, and double-blind trials have demonstrated efficacy in men with "mixed" erectile dysfunction [1]. It is of considerable interest to those performing pelvic surgery, especially whether post-proctectomy impotence responds to sildenafil to the same extent as general impotent patients.

Female sexual dysfunction

Not a great deal is known about female sexual dysfunction (FSD) after proctectomy. The functional anatomy of female pelvic nerves is not well understood and the role of pelvic nerve injury in the aetiology of post-proctectomy sexual dysfunction is unclear. In men, nerve injury is now more widely recognised as the underlying cause of post-proctectomy impotence. A distinct effort to excise the rectum with maximum preservation of neural integrity and function has emerged. This has yet to be duplicated in females. Post-proctectomy FSD, which might in part be related to nerve damage, has received limited attention.

Where are we now?

Incidence and pre-operative counselling

Rectal cancer

Permanent impotence in males has been reported in 17-100% after abdominoperineal excision (APE) and 0-49% after anterior resection (AR) for rectal cancer [2-19]. The wide-ranging rates reflect, among other factors, variations in case mix and evaluation of dysfunction, study design, surgical technique and expertise. Most data are retrospective and subjective, and patients who are sexually inactive are often not well accounted for. No standardised definition of impotence or instrument for its measurement has been used in the literature, making comparison between published series difficult. However, there is now a standardised, widely accepted and validated sexual function questionnaire available, the International Index of Erectile Function (IIEF) [20] (Table 1).

Anterior resection vs abdominoperineal resection

The incidence of sexual dysfunction after APE is higher than that for anterior resection (AR) (Table 2). APE is perceived to be more radical for lower tumours than sphincter-saving surgery. Santangelo et al, in a study of males under 60, described an incidence of permanent impotence of 44% after APE, and 25% after AR [9]. However, if these were divided into high and low anterior resection, the incidence was 0% and 33% respectively. In addition, the presence of a permanent stoma may have some psychological bearing on erectile function, though there is evidence to refute this [21].

Effect of radiotherapy

Primary radiotherapy for localised prostate cancer causes impotence in 5-40% of patients [22]. Although the treatment field and volume amongst other factors may be different from that for rectal cancer, anecdotal evidence suggests that radiotherapy contributes to postoperative impotence, although no good data exist to support this.

25 Erectile dysfunction

Table 1. International Index of Erectile Function (summary).

Sexual function domain	Questions/total domain score
Erectile function	6 / 30
Intercourse satisfaction	3 / 15
Orgasmic function	2 / 10
Sexual desire	2 / 10
Overall sexual satisfaction	2 / 10
Total IIEF	15 / 75

Table 2. Summary of published series of sexual dysfunction rate after conventional rectal excision for cancer: influence of type of resection.

Operation	Abdominoperineal excision	Anterior resection
No. of patients	494	224
Loss of ejaculation	99/332	51/217
(%)	29	24
Partial impotence	38/281	8/89
(%)	14	9
Complete impotence	78/301	10/109
(%)	26	9
Total impotence	250/494	63/214
(%)	51	29

Wide pelvic lymphadenectomy

Wide pelvic lymphadenectomy has enjoyed some popularity in Japan in an attempt to reduce local recurrence. Impotence has been reported in 23-100% of cases [23-30]. A modified "nerve-sparing" procedure has now been described but the incidence of impotence remains high [31]. Lateral node dissection yields positive nodes in only 10-15% [26,28] and local recurrence rates of 4% and 5-year survival of 78% in Dukes' B and C tumours, using TME have been reported [32]. It is unlikely that patients will accrue enough benefit to justify the high rates of impotence as well as bladder dysfunction.

Proctectomy for benign disease

Surgery for IBD is frequently offered to young patients for the relative indication of failed medical therapy. This is to be balanced against the risks and quality of life impact of medical therapy. Impotence is

Table 3. Summary of published series of sexual dysfunction rate after rectal excision: influence of malignant versus benign disease.

Indication	Rectal cancer	Inflammatory bowel disease
No. of patients	744	2535
Loss of ejaculation (%)	116/489 24	59/1996 3
Total impotence (%)	325/744 43	77/2535 3

a particular concern to young male patients of reproductive age and if surgery is to be an acceptable option, then the risk of nerve damage and impotence must be kept to a minimum.

The rate of impotence after rectal excision for IBD is lower than that for rectal cancer (Table 3), ranging from 0-25% [2,18,21,33-60]. Patient age is an important factor; the incidence of post-surgical sexual dysfunction increases with age, and generally the mean age of IBD patients having surgery is about 20 years younger than rectal cancer patients [2,24]. Surgical technique may differ, with the close rectal plane of dissection sometimes used in an effort to minimise the risk to the pelvic nerves [61,43,44]. More commonly, the mesorectal plane is used out of ease and familiarity.

In a retrospective evaluation of impotence after proctectomy for IBD in Oxford, we found a low rate of complete impotence (3%) but a significant rate of partial impotence (13%) [62]. These more minor degrees of erectile difficulties may have been overlooked in previous studies using less sensitive questionnaires. We found that patient age has a highly significant influence on impotence rate.

Aetiology: the role of pelvic nerve injury

Nocturnal penile tumescence (NPT) testing is the gold standard for objective assessment of impotence. The normal male undergoes episodes of NPT during rapid eye movement sleep, the amount being age-related [63]. The number of nocturnal erections considered to be normal is three to five per 8-hour recording session, and at least two nights of monitoring is required to establish the presence or absence of NPT activity. The basis for NPT testing is that if an impotent patient has NPT activity, then they retain some integrity of the neurovascular pathway responsible for governing erectile capacity. An assumption is made in NPT testing that the same physiological mechanism is responsible for both a nocturnal and sexually stimulated erection [64], though this assumption remains unproven [65].

Various methods of NPT testing have been employed, including the snap-gauge band technique [64] and Rigiscan [66]. The Nocturnal Electrobioimpedance Volumetric Assessment (NEVA) device calculates changes in penile cross-sectional area and length, measured via impedance changes (resistance to electrical current flow) [67,68], through electrodes connected to the base and tip of the penis (Figure 1). NPT measured by impedance correlates well with that measured by Rigiscan [67].

Two recent studies have for the first time objectively assessed the role of parasympathetic nerve function in post-proctectomy impotence. In the first study, 34 impotent males post-proctectomy and 28 well-matched potent controls with rectal cancer and IBD pre-operatively, underwent two consecutive nights of home NPT monitoring by NEVA [69]. The response to

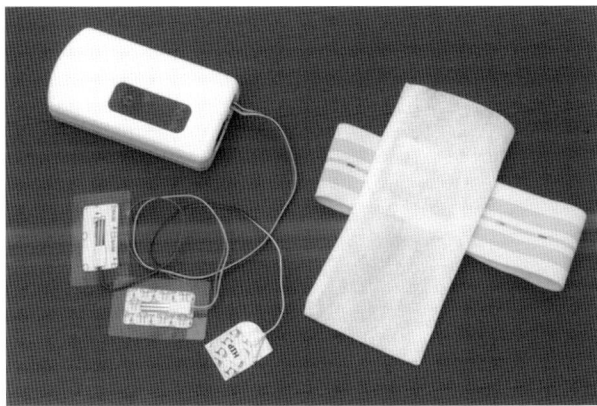

Figure 1. NEVA device and attachments.

A further study evaluated the efficacy of sildenafil in treating post-proctectomy impotence, where underlying pelvic parasympathetic nerve damage had occurred [70]. Response to sildenafil was significantly better than placebo and sildenafil improved both erectile function and total sexual function scores from pre-treatment baseline. Sildenafil is a phosphodiesterase-5 inhibitor and inhibits degradation of cyclic GMP (Figure 2). Cyclic GMP is augmented by nitric oxide released by the parasympathetic cavernous nerves, and relaxes the smooth muscle of the inflow arterioles to the cavernous corpora and thus increases cavernous blood flow and pressure.

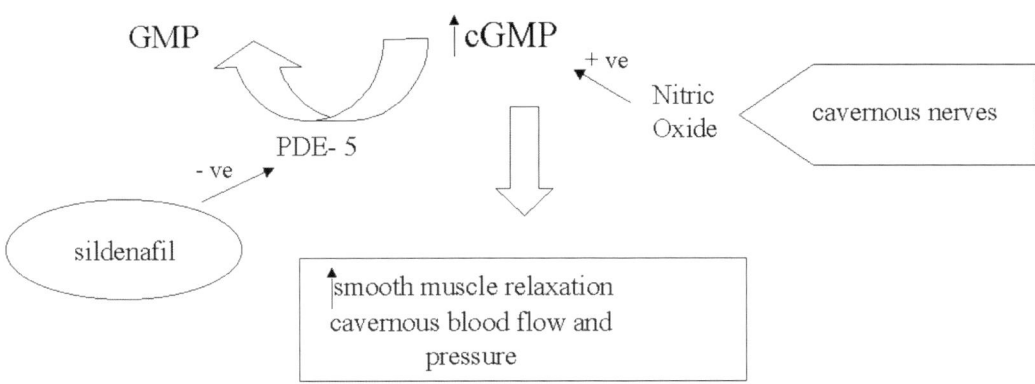

Figure 2. Mechanism of action of phosphodiesterase-5 inhibitor, sildenafil.

the phosphodiesterase (PDE)-inhibitor, sildenafil, was evaluated against nocturnal erections. The number of nocturnal erections was greater for the potent control group than the impotent study group (p=0.0004), and there was a non-significant trend to a lower mean number of nocturnal erections amongst sildenafil responders compared to non-responders (p=0.14). The conclusion was that nocturnal erections were diminished but not ablated by the trauma of surgical dissection. This suggests that some of the cavernous nerves remain intact after surgery and that the nerve injury is partial.

The effect of sildenafil is dependent upon at least partially intact cavernous nerves to produce nitric oxide.

The importance of these two studies is that they for the first time objectively place neural injury at the centre of the aetiology of post-proctectomy impotence. The studies both demonstrate intact but attenuated cavernous nerve function. NPT testing indicated persistent nocturnal function but at a reduced activity. Response to the PDE-inhibitor sildenafil, yet not to placebo, confirms a neural basis for the injury. *In vivo* injection of sildenafil into the penis fails to induce any spontaneous erectile response or a rise in intracavernous pressure. Series reporting the use of sildenafil after radical prostatectomy suggest that response to sildenafil is variable, with the response greater after bilateral nerve-sparing surgery (80%) than after unilateral (50%) or non-nerve-sparing surgery (0%) [70-72]. Animal studies have shown that bilateral cavernous nerve transection ablates whilst unilateral nerve-sparing preserves erectile function in the presence of sildenafil [74]. In the nocturnal penile tumescence study, there was a non-significant trend to fewer nocturnal erections amongst sildenafil responders compared to non-responders. Thus a response to sildenafil implies a neural injury with some intact nerve fibres, i.e. a partial nerve injury.

Pelvic anatomy

Nerves

Sympathetic nerves

The superior hypogastric plexus is a network of sympathetic fibres situated just below the aortic bifurcation. Just above the pelvic brim the midline plexus coalesces into two diverging sympathetic hypogastric nerves on the postero-lateral wall of the pelvis between the peritoneum and the endopelvic fascia [75]. The nerves are tethered to the postero-lateral aspect of the mesorectum by small rectal branches and are at risk of injury at the beginning of rectal mobilisation. The hypogastric nerves eventually leave the mesorectum for the pelvic sidewall, coming to lie deeper in relation to the peritoneum.

Nervi erigentes

The pelvic parasympathetic (splanchnic) nerves (nervi erigentes) arise from the sacral roots of S2, S3 and S4. They pierce the endopelvic fascia from behind to enter the plane of the pelvic plexus. The pelvic parasympathetics join the sympathetic hypogastric nerve in a Y-shaped connection to form the pelvic plexus [76].

Pelvic plexus

The pelvic plexus is a network of nerves forming a sheet of neural tissue that lies quite lateral in the pelvis, lateral to the lower third of the rectum [77]. The

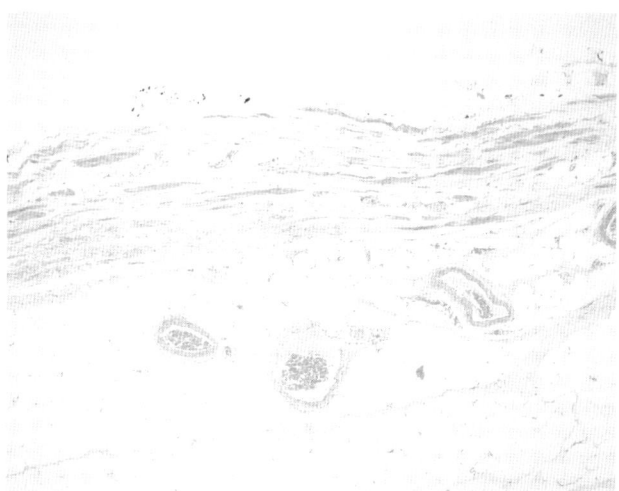

Figure 3. H & E stain of high power view of a transverse section through extraperitoneal rectum dissected anteriorly in the extramesorectal plane: Denonvilliers' fascia present.

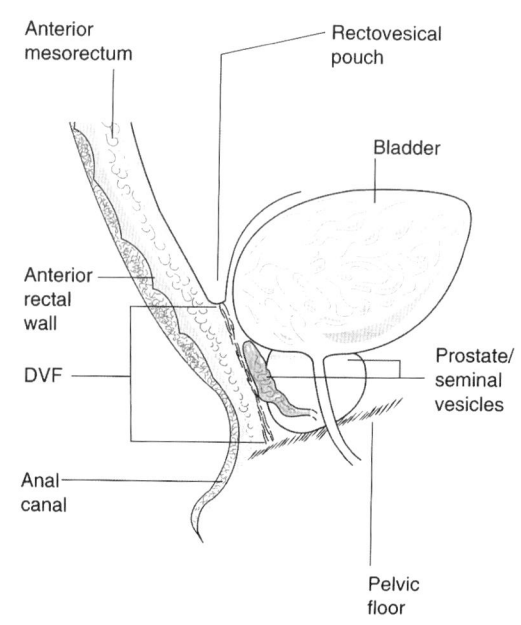

Figure 4. Lateral view of Denonvilliers' fascia (DVF) and its relationships.

lateral ligament of the rectum is described in textbooks as arising from the endopelvic fascia of the sidewall and inclined anteromedially as it approaches the rectum. In recent years, colorectal surgeons have recognised the lack of discrete anatomical lateral ligaments [78].

Cavernous nerves

Nerve fibres pass from the pelvic plexus to the bladder and sexual organs. The cavernous nerves run in neurovascular bundles at the lateral border of Denonvilliers' fascia [79-81]. These small, terminal parasympathetic fibres regulate the calibre of the inflow choke vessels to the corpora cavernosa, the erectile chambers of the penis.

Urological research into impotence after radical prostate surgery has produced a more refined understanding of the anatomy of the pelvis plexus and cavernous nerves [80,82,83] - previously the precise anatomy of these nerves was unknown. A prominent neurovascular bundle is located at the posterolateral border of the apex and base of the prostate. The visible nerves in this bundle branch to give rise to the microscopic cavernous nerves. These neurovascular bundles are consistently found in the leaves of the lateral pelvic fascia outside the prostatic capsule, at the lateral edge of Denonvilliers' fascia.

Denonvilliers' fascia

The anatomy of Denonvilliers' fascia is important because it lies in close proximity to the cavernous nerves. Its operative appearance varies considerably, but it is more obvious and substantial than the fascia propria of the rectum [84]. It is composed of dense collagen, smooth muscle fibres and coarse elastic fibres (Figure 3), and is related to the prostate and seminal vesicles anteriorly and the rectal wall, the thin anterior mesorectum and the fascia propria posteriorly (Figure 4).

There is debate about whether it is more intimate with the rectum or prostate. Some claim it is more closely adherent to the rectum [61,85,86]; others, including urologists, agreeing that the fascia is more densely applied to the prostate [84,87,88]. To answer this question, a histological study of the presence or absence of Denonvilliers' fascia on operative specimens for anterior and non-anterior lower rectal cancers was performed [89]. In non-anterior tumours, the fascia was absent, because a standard anatomical dissection was conducted. It was almost exclusively found in anterior cancers, taken by a deliberately radical anterior dissection (Figure 5). Therefore, Denonvilliers' fascia is more closely adherent to the prostate than the rectum.

Figure 5. H & E stain of low power view of a transverse section through extraperitoneal rectum dissected anteriorly in the extramesorectal plane: Denonvilliers' fascia present.

Anterior surgical planes

There are three planes available, involving the structures lying between the anterior rectal wall and the prostate/seminal vesicles (anterior mesorectum, fascia propria of the rectum and Denonvilliers' fascia). The close rectal plane, (previously perimuscular) (Figure 6) is immediately on the rectal musculature, within the anterior mesorectum. It is not an anatomical plane and dissection may be difficult and bloody [43]. The mesorectal plane, immediately outside the fascia propria, is an anatomical plane, and dissection in it separates the fascia propria and enclosed anterior mesorectum from Denonvilliers' fascia, which is left intact on the prostate and seminal vesicles. Dissection in the extra-mesorectal plane exposes the prostate and seminal vesicles and resects Denonvilliers' fascia.

Prevention: site of nerve injury and influence of the surgeon

Site of nerve injury

It is difficult to be specific about where most injuries take place, but the risk is thought to be in four key zones [90]. In the abdomen, the sympathetic hypogastric nerves are vulnerable during ligation of the pedicle of the inferior mesenteric artery. In the pelvis, high in the posterior plane of rectal dissection, the damage is purely sympathetic because the nervi erigentes has not yet joined the bundle.

During lateral dissection, straying laterally may injure the pelvic plexus, particularly if excess traction on the rectum tents the plexus superiorly and medially [91] or the middle rectal "pedicle" is clamped [92]. Damage to the pelvic plexus produces a mixed sympathetic and parasympathetic injury. Finally, during anterior rectal dissection, the cavernous branches of the pelvic plexus are at risk. There is a very narrow space between the rectum and prostate/seminal vesicles, deep in the pelvis, often under poor vision, with sometimes troublesome bleeding. It is likely that this is the zone at highest risk for nerve damage.

Influence of the surgeon: choice of planes

Proctectomy for IBD

Close rectal dissection is a surgical technique first described by Dowling and Lee in 1972 [43]. By convention, the mesorectal plane is used for rectal cancer surgery and by some surgeons for IBD. Close rectal dissection is conducted in the non-anatomical perimuscular plane (Figure 6) and theoretically should protect the pelvic nerves lying immediately outside the mesorectal plane. This remains unproven; it is a more challenging dissection and it remains open to question whether the extra time and effort is justified in terms of a reduction in morbidity. As both techniques are employed in Oxford by two different surgeons, it was natural to study the influence of mesorectal and close rectal dissection on impotence.

There was no significant difference in the rates of complete or partial impotence between those undergoing mesorectal and those undergoing close rectal dissection; close rectal dissection did not especially protect the pelvic nerves [62]. This is important, since many surgeons operate in the mesorectal plane out of familiarity - surgeons are not disadvantaging their patients by using this plane. In one very important aspect, the two techniques are the same: the anterior dissection immediately behind the prostate and seminal vesicles was conducted in the same close rectal dissection plane. This provides a clue as to the most important site of parasympathetic nerve damage, lateral or anterior dissection. The use of the close rectal plane anteriorly for both techniques, and their similar rates of impotence, is consistent with the anterior dissection having a prevailing importance as a potential site of nerve damage.

Rectal cancer

Tumours involving the anterior rectal quadrant threaten the anterior circumferential margin earlier than tumours involving other quadrants threaten their corresponding margins, because the anterior mesorectum is very thin. In an effort to ensure a clear anterior margin with an anterior tumour, surgeons usually dissect anterior to Denonvilliers' fascia, staying immediately on the seminal vesicles and prostate [88,93]. And this proved to be the case: Denonvilliers' fascia was more commonly found on rectal cancer specimens when tumours involved rather than spared the anterior rectal quadrant [89] (Figure 5).

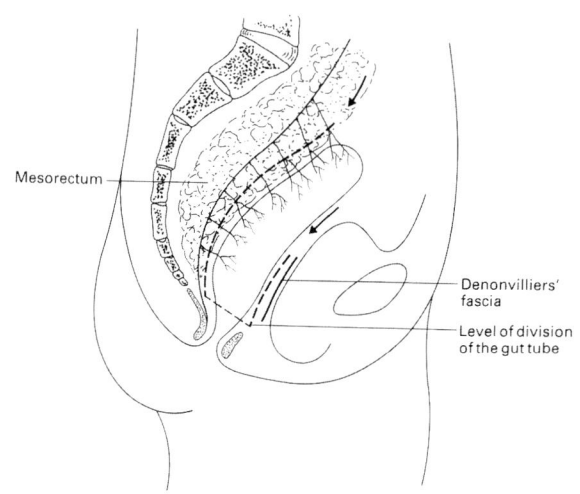

Figure 6. The close rectal dissection plane.

Table 4. Comparative efficacy of sildenafil.

Indication	Response rate (%)	
	Sildenafil	Placebo
Radical prostatectomy		
bilateral nerve-sparing	50-80	-
unilateral/non-nerve-sparing	0	-
'Mixed aetiology'	77	20

This radical anterior dissection takes the surgeon closer still to the cavernous nerves, and therefore the risk of erectile dysfunction for tumours involving the anterior quadrant is likely to be higher than for those not doing so. The risk of impotence for tumours that involved the anterior rectal quadrant was more than twice as high as those tumours that do not [94]. However, it is not necessary to expose the patient to the higher risks of nerve injury when the anterior margin is not threatened [88]. In this circumstance, an anterior mesorectal dissection should be used.

Treatment

No background information is available on the likely response of colorectal patients, but it might be expected to be similar to that reported in urology patients after prostatectomy who similarly have a major element of parasympathetic nerve damage. Recent small series reporting the use of sildenafil after radical prostatectomy suggest that response to sildenafil is less impressive than in patients with mixed erectile dysfunction, with the response greater after bilateral nerve-sparing surgery than after unilateral or non-nerve-sparing surgery (Table 4) [71-73]. Animal studies have shown that bilateral cavernous nerve transection ablates whilst unilateral nerve-sparing preserves erectile function in the presence of sildenafil [74].

This led to a trial aiming to determine whether sildenafil would improve erectile function in male patients with complete or partial impotence following rectal excision for rectal cancer and IBD [70]. The hypothesis was that the response would be similarly modest as that seen after radical prostatectomy, where cavernous nerve damage is causal. Subgroup analysis on the influence of disease group and severity of impotence was planned.

Thirty-two patients were randomised double-blind to sildenafil or placebo. After unblinding, placebo patients crossed over to sildenafil. The endpoints were improvement in erectile function and side effects. Response to sildenafil (79%) was significantly better than placebo (17%, p=0.0009). Sildenafil improved both erectile function scores (p=0.0001) and total sexual function scores (p<0.0001) from pre-treatment baseline, but placebo failed to do so (p=0.16 and p=0.10, respectively). All crossover patients not responding to placebo did so to sildenafil (p<0.0001). Sildenafil patients experienced a trend to more side effects (50%) compared to placebo (22%) but these were mostly mild and well tolerated.

Female sexual dysfunction

There have been a few reports on female sexual functioning following restorative proctocolectomy. In one questionnaire study on sexual function following restorative proctocolectomy, there was a significant increase in vaginal dryness, dyspareunia and avoidance of sexual activity because of concerns of stool leakage [95]. There was no significant change in desire, arousal or orgasm. Another study of sexual function following restorative proctocolectomy found that 15% complained of persistent dyspareunia [96]. Others have related this complaint to alterations in pelvic gynaecological alignment [97].

This led to another study aimed to determine the frequency and patterns of post-proctectomy FSD and attempted to characterise these in terms of specific disturbances of pelvic neurogenital physiology [98]. The incidence of sexual difficulties in previously normal patients undergoing restorative proctocolectomy was found to range from 5% (reduced clitoral sensitivity) to 54% (dyspareunia) and the incidence of most dysfunctions was about 10%. However, two particular problems occurred frequently: increased vaginal dryness (27%) and dyspareunia (54%). These two dysfunctions were 2 of only 3 in the Cleveland Clinic series that reached statistical significance [95]. Few studies have addressed possible neurological damage as an important cause for problems such as inability to attain orgasm, and reduced vaginal sensitivity and lubrication.

Studies of sildenafil in FSD have demonstrated modest results, despite being effective in male impotence. However, patients with symptoms suggesting pelvic parasympathetic nerve damage may be more responsive. Studies of the neurogenic mediators of the physiology of the female sexual response (particularly vaginal and clitoral blood flow) suggest a role for nitric oxide as a mediator of vaginal and clitoral smooth muscle relaxation. Sildenafil has been shown to enhance vaginal engorgement during erotic stimulation in healthy women [99]. One study has demonstrated changes in vaginal lubrication and clitoral sensitivity with sildenafil [100]. In another study, symptomatic and physiological parameters of the female sexual response were improved with 6 weeks' home use of 100mg of sildenafil [101]. No trial has yet examined the efficacy of sildenafil for post-proctectomy FSD.

Where are we going?

Better steps to prevent nerve injury during pelvic dissection need to be explored. Because the cavernous nerves are too small to see, a method of intra-operative localisation could be helpful. This has already proved useful in urology [102]. Using Cavermap, intra-operative nerve stimulation and localisation can help to identify pelvic nerve anatomy and confirm integrity of the parasympathetic nerves and postoperative erectile function [103].

More studies will explore the pelvic neural anatomy in females and relate this to the corresponding anatomy in males. A therapeutic trial of PDE-inhibitors for post-proctectomy FSD is likely to be undertaken. This would not only prove helpful to patients but could improve our understanding of post-proctectomy FSD.

Cavernous nerve grafting has begun to be studied in the urological field [104]. Whilst this seems more feasible in impotence after radical prostate surgery, where the cavernous nerve bundles are directly identified and rates of impotence are very high, this may have a role in the future for selected young patients undergoing proctectomy. There is some evidence that prophylactic sildenafil protects cavernous nerve function and aids postoperative nerve recovery after radical prostatectomy [105]. This is likely to be studied in the colorectal setting in time.

In the future, sexual dysfunction is likely to be an auditable, reportable outcome, a marker of surgical excellence that might allow better comparison between series.

References

1. Goldstein I, Lue T, Padma-Nathan H, et al. Oral sildenafil in the treatment of erectile dysfunction. *N Engl J Med* 1998; 338: 1397-1404.
2. Fazio VW, Fletcher J, Montague D. Prospective study of the effect of resection of the rectum on male sexual function. *World J Surg* 1980; 4: 149-52.
3. Leveckis J, Boucher NR, Parys BT, et al. Bladder and erectile dysfunction before and after rectal surgery for cancer. *Br J Urol* 1995; 76: 752-6.
4. Kinn AC, Ohman U. Bladder and sexual function after surgery for rectal cancer. *Dis Colon Rectum* 1986; 29: 43-8.
5. Williams JT, Slack WW. A prospective study of sexual function after major colorectal surgery. *Br J Surg* 1980; 76: 772-4.
6. Danzi M, Ferulano GP, Abate S, et al. Male sexual function after abdominoperineal resection for rectal cancer. *Dis Colon Rectum* 1983; 26: 665-8.
7. Hjortrup A, Kirkegaard P, Friis J, et al. Sexual dysfunction after low anterior resection for midrectal cancer. *Acta Chir Scand* 1984; 150: 687-8.
8. Weinstein M, Roberts M. Sexual potency following surgery for rectal carcinoma. *Ann Surg* 1977; 185: 295-300.
9. Santangelo ML, Romano G, Sassaroli C. Sexual function after resection for rectal cancer. *Am J Surg* 1987; 154: 502-4.
10. Balslev I, Harling H. Sexual dysfunction following operation for carcinoma of the rectum. *Dis Colon Rectum* 1983; 26: 785-8.
11. Goligher JC. Sexual function after excision of the rectum. *Proc R Soc Med* 1951; 44: 824-6.
12. Williams NS, Johnston D. The quality of life after excision for low rectal cancer. *Br J Surg* 1983; 70: 460-2.
13. Cunsolo A, Bragalia RB, Manara G, et al. Urogenital dysfunction after abdominoperineal resection for carcinoma of the rectum. *Dis Colon Rectum* 1990; 33: 918-22.
14. Bernstein WC, Bernstein EF. Sexual dysfunction following radical surgery for cancer of the rectum. *Dis Colon Rectum* 1966; 9: 328-32.
15. Yeager ES, Van Heerden JA. Sexual dysfunction following proctocolectomy and abdominoperineal resection. *Ann Surg* 1980; 191: 169-70.
16. Fegiz G, Trenti A, Bezzi M, et al. Sexual and bladder dysfunctions following surgery for rectal carcinoma. *Ital J Surg Sci* 1986; 16: 103-9.
17. Koukouras D, Spiliotis J, Scopa CD, et al. Radical consequence in the sexuality of male patients operated on for colorectal carcinoma. *Eur J Surg Oncol* 1991; 17: 285-8.
18. Filiberti A, Audisio RA, Gangeri L, et al. Prevalence of sexual dysfunction in male cancer patients treated with rectal excision and coloanal anastomosis. *Eur J Surg Oncol* 1994; 20: 43-6.
19. La Monica G, Audisio RA, Tamburini M, et al. Incidence of sexual dysfunction in male patients treated surgically for rectal malignancy. *Dis Colon Rectum* 1985; 28: 937-40.
20. Rosen RC, Riley A, Wagner G, et al. The International Index of Erectile Function (IIEF): a multidimensional scale for assessment of erectile dysfunction. *Urology* 1997; 49: 822-30.
21. Burnham WR, Lennard-Jones JE, Brooke BN. Sexual problems among married ileostomists. *Gut* 1977; 18: 673-7.
22. Wasson JH, Cushman CC, Brushewitz RC, et al. A structured literature review of treatment for localised prostate cancer. *Arch Fam Med* 1993; 2: 487-93.
23. De Bernardinis G, Tuscano D, Negro P, et al. Sexual dysfunction in males following extensive colorectal surgery. *Int Surg* 1981; 66: 133-5.
24. Enker WE. Potency, cure and local control in the operative treatment of rectal cancer. *Arch Surg* 1992; 127: 1396-1402.
25. Maas CP, Moriya Y, Steup WH, et al. Radical and nerve-preserving surgery for rectal cancer in the Netherlands: a prospective study on morbidity and functional outcome. *Br J Surg* 1998; 85: 92-7.
26. Hojo K, Vernava AM, Sugihara K, et al. Preservation of urine voiding and sexual function after rectal cancer surgery. *Dis Colon Rectum* 1991; 34: 532-9.
27. Michelassi F, Block GE. Morbidity and mortality of wide pelvic lymphadenectomy for rectal adenocarcinoma. *Dis Colon Rectum* 1992; 35: 1143-7.
28. Enker WE. *En bloc* pelvic lymphadenectomy and sphincter preservation in the surgical management of rectal cancer. *Ann Surg* 1986; 203: 426-33.
29. Masui H, Ike H, Yamaguchi S, et al. Male sexual function after autonomic nerve-preserving operation for rectal cancer. *Dis Colon Rectum* 1996; 39: 1140-5.
30. Koyama Y, Moriya Y, Hojo K. Effects of extended systemic lymphadenectomy for adenocarcinoma of the rectum - significant improvement of survival rate and decrease of local recurrence. *Jpn J Clin Oncol* 1984; 14: 623-32.
31. Moriya Y, Sugihari K, Akasu T, et al. Nerve-sparing surgery with lateral node dissection for advanced lower rectal cancer. *Eur J Cancer* 1995; 31A: 1229-32.
32. Macfarlane JK, Ryall RDH, Heald RJ. Mesorectal excision for rectal cancer. *Lancet* 1993; 341: 457-60.
33. Corman ML, Veidenheimer MC, Coller JA. Impotence after proctectomy for inflammatory bowel disease. *Dis Colon Rectum* 1978; 21: 418-9.
34. Watts J McK, de Dombal FT, Goligher JC. Long-term complications and prognosis following major surgery for ulcerative colitis. *Br J Surg* 1966; 53: 1014-23.
35. Donovan MJ, O'Hara ET. Sexual function following surgery for ulcerative colitis. *N Engl J Med* 1960: 262(14): 719-20.
36. Stahlgren LH, Ferguson LK. Influence on sexual function of abdominoperineal resection for ulcerative colitis. *N Engl J Med* 1958; 259(18): 873-5.
37. Prohaska JV, Siderius NJ. The surgical rehabilitation of patients with chronic ulcerative colitis. *Am J Surg* 1962; 103: 42-6.
38. Bauer JJ, Gelernt IM, Salky B, et al. Sexual dysfunction following proctocolectomy for benign disease of the colon and rectum. *Ann Surg* 1983; 197: 363-7.
39. Turnbull RB jnr. Discussion. *Arch Surg* 1956; 73: 651.

40. Bacon HE, Bralow SP, Berkley JL. Rehabilitation and long-term survival after colectomy for ulcerative colitis. *JAMA* 1960; 172: 324-8.
41. May RE. Sexual dysfunction following rectal excision for ulcerative colitis. *Br J Surg* 1966; 53: 29-30.
42. Davis LP, Jelenko C. Sexual function after abdominoperineal resection. *South Med J* 1975; 68: 422-6.
43. Lee ECG, Dowling BL. Perimuscular excision of the rectum for Crohn's disease and ulcerative colitis. A conservative technique. *Br J Surg* 1972; 59: 29-32.
44. Lyttle JA, Parks AG. Intersphincteric excision of the rectum. *Br J Surg* 1977; 64: 413-6.
45. Leicester RJ, Ritchie JK, Wadsworth J, et al. Sexual function and perineal wound healing after intersphincteric excision of the rectum for inflammatory bowel disease. *Dis Colon Rectum* 1984; 27: 244-8.
46. Meagher AP, Farouk R, Dozois RR, et al. J ileal pouch-anal anastomosis for chronic ulcerative colitis: complications and long-term outcome in 1310 patients. *Br J Surg* 1998; 85: 800-3.
47. Fazio VW, Ziv Y, Church JM, et al. Ileal pouch-anal anastomoses complications and function in 1005 patients. *Ann Surg* 1995; 222(2): 120-7.
48. Marcello PW, Roberts PL, Schoetz DJ, et al. Long-term results of the ileoanal pouch procedure. *Arch Surg* 1993; 128: 500-3.
49. Becker JM, Raymond JL. Ileal pouch-anal anastomosis: a single surgeon's experience with 100 consecutive cases. *Ann Surg* 1986; 204(4): 375-81.
50. Damgaard B, Wettergren A, Kirkgaard P. Social and sexual function following ileal pouch-anal anastomosis. *Dis Colon Rectum* 1995; 38: 286-9.
51. Öresland T, Fasth S, Nordgren S, et al. The clinical and functional outcome after restorative proctocolectomy: a prospective study in 100 patients. *Int J Colorectal Dis* 1989; 4: 50-6.
52. Pescatori M, Mattana C, Castagneto M. Clinical and functional results after restorative proctocolectomy. *Br J Surg* 1988; 75: 312-4.
53. Poppen B, Svenberg T, Bark T, et al. Colectomy-proctomucosectomy with S-pouch: operative procedures, complications and functional outcome in 69 consecutive patients. *Dis Colon Rectum* 1992; 35: 40-7.
54. Tiainen J, Matikainen M, Hiltunen K-M. Ileal J-pouch-anal anastomosis, sexual dysfunction and fertility. *Scand J Gastroenterol* 1999; 34: 185-8.
55. Michalessi F, Stella M, Block GE. Prospective assessment of functional results after ileal J pouch-anal restorative proctocolectomy. *Arch Surg* 1993; 128: 889-95.
56. Keighley MRB, Grobler S, Bain I. An audit of restorative proctocolectomy. *Gut* 1993; 34: 680-4.
57. Setti-Carraro P, Ritchie JK, Wilkinson KH, et al. The first 10 years' experience of restorative proctocolectomy for ulcerative colitis. *Gut* 1994; 35: 1070-5.
58. Emblem R, Bergan A, Flatmark A. Mucosal proctectomy with straight ileoanal anastomosis. *Scand J Gastroenterol* 1988; 23: 1165-72.
59. Skarsgard ED, Atkinson KG, Bell GA, et al. Function and quality of life results after ileal pouch surgery for chronic ulcerative colitis and familial polyposis. *Am J Surg* 1989; 157: 467-71.
60. Wexner SD, Jensen L, Rothenberger DA, et al. Long-term functional analysis of the ileoanal reservoir. *Dis Colon Rectum* 1989; 32: 275-81.
61. Goligher JC. Anterior resection. In: *Operative Surgery of the Colon, Rectum and Anus*, 3rd edition. Goligher JC. Butterworths, London, 1980: 143-56.
62. Lindsey I, George BD, Mortensen NJ, et al. Impotence after mesorectal and close rectal dissection for inflammatory bowel disease. *Dis Colon Rectum* 2001; 44: 831-35.
63. Fisher C. Dreaming and sexuality. In: *Psychoanalysis - a general psychology*. Loewenstein RM, Newman LM, Schur M, et al, Eds. International University Press, New York, 1966: 537.
64. Ek A, Bradley WE, Krane RJ. Nocturnal penile rigidity measured by the snap-gauge band. *J Urol* 1983; 129: 964-6.
65. Chung WS, Choi HK. Erotic erection versus nocturnal erection. *J Urol* 1990; 143: 294-7.
66. Bradley WE, Timm GW, Gallagher JM, et al. New method for continuous measurement of nocturnal penile tumescence and rigidity. *Urology* 1985; 26: 4-9.
67. Knoll DL, Abrams JH. Application of nocturnal electrobioimpedance volumetric assessment: a feasibility study in men without erectile dysfunction. *J Urol* 1999; 161: 1137-40.
68. Knoll DL, Abrams JH. Nocturnal electrobioimpedance volumetric assessment of patients with erectile dysfunction. *Urology* 1999; 53: 1200-4.
69. Lindsey I, Cunningham C, Mortensen NJMcC, et al. Nocturnal penile tumescence is diminished but not ablated in post-proctectomy impotence. *Dis Colon Rectum* 2003; 46: 14-20.
70. Lindsey I, George BD, Mortensen NJ, et al. Randomised, double-blind, placebo-controlled trial of sildenafil (Viagra) for erectile dysfunction after proctectomy for rectal cancer and inflammatory bowel disease. *Dis Colon Rectum* 2002; 45: 727-32.
71. Lowentritt BH, Scardino PT, Miles BJ, et al. Sildenafil citrate after radical retropubic prostatectomy. *J Urol* 1999; 162: 1614-7.
72. Zippe CD, Kedia AW, Kedia K, et al. Treatment of erectile dysfunction after radical prostatectomy with sildenafil citrate (Viagra). *Urology* 1998; 52: 537-42.
73. Marks LS, Duda C, Dorey FJ, et al. Treatment of erectile dysfunction with sildenafil. *Urology* 1999; 53: 19-24.
74. Carrier S, Zvara P, Nunes L, et al. Regeneration of nitric oxide synthetase-containing nerves after cavernous nerve neurotomy in the rat. *J Urol* 1995; 153: 1722-7.
75. Lee JF, Maurer MV, Block GE. Anatomic relations of pelvic autonomic nerves to pelvic operations. *Arch Surg* 107: 324-8.
76. Ashley FL, Anson BJ. The pelvic autonomic nerves in the male. *Surg Gynaecol Obstet* 1946; 82: 598-608.
77. Nano M, Levi AC, Borghi F, et al. Observations on surgical anatomy for rectal cancer surgery. *Hepatogastroenterology* 1998; 45: 717-26.

78. Jones OM, Smeulders N, Wiseman O, et al. Lateral ligaments of the rectum: an anatomical study. *Br J Surg* 1999; 86: 487-9.
79. Myers RP. Practical pelvic anatomy pertinent to radical retropubic prostatectomy. AUA update service 1994; 13: 26.
80. Lepor H, Gregerman M, Crosby R, et al. Precise localisation of the autonomic nerves from the pelvic plexus to the corpora cavernosa: a detailed anatomical study of the adult male pelvis. *J Urol* 1985; 133: 207-12.
81. Kourambas J, Angus DG, Hosking P, et al. A histological study of Denonvilliers' fascia and its relationship to the neurovascular bundle. *Br J Urol* 1998; 82: 408-10.
82. Walsh PC, Donker PJ. Impotence following radical prostatectomy: insight into etiology and prevention. *J Urol* 1982; 128: 492-7.
83. Lue TF, Zeineh SJ, Schmidt RA, et al. Neuroanatomy of penile erection: its relevance to iatrogenic impotence. *J Urol* 1984; 131: 273-80.
84. Church JM, Raudkivi PJ, Hill GL. The surgical anatomy of the rectum - a review with particular relevance to the hazards of rectal mobilisation. *Int J Colorectal Dis* 1987; 2: 158-66.
85. Heald RJ, Moran BJ. Embryology and Anatomy of the Rectum. *Sem Surg Oncol* 1998; 15: 66-71.
86. Heald RJ, Moran BJ, Brown G, Daniels IR. Optimal total mesorectal excision for rectal cancer is by dissection in front of Denonvilliers' facsia. *Br J Surg* 2004; 91: 121-3.
87. Huland H, Noldus J. An easy and safe approach to separating Denonvilliers' fascia from the rectum during radical retropubic prostatectomy. *J Urol* 1999; 161: 1533-4.
88. Lindsey I, Warren BF, Mortensen NJMcC. Optimal total mesorectal excision for rectal cancer is by dissection in front of Denonvilliers' facsia. *Br J Surg* 2004; 91: 897.
89. Lindsey I, Warren BF, Mortensen NJMcC, et al. Denonvilliers' fascia lies anterior to the anterior plane of rectal dissection in total mesorectal excision. *Colorectal Dis* 2000; 2 (Suppl.): 42.
90. Lindsey I, Guy RJ, Mortensen NJ, et al. Anatomy of Denonvilliers' fascia and pelvic nerves, impotence and implications for the colorectal surgeon. *Br J Surg* 2000; 87: 1288-99.
91. Pearl RK, Monsen H, Abcarian H. Surgical anatomy of the pelvic autonomic nerves. A practical approach. *Am Surg* 1986; 52: 236-7.
92. Mundy AR. An anatomical explanation for bladder dysfunction following rectal and uterine surgery. *Br J Urol* 1982; 54: 501-4.
93. Lindsey I, Mortensen NJ. Iatrogenic impotence and rectal dissection. *Br J Surg* 2002; 89: 1493-4.
94. Lindsey I, George BD, Mortensen NJMcC, et al. Erectile dysfunction after rectal cancer surgery: anterior tumours at greater risk. *Colorectal Dis* 2001; 2 (Suppl.): 27.
95. Bambrick M, Fazio VW, Hull TL, et al. Sexual function following restorative proctocolectomy in women. *Dis Colon Rectum* 1996; 39: 610-4.
96. Counihan TC, Roberts PL, Schoetz DJ, et al. Fertility and sexual and gynecologic function after ileal pouch-anal anastomosis. *Dis Colon Rectum* 1994; 37: 1126-9.
97. Öresland T, Palmblad S, Ellström M, et al. Gynaecological and sexual function related to anatomical changes in the female pelvis after restorative proctocolectomy. *Int J Colorect Dis* 1994; 9: 77-81.
98. Lindsey I, Finlay T, Mortensen NJMcC. Female sexual dysfunction after ileal pouch-anal anastomosis: is there an identifiable neurogenital lesion? *Colorectal Disease* 2003; 5 (Suppl. 1): 5.
99. Laan E, van Lunsen RH, Everaerd W, et al. The enhancement of vaginal vasocongestion by sildenafil in healthy premenopausal women. *J Womens Health Gend Based Med* 2002; 11: 357-65.
100. Basson R, McInnes R, Smith MD, et al. Efficacy and safety of sildenafil citrate in women with sexual dysfunction associated with female sexual arousal disorder. *J Womens Health Gend Based Med* 2002; 11: 367-77.
101. Berman JR, Berman LA, Lin H, et al. Effect of sildenafil on subjective and physiologic parameters of the female sexual response in women with sexual arousal disorder. *J Sex Marital Ther* 2001; 27: 411-20.
102. Walsh PC, Marschke P, Catalona WJ, et al. Efficacy of first generation Cavermap to verify location and function of cavernous nerves during radical prostatectomy: a multi-institution evaluation by experienced surgeons. *Urology* 2001; 57: 491-4.
103. Hanna NN, Guillem J, Dosoretz A, et al. Intraoperative parasympathetic nerve stimulation with tumescence monitoring during total mesorectal excision for rectal cancer. *J Am Coll Surg* 2002; 195: 506-12
104. Chang DW, Wood CG, Kroll SS, et al. Cavernous nerve reconstruction to preserve erectile function following non-nerve-sparing radical retropubic prostatectomy: a prospective study. *Plast Reconstr Surg* 2003; 111: 1174-81.
105. Schwartz EJ, Wong P, Graydon RJ. Sildenafil preserves intracorporeal smooth muscle after radical retropubic prostatectomy. *J Urol* 2004; 171: 771-4.